Occupational Therapy and Vocational Rehabilitation

Occupational Therapy and Vocational Rehabilitation

JOANNE ROSS

BICENTENNIAL
1807
WILEY
2007
BICENTENNIAL

John Wiley & Sons, Ltd

Other Wiley Editorial Offices

John Wiley & Sons Inc., 111 River Street, Hoboken, NJ 07030, USA

Jossey-Bass, 989 Market Street, San Francisco, CA 94103-1741, USA

Wiley-VCH Verlag GmbH, Boschstr. 12, D-69469 Weinheim, Germany

John Wiley & Sons Australia Ltd, 42 McDougall Street, Milton, Queensland 4064, Australia

John Wiley & Sons (Asia) Pte Ltd, 2 Clementi Loop #02-01, Jin Xing Distripark, Singapore 129809

John Wiley & Sons Canada Ltd, 6045 Freemont Blvd, Mississauga, ONT, L5R 4J3, Canada

Wiley also publishes its books in a variety of electronic formats. Some content that appears in print may
not be available in electronic books.

Anniversary Logo Design: Richard J. Pacifico

Library of Congress Cataloguing-in-Publication Data

Ross, Joanne.
    Occupational therapy and vocational rehabilitation / by Joanne Ross.
        p. ; cm.
    Includes bibliographical references.
    ISBN 978-0-470-02564-2 (cloth : alk. paper)
    1. Occupational therapy. 2. Vocational rehabilitation. I. Title.
    [DNLM: 1. Occupational Therapy. 2. Rehabilitation, Vocational. WB 555 R835o 2007]
    RM735.R65 2007
    615.8'515–dc22
                                        2007022437

British Library Cataloguing in Publication Data

A catalogue record for this book is available from the British Library

ISBN 978-0-470-02564-2

Typeset by Aptara, New Delhi, India.
Printed and bound in Great Britain by TJ International Ltd, Padstow, Cornwall

This book is printed on acid-free paper responsibly manufactured from sustainable forestry in which at
least two trees are planted for each one used for paper production.

Contents

Introduction

The cover design of this book shows part of a jigsaw puzzle, which is a fitting analogy with which to begin our exploration of the subject of occupational therapy (OT) and vocational rehabilitation (VR). As we piece together the various bits, using something of a trial and error approach, we begin to build up a picture of VR. Anticipating what the finished picture will look like is a vital aspect of knowing where each piece is likely to fit. With each bit added to its rightful place we increase our understanding of the role and contribution which it makes to the emerging image. Some pieces will be easy to identify and to place. Others perhaps more obscure. And so it is with VR.

Each of us reading this book will be doing so because we want to learn more about VR. We will already have created our own picture, or impression, of what VR is, or what it might look like. Some ideas will, perhaps, be well-formed, others still incomplete. The purpose of this book is to add a few more pieces to this emergent picture. To challenge and extend our existing knowledge about occupation, work and rehabilitation. To build on and improve our skills in enabling our clients to meet their work goals. There is no blueprint or completed image to guide us in this task. So our puzzle will require much creative thought and ingenuity if we are to be successful in our quest!

Taking this comparison no further, let us move on to discuss the layout of the book. Outside of this Introduction the text is divided into ten chapters, with each one exploring and discussing a different topic. In the first chapter we will begin by examining what is meant by the term 'vocational rehabilitation' and the definitions that have been attached to it. We will also look broadly at the various sources of knowledge which we may draw from to enhance our understanding in this field. The foundations of our knowledge base include, for example, social equity, occupational knowledge, and the impact of disability on functional performance. We will return to these, although perhaps in somewhat different guises, throughout the course of the book.

The second chapter takes us along a fascinating journey back in time. It describes how work activities have been used therapeutically since the earliest origins of the OT profession. It also charts the rise and fall of VR, and the place of disabled people in the labour force, at different points in history. We will read about the changing nature of work and work patterns, the causes of illness, the impact of wars, economic recessions and other major influencing societal events, including political pressures. Following this historical story through will add to your understanding of how OT in VR has emerged, evolved and resurged over time. It may also allow us to reflect on possible outcomes from the renaissance of attention which is currently being directed towards this intervention.

The third chapter is all about work. Existing OT literature does not currently provide us with a well-articulated perspective of this occupation. Nor is an occupation-focused perspective of work and productivity especially well-rooted (Lysaght and Wright, 2005), or delineated (Ross, 2006), in undergraduate curricula. However, in order to practice VR effectively, it is my firm belief that we need to have a solid understanding of what work is. Are you able to describe an OT perspective of work? How might we begin to conceptualise the different forms of work which exist in society today? These are key questions which will be addressed in Chapter 3.

Within our modern society, the term 'work' has largely become associated with paid employment. This chapter will encourage you to consider work in a far wider sense. Other forms of activity, such as care-giving, child rearing and home maintenance may be seen as different, but no less important, work functions. In addition, we will also explore some of the meanings that individuals and societies attach to work and the qualities and characteristics which may separate it out from leisure or self-care. We will consider how work might fit into an individuals' wider pattern of everyday occupations. We will also seek to understand work from different perspectives. We will explore a socio-economic, sociological, psychological, and an occupational view of this activity. We will also examine its links to social inclusion, as well as the various standpoints of disabled people, employers and health professionals.

Chapter 4 examines theoretical frameworks which can be drawn upon to guide and underpin occupational therapists' practice in VR. Models of practice and other such conceptual scaffolding can usefully be brought into play to help justify, support and explain our practice. We will begin with two well-known generalist models, both drawn from within the existing OT knowledge base, which are likely to already be familiar to many occupational therapists. The Canadian Model of Occupational Performance (Townsend, 2002) and the Model of Human Occupation (Kielhofner, 2002), can both be successfully applied to enhance our understanding of the worker in his or her workplace. During this chapter, and throughout this book, case examples will be used to illustrate how we may potentially utilise this knowledge in a real-life situation.

We will also look outside of recognised OT frameworks as well. We will include the biopsychosocial model, originally from within our own discipline, which now has widespread popular support within the VR sector. Further discussions will centre on the International Classification of Functioning, Disability and Health; the social model of disability; and the notion of the healthy workplace. The disability management model is perhaps better known in Canada, but nevertheless offers valuable insights, particularly with people who have sustained a workplace injury. Our final theoretical framework will be one which clearly demonstrates the cycles of vulnerability faced by people who are in work, with a disability. Each of the various theories and conceptual frameworks which we will be discussing here are congruent with the philosophy of OT. As such, they can assist us, as novice practitioners, to significantly enhance our understanding of this field.

In the fifth chapter we will be seeking to enhance our knowledge of different service models in VR. Unfortunately, there is no escaping the fact that the vast array of state, voluntary and private sector involvement in the work sphere contributes to the complexity of the field. Services are fragmented and cross-organisational working is complicated. They may be available to people with certain types of conditions, but not with others. They may exist in one area, but not in another. Some will only be for people with the right type of insurance, others on the correct state benefit. Access routes into many types of provision are no less complicated. This book does not try to avoid or make light of these complexities, rather it takes the view that occupational therapists are used to addressing complex needs often in complex situations, and that their skills are ideally suited to doing so.

However, so as to create some order, and begin to make sense of these complications, we will take a view of VR activities as occurring along a continuum. By taking a step away from the intricacies of the existing situation we may, somewhat hypothetically, arrange these services according to a more person-centred approach, thereby allowing us to more easily navigate our way through the maze.

Our hypothetical continuum consists of three possible stages. The first begins with the person who is 'out of work'. Under this heading we will examine what it means to be out of work, including concepts such as worklessness, unemployment, and economic inactivity. We will then examine the notion of 'moving into work' and the sorts of services which may be available to help those who need assistance with gaining a worker role. We will introduce organisations such as Jobcentre Plus, as well as examining a range of different service models for people with disabilities, or health conditions, who are currently not in work. These include, amongst others, sheltered and supported employment, individual placement and support, social firms, and clubhouses. We will also learn more about current Government initiatives specifically designed to help disabled people move into work, including the New Deal for Disabled People and the Pathways to Work programme. The third stage on our continuum is 'keeping in work'. This will examine the ideas behind job retention and prevention of job loss, for people who may be at risk, particularly because of a chronic health condition. We will also explore the process of sickness certification, sickness absence and how absence may be managed by employers. The role played by occupational health services will be introduced, as will new Government initiatives, such as Workplace Health Connect.

The role of the occupational therapist within some of the services outlined will be discussed and illustrated using case studies and examples. While the number of occupational therapists working within settings such as occupational health in the United Kingdom is still relatively small, the scope and opportunities are clearly demonstrated by those who have moved into these areas of practice. We will also draw on the international evidence base here, to highlight potential areas for occupational therapists' future involvement as the sector becomes more firmly established.

As occupational therapists, we have a firm belief in the positive relationship which exists between health and occupation. However, this chapter should dispel any possible myth that every form of employment is good for your health. Worldwide, the statistics for injury and death caused directly by work are alarming. Even within our own country, there remains a very real need to improve work conditions and the quality of jobs available, particularly for those in lower paid jobs, which, as we will discover, frequently includes people with disabilities.

Chapter 6 will move away from theoretical concepts and service structures, to provide more specific details on how we might actually **do** VR. It will describe, at length, the VR process, and you will notice, as you work your way through this chapter, the similarities and differences to the more familiar, traditional OT process. Beginning with the receipt of a referral, it takes us through the initial assessment and provides a sample assessment form to help gather the necessary information. It examines how we might, together with our client, assess their work readiness. We will then discuss the optional pre-vocational phase, along with building work tolerance and assisting the person to retain a worker identity. We also examine vocational exploration for the person who is out of work, or needs to explore an alternative career path.

As we progress through the VR process, we enter the worksite visit stage, during which we will increase our understanding of the different types of jobs, and how to go about undertaking a workplace assessment. We will examine the documentation needed, including the process of drawing up a return to work plan, and what we may want to include in it. With our return to work plan in place, we will next look at a range of possible interventions to support our return to work, including working collaboratively with others, as well as alternative interventions widely used in other countries, such as work hardening and occupational rehabilitation. Finally, as we reach the end of our VR process, we will touch on evaluation, outcomes and discharge.

In Chapter 7, we deal with conditions which are commonly seen by the occupational therapists in VR. While VR is not illness or disability specific, it is important to recognise that occupational therapists are often based in services which are targeted at clients with a particular condition. This chapter acknowledges this reality. It therefore draws on current knowledge and best practice regarding key interventions for people with particular conditions. It will also discuss work-related factors that may impact on these conditions, and ways in which specific difficulties may be addressed.

This chapter may, perhaps, serve as a useful starting point for readers who wish to gain a brief overview of information about VR with their client group, as well as any salient issues which may surround the area of practice within their field. The conditions included have been grouped under four broad headings, the first of which is mental health conditions. Under this heading we will examine the needs of those with both common, and more severe, mental health problems as well as those who have a substance addiction. We will discuss the need for interventions such as combating stigma and promoting self-management and recovery.

The second group of conditions is centred on common musculoskeletal disorders. We will include upper limb disorders, arthritis and back pain in our discussions. We will also examine the use of functional capacity assessments, a common tool used by therapists working in some settings. The role of computers, how to go about undertaking a simple workstation assessment, and the importance of posture and seating will also be addressed.

Moving on to examine the third group, cardio-respiratory conditions, we will touch on possible work interventions for people with these types of illnesses. In the fourth and final group of this chapter, we will be briefly discussing various neurological conditions and some ways in which work opportunities may be provided for this group of individuals. We will conclude with the views of disabled workers themselves, with regard to the value and effectiveness of a selection of disability management strategies in the workplace.

Finally, Chapter 8 describes the team and team structures in VR and goes on to introduce the notion of a VR team built around each work seeker or work returner. This discussion identifies members who may be part of a core VR team, including the return to work facilitator, perhaps acting as a case manager, the client and others. Within an extended VR team, team members may be drawn from across the boundaries of different agencies. In order to learn about the roles of some different people who may potentially be involved in the VR process, we will be introduced to individuals such as the claims manager, the safety practitioner, the occupational physician, the occupational health nurse, an occupational hygienist, a personal advisor and a work psychologist.

Chapter 9 examines the legal framework within which VR must be delivered. Occupational therapists are not expected to have an in-depth understanding of the law, however this area is a common source of concern for therapists who are new to the field. Therefore, within this chapter we will outline key legislation which has direct relevance to the field, focusing in particular on health and safety and disability rights. We will also discuss potential implications of the various regulations and Acts for occupational therapists. We will also be introduced to other organisations of relevance in the field, including, for example, the Industrial Injuries Advisory Council (IIAC) and the Advisory, Conciliation and Arbitration Service (ACAS).

The final chapter, Chapter 10, will look to the future. In it we will examine the challenges facing occupational therapists, with a particular emphasis on education, anticipated accreditation, and priorities for research.

1 Understanding Vocational Rehabilitation

In this first chapter we want to start the process of demystifying what vocational rehabilitation (VR) is, and move forwards with a shared understanding of the activities and interventions which may come together under its umbrella. We also want to reflect on how we might draw on existing knowledge sources, some of which will already be very familiar to occupational therapists, in order to begin working towards creating a uniquely occupation-focused perspective of work and VR.

As we do so, let us remind ourselves that the essence of occupational therapy (OT) is built on a belief in the necessity and value of occupations. Each of us strives, throughout our life, to achieve a balance of meaningful and purposeful work, rest, self-care and leisure activities. Of all the occupations in which we engage across our lifespan, work arguably occupies the most central position. Work provides us with a significant life role that accounts for up to a third of the life of an average adult. Furthermore, the links between work and health, well-being and longevity, have already been well-argued (Wilcock, 1998). Despite this understanding, far too few occupational therapists in the UK today, ask the 'work question', even when they have clients who are of working age. Fewer still are involved, to any great extent, in addressing the actual work or employment needs of their clients. People outside of the profession could be forgiven for questioning why **occupational** therapists don't deal with, perhaps, the most commonly recognised occupation.

But all this is changing. A growing recognition of the potential roles for occupational therapists within VR in the UK is fueling interest in learning more about this topic. The starting point must, of course, be with our shared understanding of VR itself, so let us examine what is meant by this.

DEFINING VOCATIONAL REHABILITATION

It is fair to say that, to many, 'vocational rehabilitation' is an unfamiliar term. It is also unpopular, with somewhat dated, value-laden connotations attached to it. The notion of a 'vocation' conjures, perhaps for some, images of religion. In popular language the word has often been associated with a calling to a certain profession – your vocation in life. 'Rehabilitation' fares little better, since nowadays it is frequently applied to strategies aimed at reducing criminal behavior and offending rates. It is also increasingly used in connection with expensive clinics, where celebrities enter 'rehab' to go through detoxification for a substance addiction. These images are unfortunate, since the terminological confusion which they create hinders understanding, as well as having the effect of positioning VR away from ordinary, everyday problems and interventions.

With the perceived unsuitability of this terminology, it is probably unsurprising that occupational therapists have sought out alternatives. This has resulted in a plethora of terms which largely describe a similar range of interventions, none of which seems to have successfully captured the essence of practice in this field. In the American literature we find frequent references to 'work rehabilitation', in Australia and New Zealand we find 'occupational rehabilitation' and 'injury management', in Canada 'vocational practice' and 'disability management'. Attempts have been made in the UK to group the range of interventions which make up VR under the broader heading of 'work practice' (Pratt and Jacobs, 1997). In some countries 'vocational rehabilitation' is used to describe interventions only undertaken with those who are returning to work, since, strictly speaking, job seekers who have never worked, would more aptly be participating in habilitation, rather than rehabilitation. Confusingly, in yet other countries, VR is predominantly undertaken with those who are currently **out** of work, but may perhaps have worked in the past.

Unfortunately, if we extend our discussion beyond OT, the situation becomes even more complicated, since 'vocational rehabilitation' has different meanings to different groups of people. As well as the perceptions of the general public, others such as employers, insurers, health professionals, and politicians, each have their own take on what VR is, the purpose it serves, and frequently their own associated jargon.

Not only are there terminological differences, but there are similar disagreements about what VR actually entails. Some may describe it as a type of process. Kumar (2000), for example, introduces it as a multi-disciplinary process. Others may view it narrowly as a particular type of service model, which takes its place alongside work hardening and injury management programmes, or sheltered employment provisions (Perron and McKay, 1997). Alternatively, it may be used to describe an array of services. Commonly it is seen as a form of intervention, perhaps directed towards assisting somebody back to work. We will not resolve these terminological or ideological conflicts, nor will we attempt to try. The reader who consults the international literature does, however, need to be aware that these idiosyncrasies exist.

In acknowledging these global difficulties, let us now look at two of the, perhaps, most widely accepted definitions of 'vocational rehabilitation' within the UK context. The first was put forward by the Department for Work and Pensions (DWP) as part of a document entitled *Building Capacity for Work: A UK framework for vocational rehabilitation* (2004, p.14), and describes it as follows:

- *Vocational rehabilitation is a process to overcome the barriers an individual faces when accessing, remaining or returning to work following injury, illness or impairment. This process includes the procedures in place to support the individual and/or employer or others (for example, family and carers) including help to access VR and to practically manage the delivery of VR; and*

- *in addition, VR includes the wide range of interventions to help individuals with a health condition and/or impairment overcome barriers to work and so remain in, return to, or access employment. For example, an assessment of needs, re-training and capacity building, return to work management by employers, reasonable adjustments and control measures, disability awareness, condition management and medical treatment.*

The second is from the British Society of Rehabilitation Medicine (BSRM) (2003, p.1) who describe it as:

> *...a process whereby those disadvantaged by illness or disability can be enabled to access, return to, or remain in, employment, or other useful occupation.*

You will note from these definitions, that they share a common perspective of VR as a process, designed to assist those with work goals, regardless of whether they are seeking to enter or remain in work. In addition, according to the first definition, it also covers a range of possible interventions as well, thus allowing the term to be used interchangeably. The DWP definition does, however, focus specifically on employment, whereas the BSRM suggests a wider understanding of work.

Having reached an understanding on what we mean when we talk about 'vocational rehabilitation', let us now briefly consider the sources of knowledge which we may draw on in order to effectively practice within it.

Figure 1.1 broadly depicts the main types of knowledge that occupational therapists may use in this field. Some will already be familiar, others perhaps less so. At the top of the figure there are two rows of boxes. We can see that the five boxes in the top row identify the sources of knowledge which occupational therapists may use in their VR practice. These include knowledge of work and the workplace, and knowledge

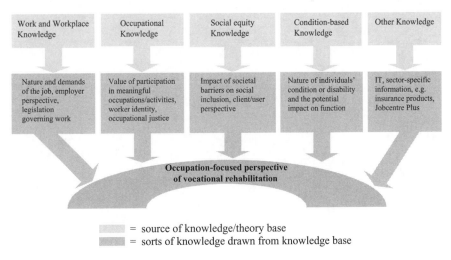

= source of knowledge/theory base
= sorts of knowledge drawn from knowledge base

Figure 1.1. An occupation-focused perspective of vocational rehabilitation

about human occupation, drawn mostly from the occupational science paradigm. They also include social equity knowledge which helps us think about issues such as environmental barriers and the stigma which often faces disabled people who want to work. In addition, condition-based knowledge helps the practitioner to understand the nature of an individual's illness or disability and the impact of this condition on their functional performance. Finally, the occupational therapist must draw on other sources of knowledge, such as information technology, as well as knowledge specific to the sector in which they are practising. For example, an occupational therapist working in the insurance sector may need to understand insurance products and the claims management process, whereas a practitioner in the voluntary sector, or in a condition management programme, would not. In the second row of boxes, we are given examples of the sorts of knowledge which occupational therapists may potentially draw from these respective knowledge bases.

All these sources of knowledge collectively contribute to what has been termed 'occupation-focused practice'. Occupation-focused practice is represented in this diagram by an arc. The arc itself represents the way in which OT may act as a bridge between employers, doctors, clients and others involved in the VR process. Occupation-focused practice draws on these different forms of knowledge so as to support the client to engage in the occupation of work in a way which is meaningful and purposeful to them. It is tempered by the need to have a commercial awareness of the realities of the workplace and the barriers which may act as obstacles to achieving this. Each of the different forms of knowledge identified here will be discussed further, in detail, in later chapters of this book. It may be worth reflecting at this point, on the key areas in which you wish to boost your own understanding of occupation-focused practice in VR.

2 The Evolution of Vocational Rehabilitation

This chapter begins with the earliest uses of occupation, and work, as therapy. Over the course of time there have been dramatic changes both to the role of the worker and the nature of work. The ways in which we, as a society, have organised, structured and performed this work, have also seen great transformations. Once considered to pose a significant risk to health, and even to life itself, work is now seen to have a positive effect on health and well-being. This short journey through time illustrates the ever-shifting relationship between the occupational therapy (OT) profession and the world of work.

The link between therapy, work and health, has always been influenced by wider societal attitudes to work, leisure, unemployment, poverty and health (Jackson, 1993). By gaining a clearer perspective of factors such as the health of the workforce and of the population at large, changing gender roles, economic and social issues, and public health priorities, we can gain a greater understanding of the interwoven history between OT and work. The purpose of this chapter, then, is to illustrate how these factors, and others, have impacted on the practice of OT in vocational rehabilitation (VR) in the past. In later chapters we can then explore how these factors may continue to influence our practice today.

Throughout this chapter, the challenges faced by previous generations of occupational therapists are clearly evident. Addressing the health needs of workers was not easy for the women who were the pioneers of OT. The injuries and health conditions which they were faced with were often very different from those seen today. The availability and range of treatments was very limited – there were few effective medicines and the cost of healthcare was beyond the reach of many. Work was risky and there were few safe-guards for workers. Over the course of time, OT has, out of necessity, had to evolve to meet the changing demands and needs of different client groups in different settings, as it continues to do today.

This chapter demonstrates how, at certain times in our history, there has been a strong OT focus on assisting disabled or ill workers. At other times, as seen in recent decades in the UK, there has been little or no involvement at all. This shifting emphasis has societal, political, and economic roots. By exploring these origins and influences, we may begin, perhaps, to anticipate potential future trends which may impact on the growth, and perhaps even the survival, of the profession in the future. You will note, as this chapter unfolds, how early occupational therapists faced particular challenges because of the established gender roles of the time. The dominance of the medical profession, together with tremendous medical advances, has exerted a particularly strong influence on the direction taken by OT. However other events, such as two world wars, economic recessions, and the advent of the welfare state, have also played a part in determining the involvement of occupational therapists in workplace health and workers' rehabilitation.

The chapter will conclude by outlining how changes in the political and economic climate have, once again, put VR firmly on the agenda. These favourable conditions mean new and exciting opportunities. The challenge for occupational therapists is, once again, to refocus. In order to make effective use of the growing body of professional knowledge about human occupation, and the value of decent work to health, occupational therapists need to be ready to meet societies' growing requirement to address the work needs of ill and disabled people.

THE EARLIEST USES OF OCCUPATION AS THERAPY

It has been suggested that the early use of occupation as therapy began alongside the introduction of moral treatment to mental asylums in the mid-16th to mid-19th centuries (Barris *et al.*, 1988). This is not strictly true, since the use of activity to enhance physical and mental health, and well-being, stretches back to far earlier times. In fact, the therapeutic use of occupation can be traced back through the ages (MacDonald, 1970). Occupations such as work, exercise and recreation have been used in both Eastern and Western cultures to improve health and well-being (Paterson, 1997a). In ancient Chinese cultures, for example, physical training was used for the promotion of health. The Greeks reportedly made use of remedies such as music, wrestling and riding. Even as early as 30BC, employment was recommended for mental agitation. Alternating work and play was recognised as improving dysfunctional thought patterns as well as creating a sense of well-being (Primeau, 1996).

Many more examples of past uses of the healing powers of therapeutic activity can be found in the literature. The purpose of this chapter, however, is not to delve into the use of occupation as therapy, nor to expand on the origins of OT itself. Instead, it charts the relationship across time, between OT and the occupation of work. It begins with the therapeutic use of work in 18th century asylums.

MORAL TREATMENT, OCCUPATION AND WORK

In western Europe, towards the end of the 18th century, a new political agenda emerged in response to changing societal attitudes and reforms (Quiroga, 1995). A clear example of this shift in attitude was seen in the way mentally ill people were treated. They had previously been subjected to harsh medical remedies, such as regular bleeding, vomiting and purging, and were chained up in prison-like institutions. Then a new era of 'moral treatment' emerged (Paterson, 1997a). Society began to believe that there was a moral obligation to care for the mentally ill. People with mental illness deserved compassion and could not be held responsible for their actions. They were deemed as needing a cultural way of life, and opportunities for involvement in their everyday world, regardless of having a mental illness (Barris *et al.*, 1988). The strong puritan influence of the time supported the use of work; viewing it as a positive and beneficial activity (Harvey-Krefting, 1985).

These contemporary perspectives brought about significant changes within asylums. Patients were freed from restraining chains and physical exercise and manual occupations were prescribed as innovative, new forms of treatment. These changes were implemented across the western world. For example, work treatment programmes were introduced into an asylum for the insane near Paris, France. Similarly, The Retreat, a psychiatric hospital in York, England, used employment to restore order within the asylum (Morrison, 1990). As these moral treatment approaches became more widespread, so too did the range and breadth of the occupations available to patients. This was particularly so in private institutions which served more affluent patients, since moral treatment did not extend to those who were considered paupers (Harvey–Krefting, 1985). Sir William Ellis, an English psychiatrist who was ahead of his time, highlighted the link between poverty, unemployment and insanity in the mid-1830s. In an attempt to combat this destructive cycle, he introduced the 'gainful employment' of patients in his asylum on a large scale. He recognised that individuals needed to be prepared for employment after discharge, so as to prevent relapse (Paterson, 1997b). Much of modern day thinking around social inclusion reflects similar values and ideals.

Early use of work activities was largely in keeping with class and gender norms of the time (Bracegirdle, 1991). Women tended to be occupied by domestic work in the kitchens or sewing, knitting or crochet. Garments made were often sold. Men were involved in manual work such as horticulture, bricklaying, blacksmith work, basket making and tailoring. These work activities had a primarily restorative purpose and any economic benefits to the institution were, at that time, of only secondary importance (Hanson and Walker, 1992). Indeed, occupation was not only used in the treatment of the mentally ill. The ideals behind moral treatment extended beyond the asylum and so there was widespread interest in employment opportunities for physically disabled people too. Trade schools and other training workshops were developed, and served much the same purpose as sheltered workshops of more recent times. Workshops for blind people offered music, crafts and work projects. Products made were sold, but the main purpose was to give structure and purpose to the lives of individuals, rather than financial independence (Harvey-Krefting, 1985).

Unfortunately, however, the progressive changes of the moral treatment era were short-lived:

- Increasing urbanisation and industrialisation contributed to growing numbers of chronic patients entering asylums. By the mid- to late 1800s, asylums had increased to such a size that they had become unwieldy. There were over 100,000 inmates, and still more in workhouse infirmaries (Hardy, 2001).

- At around this time, public attitudes began to change. The humanist values underpinning moral treatment were replaced by a philosophy which emphasised the personal responsibilities of the individual.
- Medical opinion of mental illness became dominated by a biological perspective. This led to pessimistic beliefs about the poor long-term prognosis of what was, at the time, viewed as a disease of the brain (Harvey-Krefting, 1985).

Given these pressures, reform could not be sustained. By the turn of the century, many institutions were unable to provide much more than custodial care. As moral treatment died out, so too did much of the early promise of the use of work and occupation as forms of therapy. It wasn't until after the First World War that productive work returned to asylums on a large scale.

WORK IN THE 18TH AND 19TH CENTURIES

In this section we will turn our attention to exploring what work was like in the past. In doing so, we learn that work was a very different experience from that of nowadays. Although accurate records do not exist, estimates suggest that in Britain before 1755, the occupational structure was quite stable. The pace of work was relatively slow and up to a third of the year consisted of holidays for religious celebrations, festivals, weddings, carnivals and funerals. Change began with a rapid increase in the two largest industries, agriculture and manufacturing, during the second half of the 18th century. Other economic activity took place in the smaller industries of commerce, building and mining. At about the same time religious reformers, such as Puritans, began to reject existing work patterns and introduced a harsher regime, consisting of six days of work and one of rest. It was believed this was an essential way to improve humanity (Primeau, 1996). It is important to bear in mind that although work has come to be associated with dignity and status in modern times, in the past it used to invariably involve pain and degradation (Berg, 1987) and was very much used as a means of social control. Workers were afforded few protections and industrial accidents were commonplace. The risks of injury and even death were very real. Many of these issues still confront workers in developing countries today.

THE PLACE OF WOMEN IN THE WORKFORCE

Work at this time was traditionally divided by gender. Women and children made up a large percentage of the workforce in some industries. For example, in late 18th century Britain the largest, most dominant sector within manufacturing was the textile industry. Textiles produced included wools, linen, silk, lace, hand and framework knits, and cotton. Across this sector, women and children did most of the work tasks. This type of work took place in small, individual textile industries and in the home, within the family economy. Other significant manufacturing industries included leather trades and metalwork industries. These, together with the building and coal industries, were the domain of men. Mixed trades did, however, exist within the iron and brewing sectors (Gray, 1987).

As mechanisation increased, there were reduced opportunities in many industries, and a drop in earnings followed. It is recorded that a good spinner in the linen industry in Scotland, working a 12-hour day, could produce $1\frac{1}{2}$ spindles per week. But even working these long hours, she wasn't able to cover the price of her food, clothing and rent. Whereas during the pre-industrial and early industrial periods, the employment of women in the trades was widespread (Gray, 1987), this all changed with high levels of male unemployment and a glut of trades. Work shortage resulted in the barring of women from many trades, as well as from higher-paid work in the textile industry. In addition, increasing industrialisation led to much of the available employment moving away from the home. This shift, combined with restricted roles within the trades, produced a far greater split in the division of labour than had previously existed. The changes also contributed to widening pay inequities. Domestic labour became the forced option for many women, particularly in more rural areas (Berg, 1987).

TECHNOLOGICAL CHANGE

Across these two centuries, division of labour was also influenced by new, emerging technologies. For example, in some industries the need for strength in manual labour decreased, so that boys, as young as six or eight, could be as capable as men (Gray, 1987). In contrast, the large engineering companies which emerged in the early 1870s employed thousands of skilled men in industries such as shipbuilding (McClelland, 1987). The increasing use of mechanisation also introduced other new forms of work, such as tailoring, glove-making and shirt-button making. Much of this delicate work was considered to be best suited to women and girls, since they had smaller hands, and many had already gained similar skills doing needlework in the home.

Despite these technological advances, work conditions remained extremely poor. For example, a typical lacquering room, used by five to six women workers at a time, would be no more that 12ft by 15ft in size. It would house a couple of iron plate stoves (Gray, 1987) and the heat and fumes were quite overpowering. During the mid-19th century, many factory employees worked for more than 70 hours a week. Few religious holidays were observed, and paid holidays did not exist (Deem, 1988). The need for reform was highlighted by rising levels of distress and unrest. Attempts were made to reduce exploitation and cruelty by giving employers increased responsibility for improved conditions and events which took place at the factory. The Ten Hours Act and the Factory Acts brought about slight improvements in conditions for workers (McClelland, 1987). In the same way that the moral era, discussed earlier, had heralded changes in the conditions in the mental asylums, these reforms set out basic moral responsibilities that were expected of employers.

Most notably from these times, a link was created, which still exists to this day, between work and social inequalities. The shift from agricultural to industrial production, together with the growth of bureaucratic workplaces away from the home, brought lasting change to the place of work in individuals' lives, and to the narrower ways in which work was understood, valued and rewarded (Deem, 1988).

THE 20TH CENTURY

1900s–1910s: WAR AND RECONSTRUCTION

Towards the end of the first decade of the new century, an economic crisis loomed. Workers in the key industries of mining, railways and transport were threatening a mass strike, demanding improved working conditions and union representation. Unemployment remained a major concern, and the Unemployed Workmen Act of 1905 was passed to prevent men without a job being subjected to the stigma of the Poor Laws. The National Insurance Act (1911) was introduced in recognition of the inevitability of periods of unemployment, because of the cyclical nature of work (Beveridge, 1960). Shortly thereafter, a century of almost uninterrupted peace was shattered by the outbreak of war in 1914. The onset of the war put domestic problems on the backburner and for a time there was a strong sense of united purpose. Manufacturing and commercial enterprises worked hard to maintain a 'business as usual' ethic (Morgan, 2000). The whole population became involved in the war effort and, in the early years at least, many patriotically upheld the view that it was a right and just war. Large numbers of men volunteered to join the armed services, despite the extremely poor physical state of those from the slums and the factories (Doyle, 2003).

As the war dragged on, it produced an unprecedented number of casualties. In Britain alone, over half the generation of young men, some 750,000, were killed. A further 2.5 million were wounded, and many of them were permanently disabled (Morgan, 2000). It is important to bear in mind that the treatment of those injured in the war, and others in civilian hospitals with tuberculosis and polio, was often a lengthy process. In many instances, there was seldom much hope of recovery. The despair of wounded soldiers in military hospitals, in particular, caused widespread concern. There was an urgent need to get the hundreds of thousands of men back into society (Bloom Hoover, 1996). This desperation heralded the introduction of occupation into the wards in the form of reconstruction programmes. While the earlier beginnings of OT had been confined to psychiatric treatment, the war brought about its rapid expansion into the field of physical medicine.

Reconstruction programmes for disabled soldiers were set up around the world. The English reconstruction model, put in place before America even entered the war, comprised orthopaedics, OT (then known as bedside occupations and curative workshops), physiotherapy and vocational re-education. These teams were led by orthopaedic physicians who prescribed reconstruction in a similar way to medication. The physicians decided who received treatment, its type, duration and the time of discharge. American post-war programmes consisted of three clearly identified stages.

In the first, reconstruction aides in OT, as they were known, provided diversional occupations at the bedside (Gutman, 1995).

These reconstruction aides are recognised as having made a significant contribution to the war effort, at critical stage in the infancy of OT. Many of the women (only women were allowed to be reconstruction aides) already had a degree, which was unusual for the time. In addition, a number came to the role with first-hand experience of caring for someone with a disability (Gutman, 1995). Reconstruction aides came from backgrounds such as craftspersons, teachers and artists, but they lacked any medical knowledge (Spackman, 1968; Low, 1992). Basic training was provided to equip them to teach simple crafts to patients in military hospitals. They were civilians who did not receive military rank and were therefore at the lowest level in the hierarchy of the military. Initially, there was fierce opposition to their introduction, because it was considered to be 'not desirable to employ women in this type of work in military hospitals' (Crane, 1927, p.81 cited in Gutman, 1995, p.257).

Purposeful occupation

Although the ways in which work was used by the OT pioneers was diversional, at the same time it was purposeful and therapeutic. Participation was intended to 'divert the mind, exercise some part of the anatomy, or to relieve the monotony and boredom of illness' (Barton, 1999 cited in Harvey-Krefting, 1985, p.303). The rationale for the diversional occupations was to draw the soldiers' attention away from their pain and suffering. Men could spend many months in hospital, so crafts were used to give meaning to life and encourage intrinsic motivation. In these early days, little attention was paid to the meaningfulness or relevance of the occupations to the individual and popular choices included knitting, basket weaving, raffia work, bead work, rug making, toy making and crochet (Bloom Hoover, 1996; Hanson and Walker, 1992). When the patient was sufficiently recovered to leave the ward, he attended the curative workshop during the second stage of the reconstruction programme.

Curative workshops, attached to special military hospitals, were established on both sides of the Atlantic. OT in the workshops involved the manufacture of appliances, such as splints and other orthopaedic devices, or maintenance work within the hospital setting (Spackman, 1968). This therapeutic work served as an important bridge between physical restoration and return to work (Matheson et al., 1985). It established a foundation for the third and final stage of the reconstruction programme known as vocation education, which was considered, at the time, to be beyond the scope of OT. This vocational training, which also took place in workshops in the military hospitals, was provided by men with the expertise to teach returning soldiers a vocation. The vocational education worker studied each individual so as to identify a suitable training, with a view to future placement in a trade or profession (Hall, 1918 cited in Spackman, 1968, p.69).

It is clear from these historical accounts that the women who were the early OT pioneers played a pivotal role in assisting injured soldiers toward recovery and re-integration into civilian life. These achievements were made all the more remarkable in the context of the strong male dominance within both medicine and the military at the time.

War and mental illness

Until the Great War, psychiatrists continued to hold a firm belief in the organic nature of mental illness. They also remained strong supporters of the clear distinction in English law between the sane and the insane. However, the mental distress caused by the horrors and destruction of war gave rise to illnesses which they had not previously encountered. These illnesses included deep depression, convulsive shaking, nightmares, mutism and paralysis. These mental conditions collectively became known as 'shellshock'. However, shellshock could not be associated with an identifiable brain lesion. Doctors were faced with the stark choice of deciding if the patient did indeed have an illness, and should therefore be sent for treatment, or, if not, sent back to the military to be shot for cowardice. Previously unshaken public expectations, that soldiers should show their bravery through stoicism, faltered, as this new form of illness emerged on a large scale. The eventual acknowledgement of the psychological nature of this condition led to the re-introduction of more psychotherapeutic treatments. Although these changes initially took place in the military hospitals, they eventually spread to civilian treatment centres as well (Hardy, 2001).

Illness in civilian life

Despite the human toll, the war years were a catalyst for widespread industrial and social reform. War also brought with it new freedoms and new employment opportunities for civilians. Since much of industrial and agricultural production was directed into the war effort, there was practically no unemployment. Basic education was made free and social housing policy introduced. Women in particular were beneficiaries of these developments. Many served in field hospitals and new opportunities became available in clerical and administrative work. Others took up jobs, which had previously been reserved for men, in munitions and engineering factories (Morgan, 2000).

However, not all these freedoms were as positive. Excessive drinking, already an established problem before the war, was blamed for high levels of absenteeism amongst munitions workers. As a result, they were subject to criticism for failing to keep up with army requirements. The Government intervened with legislation to regulate the trade in liquor, and this action reduced the number of deaths from cirrhosis of the liver. Unfortunately, however, the decreased availability of alcohol produced a rapid rise in cigarette smoking, amongst both men and women, but the negative health effects of this substitute substance were only to become apparent many years later.

Infectious illnesses also remained a deadly killer during this era. Meningitis, then known as cerebrospinal fever, was responsible for 2,000 deaths in 1915 and the same number again died from scarlet fever. Measles caused the death of 16,000 young people, 6,000 died from whooping cough and a further 5,000 from diphtheria. The incidence of respiratory tuberculosis among young women was rising, and was thought to be related to poor nutrition combined with stressful conditions at home and work (Hardy, 2001). The largely palliative nature of care for these, and other conditions, meant that patients in civilian hospitals were often too unwell for work activities to be realistic (Cromwell, 1985). OT did, however, take place within sanatoria for patients with tuberculosis. Work programmes were run from workshops located nearby (Mosey, 1986). Patients produced articles such as pottery, weaving, basketry and wood-carving. The cost of transport to the workshop, and the instruction received, were offset against the proceeds from the sale of items produced (Hanson and Walker, 1992).

1920s–1930s: ECONOMIC DECLINE AND UNEMPLOYMENT

The early post-war years produced an economic boom. The working week was reduced to 48 hours and this allowed more leisure time. Paid holidays were introduced by many employers. Families were able to enjoy outings on the cheap transport provided by the newly introduced bus. However, this period of relative wealth was short-lived. By the early 1920s, many parts of Britain were experiencing depression and rising levels of unemployment. In particular, Wales and the north of England were hard hit, with three quarters of unemployed families living below the poverty line. In these areas, deaths from conditions such as diphtheria, heart disease, tuberculosis, bronchitis and pneumonia were also significantly higher than elsewhere (Constantine, 1980). The Great Depression, following the collapse of the Wall Street stock market, produced a jump in unemployment from one to three million within two years. As the state struggled to cope with rising demand, unemployment benefits were cut in response. The areas worst hit by this economic downturn were the old industrial areas. Coal mining, ship-building and steel industries went into a rapid and steep decline. In some areas, unemployment rose to over 70 per cent. Those parts of the country with new, light manufacturing industries, such as electricity, car and radio production, were less affected by these events (Hardy, 2001).

Basic improvements in the working conditions of employees introduced during and after the war, had however failed to address the extensive health and social problems existing in the population at large. Unemployment, combined with poor housing and nutrition, and high levels of pollution, contributed to ongoing poor health for many. It was estimated that over 80 per cent of the children of this generation showed signs of rickets (Hardy, 2001). In America, dramatic cuts in spending on medical care meant that it could barely be afforded by many (Rerek, 1971). The difficulties in gaining employment during the depression of the inter-war years also placed a heavy burden on families. In the wool textile industry, for example, it was commonplace for employers to include the labour and skills of a wife and unmarried daughters as a condition of employment for any male workers. Girls were taken out of school to work on the looms. Working conditions were extreme, with very high temperatures, poor air quality since it was thick with dust, and little clean drinking water. For the vast majority of workers of these times, the conditions under which they worked remained outside of their control, so these practices remained well into the 1950s (Allen, 1997).

Occupational therapy and vocational rehabilitation

OT schools were established in America by the end of the war. Early schools were open only to 'refined and intelligent young women' (Partridge, 1921, p.64 cited in Woodside, 1971, p.229). Six- to 12-week courses were run for women with a background in nursing, teaching, or arts and crafts. Concepts which remain central to OT practice today, such as grading an activity according to an individual's capacity, emerged early on in the professions' history. A core element of the underpinning philosophy of OT was eloquently captured by one of its early proponents who said that 'Man learns to organize time and he does it in terms of *doing* things, and one of the many good things he does between eating, drinking and wholesome nutrition generally, and the flights of fancy and aspiration, we call *work and occupation*' (Meyer, 1922, reprinted 1977, p.642). So the link between OT and work as a significant form of human occupation was clearer then than perhaps it is nowadays.

The success of OT in military treatment centres resulted in the extension of similar programmes into civilian hospitals (Hanson and Walker, 1992). However, the tight control of OT by orthopaedic surgeons resulted in an increased emphasis on the medical application of occupation. This meant that prospective occupational therapists were required to have an aptitude for science. The shift away from central beliefs in the value of occupation for health was combined with a growing interest in disability, function and reductionism. This biomedical approach has since dominated much of professional practice in the intervening years (Friedland, 1998). Other sources of knowledge were, however also explored, and the value and relevance of ideas being developed in industrial engineering, such as motion study, also attracted the attention of occupational therapists. These new forms of knowledge contributed to the early analysis and classification of crafts for therapeutic use in both physical and mental health fields (Creighton, 1992).

In America in 1920, the Vocational Rehabilitation Act came into existence. This was an important development because it provided funds for the rehabilitation of people with a physical disability, to retrain them if necessary, and then to place them into a suitable job (Matheson *et al.*, 1985). Shortly thereafter, the Federal Industrial Rehabilitation Act (1923) required that OT should be provided in general hospitals, to those suffering from an industrial accident or illness (Hanson and Walker, 1992). While these Acts did not apply to psychiatric patients, they do seem to have helped to embed the role of OT in VR in that country, more effectively than was achieved in the United Kingdom at the time. Further amendments to the Act in 1943 and 1954 resulted in additional increases in funding, thereby ensuring the continued expansion of VR services in that country (Matheson *et al.*, 1985).

Health and medicine

At this time, illnesses such as cancer caused a rising number of deaths – over 40,000 in 1920 – and new treatments, such as radium, were being experimented with. A particularly important new medical discovery was a group of drugs which was effective against bacterial infections. The success of these new drugs, the forerunners of penicillin, was dramatic, and as a result the number of deaths from infection dropped significantly (Hardy, 2001). British spa towns increased in popularity during the 1930s, as the depreciation of sterling reduced the prospect of recuperative trips abroad. Medical advice was sought to decide on the most suitable spa for specific treatments. Hydrotherapy (or balneotherapy as it was also known) was used to treat medical disorders of the locomotor system, such as rheumatism. Medical supervision was available at hotels and hydros at seaside resorts. Prescriptions could be issued for hot sea water or seaweed baths. Woodhall Spa, in Lincolnshire, treated ailments such as arthritic and rheumatic disorders, while Cheltenham in Gloucestershire specialised in heart and circulation conditions and digestive disorders. Weston-Super-Mare treated asthma and kidney disease, while Herne Bay in Kent was considered suitable for early pulmonary tuberculosis and infantile gland and bone diseases (Meredith, 1935). The use of these natural treatment remedies for chronic conditions has retained widespread popularity and public funding in some European countries, such as France, to the present day.

The hazards of work

In the 1930s, the market for leisure activities continued to grow. Cinema, dance halls, cricket, football, horse and greyhound racing all enjoyed much popularity. Despite these newly found pleasures, work remained a hazardous occupation for many. Occupational diseases were rife, and poisoning, cancers, lung disease, deafness and blindness, as a result of work, were commonplace. In Britain, for example, 6,000 men were disabled each year by a condition known as miners' nystagmus. This is thought to have been a form of eye strain caused by poor lighting at the coal face. It is also estimated that 20 per cent of glass workers and iron workers developed cataracts from their exposure to furnace glare. Pneumatic tools caused 'dead fingers', stiffness and muscle wasting. These symptoms affected over 60 per cent of workers after just ten years in this line of work. In some severe cases, workers developed gangrene. Those who were boilermakers experienced a gradual, permanent deterioration of their hearing. No-one engaged in this sort of work escaped this impairment. In other types of work, musculoskeletal conditions abounded. For example, Covent Garden porters often developed a painful swelling, known as a hummy, on the upper part of their back. Doctors noted the similarity of the nature of this condition to 'weavers' bottom', a kind of ischial bursitis experienced by those working certain looms. Constant kneeling on hard surfaces led others to develop Housemaid's Knee (Meredith, 1935).

As well as causing various impairments, work could also be fatal. In England, about 2,000 people were exposed to the inhalation of pure asbestos dust on a daily basis. As with a number of other toxic substances, it took some time for the dangers of asbestos to become apparent. The symptoms of shortness of breath and coughing, which workers developed, led to eventual heart failure. In the cotton industry, up to 75 per cent of the workers developed asthma-like attacks and bronchitis as a result of the dust. At that time, there was no cure or even treatment for this affliction. Also in the textile industry, 1,000 cotton mule spinners developed skin cancer. This condition also affected chimney sweeps, caused by some of the substances they came into contact with through the course of their work (Hardy, 2001). A rare and mysterious disease was discovered in young women who presented with an inflammation of the jaw. As it progressed, the condition produced a severe, and finally fatal, anaemia. Their illness was found to be the result of poisoning with radium, a radio-active substance. The women had all worked, at some stage, in factories which manufactured luminous watch dials. The paint they used to inscribe the figures, and which contained the poison, was ingested when they brought the brush to a point using their mouths (Meredith, 1935).

As well as the threats posed by toxic chemicals, increasing mechanisation and powerful machinery in the workplace resulted in rising numbers of serious accidents. Some workers who sustained injuries at work in this way attended industrial workshops. Occupational therapists treated these injured workers alongside people with orthopaedic conditions, arthritis, cardiac diseases and tuberculosis in these rehabilitation workshops (Wise, 1930 cited in Hanson and Walker, 1992, p.58). A traditional gender divide existed between the types of activities that took place in the workshops. Eighty-five per cent of the patients were men, coming mostly from a manual labouring background. Therefore, woodwork was commonly used in treatment programmes. Far smaller numbers of women patients took part in textiles and needlework activities. These were seen as a typical woman's occupation from their role in homemaking. As well as having an understanding of the therapeutic nature of occupation, occupational therapists at this time were required to have a commercial knowledge as well (Hanson and Walker, 1992).

Industrial therapy programmes could also be found in the mental hospitals of the 1930s. Unlike the work programmes of the earlier moral treatment era, which were intended to restore health, these later industrial therapy programmes clearly had a much stronger economic purpose. They were defined as 'the prescribed use of activities inherent to the hospital operation planned for the mutual benefit of patient and institution' (Shalik, 1959, pp.1–7 cited in Matheson et al., 1985, p.315). Some occupational therapists, uncomfortable about the growing conflict between therapeutic and commercial objectives, moved out of these treatment environments.

1940s–1950s: WAR, EMPLOYMENT AND REHABILITATION

The rehabilitation principles underpinning the curative workshops had not been widely pursued during the peace years of the 1920s and 1930s. The limits of available treatments meant that long periods of convalescence in hospital were the norm. This approach changed out of necessity, with the second advent of global war. Unprecedented numbers of casualties meant that a far quicker return to health was demanded. To help achieve this, a rehabilitation approach was introduced. Patients with similar physical conditions were grouped together and progressed through intensive programmes of graded activities and exercises. Physiotherapy, OT and hydrotherapy formed an essential part of these programmes (Nichols, 1980). The aim of the

rehabilitation programmes was to assist patients to achieve maximal functional efficiency. Despite this goal, therapists often had to deal with low levels of motivation
as many men, who feared being sent back to fight, showed little desire to recover
(Hanson and Walker, 1992).

It is interesting to reflect on this raised emphasis on rehabilitation and recovery
for work, at this point in history. In the same way that the First World War had acted
as a catalyst for the development of OT in this field, so too did the onset of the
Second World War, when these further developments took place (Eldar and Jelic,
2003). It was not, however, only about the recovery of injured soldiers. During the
war years, disabled people were also needed to contribute to the war effort (Floyd and
Landymore, 2000), so the need for VR, to enable access to work roles, was established.
Before this, people with any form of impairment were segregated from the rest of
the population in large-scale institutions, often located far outside existing towns
and cities. After the war – realising the economic costs of institutionalisation – the
Government pursued the idea of care within, and by, the community. In the education
sector, for example, The Education Act (1944) was intended to remove the separate
education system for disabled children, and integrate them into mainstream schools.
Similarly, the Disabled Persons (Employment) Act, of the same year, was meant to
prevent exclusion from work (Drake, 1999).

At this time, American occupational therapists developed a new type of VR service. These work evaluation programmes, as they were called, were designed to assess
and rehabilitate people with physical disabilities for work, after their medical treatment had been completed (Marshall, 1985). The programme took place in simulated
industrial environments where a variety of manual 'jobs' were on offer. Initially,
the occupational therapist analysed performance, work tolerance and work skills,
including tool handling, strength and dexterity. Following this, possible options for
work were considered. The vocational interests and aspirations of the client were,
however, of secondary importance within this process, since they were taken into
account only after functional work tolerances had been determined. Work evaluation and pre-vocational programmes became an accepted OT role (Marshall, 1985),
but they had shifted the focus away from the use of occupation to maintain and develop health, to improving medical outcomes (Friedland, 1998). In this context, the
rehabilitative approach was purely concerned with achieving physical restoration
(Mosey, 1986).

Resettlement and industrial rehabilitation

Just as the previous war had been instrumental in producing social change, so too,
was this one. In 1942, new British Government plans to introduce wide-ranging social security provisions were set out in the Beveridge Report. Measures included free
medical treatment and greater financial support during any short periods of unemployment. These ambitious plans were to be achieved through full employment and
freedom from idleness (Beveridge, 1960). The Tomlinson Report in 1943 supported
these ideals and the 1944 Disabled Persons (Employment) Act came into being. This

Act made provision for the resettlement and rehabilitation of disabled people. Resettlement services were provided by disablement resettlement officers (DRO) based in job centres. They made decisions about clients' suitability for open or sheltered work and referred them on to relevant services, accordingly. At this time a dual system was in operation, since occupational therapists were carrying out very similar work within hospitals (Kennedy, 1986). In addition, some schemes were run by local authorities and the voluntary sector. However, most of the sheltered workshops set up by the Government as part of this provision, were run by an organisation called Remploy. Although it has undergone some re-branding in the intervening years, Remploy continues to provide sheltered work for disabled people to this day. The current Remploy organisation and services will be discussed further in a later chapter.

As well as sheltered workplaces, industrial rehabilitation units were set up in larger cities. Within the open labour market, companies with over 20 employees were required to follow a quota system, which meant employing a percentage (three per cent) of disabled people. The combination of measures set out in the Disabled Persons (Employment) Act (1944) helped assist many disabled people into work, in the early years (Floyd and Landymore, 2000).

Developments in healthcare and rehabilitation

As well as changes to employment services, the introduction of the National Health Service (NHS) in the late 1940s resulted in significant changes to the way in which healthcare was provided. Before this the Emergency Medical Service, which had been established during the war, continued to treat and rehabilitate both military personnel and civilians, such as injured miners (Paterson, 1998; Morrison, 1990). The creation of the state-funded NHS meant that the small numbers of occupational therapists working in the Emergency Medical Service became employees of the new NHS. During these early years, few significant changes were noted to OT practice as a result of this transition (Paterson, 1998). Tuberculosis continued to provide a significant workload for occupational therapists, since it remained a prominent cause of ill-health and death. Over 32,500 beds were needed to provide care for people with this illness, until an effective medical treatment was developed later in the 1950s.

Outside of OT, further developments in rehabilitation took place with the establishment of rehabilitation medicine. This medical specialty crossed the range of traditional specialisms and was particularly concerned with conditions such as stroke, rheumatoid arthritis, amputations, rehabilitation after surgery, spinal injuries and head injuries. It was directed towards the physical, social and organisational aspects of the after-care of those patients who needed more than just acute, short-term care (Nichols, 1980). Rehabilitation was defined as 'the whole process of restoring a disabled person to a condition in which he is able, as early as possible, to resume a normal life' (Report of the Committee of Enquiry on the Rehabilitation, Training and Resettlement of Disabled Persons, 1956, para 5 cited in Nichols, 1980, p.1).

On a more global level, the International Labour Organisation set standards for VR in 1955. These standards detailed the scope, principles and methods of VR for the disabled. They were revised in 1983, to more clearly identify the link between work and social integration, or inclusion as it is better known today. The purpose of VR was defined as 'to enable a disabled person to secure, retain or advance in suitable employment and thereby to further such person's integration or re-integration into society' (International Labour Organisation, 1983, p.1).

Occupational therapy and work programmes

Work assessment and work resettlement became crucial functions of OT in psychiatry during the 1950s. There were rising numbers of programmes concerned with work and industrial rehabilitation. Favourable conditions meant that large numbers of patients were able to return to employment. The advent of medicines, such as chlorpromazine for schizophrenia, and later lithium for mania, provided more effective treatment for people with psychosis, particularly younger patients. This was coupled with the healthy state of the post-war national economy resulting in an increased demand for manual workers (Monteath, 1983). The aim of OT in industrial rehabilitation programmes was 'to employ every patient in the hospital who is capable of, or can be made capable of employment. Its purpose is to help these patients readjust themselves to life and to guide them back to a useful life either in the outside world or in the hospital community' (Haworth and Macdonald, 1946, p.10 cited in Paterson, 1998, p.312). A survey of psychiatric hospitals in 1962 showed that most had an industrial therapy unit which was supervised by the head occupational therapist, although the financial side was generally managed by the finance department (Hill, 1967).

Towards the end of this decade, however, the main form of industry in America and much of western Europe began changing. A shift from production and manufacturing jobs towards service provision work meant less availability of industrial jobs. Greater emphasis was placed on education as the requirements of the marketplace changed. The use of work activities in rehabilitation programmes declined as unskilled and manual work became harder for patients to find. Programmes refocused away from work towards alternative forms of occupation, such as crafts. This move away from the use of work as therapy continued through much of the 60s and into the early 70s (Hanson and Walker, 1992).

1960s–1970s: WOMEN, WORK, UNEMPLOYMENT AND REFORM

In 1960 in the UK, Lord Beveridge declared that the ambition from 16 years earlier had been met: full employment had been achieved. Any celebration of this success was short lived, however, as the pace of change within the labour market continued to accelerate. Earlier, we read about how increasing mechanisation during the first half of the century led to extensive job losses within the manual labour force. Then, the information age came into being. This technological revolution threatened the established jobs and livelihoods of skilled and professional workers. New jobs were created as old ones quickly became obsolete. The impact of these changes was felt particularly amongst older workers. They were encouraged to retire early, to make way for younger, more highly skilled, workers. These practises took place before the introduction of equal opportunity legislation, when ageism in industry was at its peak. Advertisements for jobs discriminated against school leavers lacking industry experience and older workers alike.

The 1970s also saw changing gender trends in employment. The proportion of women in the paid workforce started to increase, particularly amongst mothers with pre-school children. At the same time, the numbers of working men began to decrease (Harkness, 2005). There were clear economic benefits for employers in this trend, since the wages earned by women were only around 70 per cent of the average male wage. This movement towards greater numbers of women working outside the home has continued, so that by 2004, 70 per cent of working-age women were in paid employment (Office for National Statistics, 2005).

Alongside the technological advances, and workforce changes which were taking place, there were also increasing levels of dissatisfaction with the nature of work (Green, 2005). The impersonal character of large, post-industrial, bureaucratic organisations served few beyond the needs of the organisations themselves. Many jobs were monotonous and roles were narrowly defined and prescribed. The growing complexity of jobs also demanded higher levels of specialisation. This trend was reflected in OT, as therapists started addressing particular aspects of the patient, rather than the holistic needs of the person as a human being (Diasio, 1971). There were also major changes to the main client groups of occupational therapists. The discovery of an effective treatment for tuberculosis earlier in the 1950s had dramatically cut the numbers suffering from this condition. Then later, in 1962, the introduction of an oral vaccine brought about the eradication of polio from the UK, a major cause of disability (Paterson, 1998).

Changes also began to take place within OT education. New knowledge from the behavioural sciences was embraced. Sociological, developmental and human potential approaches offered a welcome alternative framework to that of the medical model (Diasio, 1971). In pursuing these new perspectives, many occupational therapists once again began to focus their attention away from work programmes, in a similar pattern to the decades which had followed the First World War. Again, these changes coincided with an economic downturn. The country began sliding into depression and concerns about rising unemployment levels were clear. By 1976 this number was increasing by 10,000 people a month. A review of services introduced 30 years earlier, under the Disabled Persons (Employment) Act, was highly critical of their failure to keep abreast of changes, both in the nature of disability and in the labour market (Tunbridge and Mair, 1972 cited in Floyd and Landymore, 2000). Sweeping reforms to Britain's employment and training services followed. The Manpower Services Commission took over from the Department of Employment. It was split into the Employment Services Agency and the Training Services Agency.

The Employment Services division was responsible for the employment centres and job centres around the country and also employed DROs (Nichols, 1980). DROs performed a similar role to vocational educators, present in America since reconstruction programmes were set up after the First World War. They had specialist training and their main task was to place disabled people in suitable work, if necessary after employment rehabilitation or vocational training. DROs were seen to potentially have a key role at the interface between the patient, health services and industry, but this ideal was never fully realised. As mentioned earlier, these employment-related services continued to be delivered in parallel to the rehabilitation services provided in many hospitals, where physiotherapists and occupational therapists were successfully returning patients back to their own job, or other similar work. Despite their success, the employment rehabilitation centres had the advantage of being able to provide a more realistic work environment than the hospital could (Nichols, 1980).

During these years, the pace of change in the labour market continued as jobs in manufacturing, utilities, mining and agriculture gave way to increases in jobs in the service sector. This trend continued, so that by 1995, the proportion of the overall workforce involved in the service sector in Britain was over three-quarters of the number of employees. The highest growth industries were to be found in sectors such as banking, insurance, finance, hotels and catering (Noon and Blyton, 1997).

1980s–1990s: DISABILITY IN THE COMMUNITY

For patients with a mental illness, industrial therapy had long since been a central part of their OT programmes. The aim of these programmes was to foster a degree of independence through participation in occupation, as well as to maintain the individual's habits and routines (Cromwell, 1985). Work roles tended to be traditional, with women doing work indoors and men outdoors.

During this decade, however, governments in the United Kingdom, Canada and America were all similarly intent on decreasing welfare expenditure. These reforms included large-scale closure of the mental asylums, together with most of the industrial workshops attached to them (McColl *et al.*, 1993). In a review of the literature, Vostanis (1990) examined the role of work in psychiatric rehabilitation. At the time, which was at the height of the de-institutionalisation movement, work was seen as an integral component of psychiatric care for this client group. Therefore, as long-stay patients were being moved out of large asylums, and into community-based accommodation, work needs were provided for through sheltered employment. Any form of competitive employment was seen as unrealistic, in view of the discrimination and the high levels of unemployment which existed in the United Kingdom at the time.

The effects of the recession, coupled with the shift towards community living, had a significant impact on occupational therapists' ability to support the resettlement of disabled patients into work. Demographic changes also meant that less young people were admitted to psychiatric hospitals and, if they were, it was for shorter stays. Those who stayed for any length of time tended to be elderly, long-stay patients and people who were very unwell. Assessment and preparation for work were unrealistic options for this population (Monteath, 1983), so these hospital-based services began to decline.

Employment Services, too, needed to adapt to the rising numbers of disabled people who were now resident in the community, rather than in institutions. The programmes run by employment resettlement (or rehabilitation) centres, were considered to be too inflexible and intensive, particularly for people who had disabilities caused by mental illness. Therefore a sheltered placement scheme was introduced, which placed disabled people into jobs in the open labour market, with a contribution to their wages, according to their productivity levels (Floyd and Landymore, 2000).

Despite visible shifts in policy during this time, underlying attitudes to disabled people remained largely unchanged. The dominant political convictions still reflected a 'personal tragedy' model. Disabled people were seen to be disadvantaged, through no fault of their own. Increasing numbers of state-run services were established in the community to provide care and facilitate independence. In this early stage of integration, much of the provision, despite being based in the community, remained separate from the rest of society. Leisure and social needs were mainly addressed through a variety of social clubs provided by health and social services (Drake, 1999). Many day centres were established for people who were not able to find work. Occupational therapists were frequently involved in organising substitute forms of work within some of these centres. Work, for many at the time, took the form of sheltered workshops or industrial therapy (Hill, 1967). Department of Health guidelines recommended that 50 sheltered places should be provided per 100 000 population (Vostanis, 1990). Despite these measures, however, employment opportunities through the quota system, introduced in 1944, did not materialise for many. While these laws had been intended to prevent exclusion from work, they were never actively enforced, and fines or prosecutions for contravention were seldom imposed.

Up until the 1980s, developments within OT in VR had taken similar routes in America and England. However during this decade the paths began to diverge. American occupational therapists re-asserted their role in this field, supported in their efforts by changes introduced to the workers' compensation legislation in the late 1970s. Renewed interest in VR meant that work hardening programmes, as they were known, abounded. These programmes treated mainly manual labourers with back ailments and traumatic injuries. Therapists were expected to be well-informed about the types of industries in their local areas, where they undertook consultancy roles, mainly aimed at injury prevention (Hanson and Walker, 1992). In contrast, the British literature reflected therapists' concern about the decline of OT in VR (Monteath, 1983). A combination of:

- growing demands for independent living skills resulting from community care
- high levels of unemployment
- a requirement for greater skill and educational levels within the labour market, meaning less job opportunities for people with disabilities (in 1986, seven per cent of the workforce had a degree, by early 2000 that had risen to 16 per cent) (Park *et al.*, 2003)

- a changed emphasis towards knowledge rather than skills, within OT curricula, as OT schools moved into higher education

meant that over the forthcoming ten years, any real involvement in 'work', for the majority of occupational therapists, was to become a thing of the past.

1990s – TODAY: THE RISE OF WORK-INDUCED STRESS-RELATED ILLNESS

Recognition of the social exclusion faced by disabled people within society, brought with it important changes to their rights in several western countries. A shift from a 'medical model' approach to disability, to a more 'social model' approach began. In 1990, after 20 years of fierce lobbying, the Americans with Disabilities Act came into being. A few years later, Australia and Canada similarly introduced civil rights legislation for disabled people. These enforceable measures required employers to make 'reasonable accommodations' for disabled people to be able to carry out the 'essential functions' of a job. In America, discrimination was prohibited against disabled job applicants able to perform the essential functions of the job. Despite these measures, a significant gap remains to this day between the rate of employment of disabled and non-disabled people. In the UK, in contrast, the Disability Discrimination Act (1995) was met with disappointment by disabled activists. It was viewed as a 'diluted measure, hedged about with qualifications and "let out" clauses' (Drake, 1999, p.86). A further ten years passed before it was reformed, to make compliance a legal, enforceable requirement.

The introduction of the NHS and Community Care Act (1990) meant that large numbers of occupational therapists, and other health professionals, moved out of acute hospitals into community-based services. This refocusing of health service provision, away from lengthy in-patient stays, brought significant challenges and opportunities for occupational therapists. The focus of the OT profession shifted towards facilitating independent living, as more occupational therapists began to work with people in their own homes, in the community. The rolling programme of mental asylum closure was at its peak at this time and many occupational therapists worked with long-stay institutionalised patients, to help them develop the life skills that they needed for independent living in the community. A similar focus was directed towards the increasing numbers of elderly people who were being encouraged to stay at home rather than move into care or nursing homes. The sheer demand for these forms of support at the time meant that the shift away from rehabilitation for work was largely disregarded by many within the profession. These changes also meant that the facilities which had previously been used for rehabilitation in hospitals, such as heavy and light workshops, became largely redundant and these spaces were soon put to other uses.

Meanwhile, in the workplace, there was a significant decline in levels of job satisfaction during the 1990s. In Britain, this was blamed on the changing nature of work, as opportunities for personal responsibility and initiative decreased. At the same time, people experienced an increase in the intensity of work effort required, meaning they had to work harder (Green, 2005). Traditional structures within workplaces continued to change, particularly in the ways in which workers were rewarded for their work. Fewer tiers in company hierarchies led to fewer opportunities for promotion. Appraisal of individual performance and performance-related pay replaced traditional arrangements for collective bargaining and group pay awards. New appraisal systems often failed to accurately reflect worker effort or output. A greater emphasis on team working was in conflict with the way in which performance was measured and rewarded, since this was done on an individual basis (Doyle, 2003). While these changes and others, including greater job insecurity, were taking place, the incidence of stress-related illness was on the rise. Greater numbers than ever were moving out of the labour market and onto state benefits because of ill-health.

The Health of the Nation (Department of Health, 1992) policy was a strategic attempt to improve the overall health of the population. It targeted health service resources towards reducing deaths from particular diseases such as heart disease, stroke and cancer. It failed, however, to recognise the negative influences on health from factors such as social inequity, poverty and unemployment. Work was no longer recognised to produce desirable health outcomes. As a consequence, rehabilitation services were focused away from the workplace and the health needs of workers. The decline in VR services, which had begun the previous decade, continued unabated. Yet again, criticism of the Employment Services, this time from the National Audit Office, resulted in the closure of all the employment rehabilitation centres. Restructuring took place and they were replaced by placing, assessment and counselling teams (PACTs). Each PACT served a population of up to a million people. DROs were renamed disability employment advisers (DEAs). Most of the rehabilitation and training for work services which they had provided was contracted out to non-governmental organisations as part of this service reconfiguration. The number of sheltered workshops was also reduced, and the move was made towards more sheltered placements instead (Floyd and Landymore, 2000).

WELFARE TO WORK

A change of government in 1997 resulted in an extensive programme of welfare reforms. These reforms set out a new approach to welfare provision and adopted the mantle of 'work for those who can, security for those who cannot' (Department for Work and Pensions, 2000, p.5). Since that time, this principle has formed the cornerstone of many of the reforms introduced. A re-organisation meant that the Departments of Education, Employment and Social Security were restructured, and the Department for Work and Pensions was brought into existence. Since its inception, this department has taken a lead role in advancing work retention and VR. For the first time since the Second World War, work was brought back onto the political agenda.

This change in political will has resulted in several key pieces of legislation directly concerned with work, VR, disability and workplace health. Initially, the main driver of these policies was towards containment of expenditure, and the associated financial burden, as the numbers claiming disability-related benefits was spiralling out of control. Later the agenda was linked to social inclusion, reducing child poverty, and decreasing the health inequities between those who are employed and those who are out of work. The current broad message linked to this agenda is that work is good for your health. This message is based on evidence suggesting that, people who are in work live longer, and have better health, than those who do not (Waddell and Burton, 2006). We will return to some of these themes, in greater detail, later in the book.

For now, let us content ourselves with listing the key policies which have been introduced as part of these welfare reforms. The starting point was *The New Deal for Disabled People* (Department of Social Security, 1998) which was part of a wider New Deal Programme. It set out how groups, such as lone parents, older workers and people with disabilities, would be helped off benefits and into employment. It was soon recognised that these measures alone were inadequate for the large numbers of claimants with health-related conditions, and therefore *Pathways to Work: Helping people into employment* (Department for Work and Pensions, 2002), was subsequently introduced. The Government wished to involve employers in improving workers' health, and thus a long-term occupational health strategy, *Securing Health Together* (Health and Safety Executive, 2000) came into being. Furthermore, recognition of the role of insurers, as key stakeholders in the VR market, saw the inception of *Building Capacity for Work: A UK framework for vocational rehabilitation* (Department for Work and Pensions, 2004).

As mentioned earlier, the Department for Work and Pensions, through the employment sector, has been the driver behind much of the policy of relevance to occupational therapists interested in VR. Within the health sector, *National Service Frameworks in Mental Health* (Department of Health, 1999a), and *Long Term Conditions* (Department of Health, 2005a) have identified a need for work, work opportunities and rehabilitation, but have resulted in limited, if any, additional provision of on-the-ground resources to deliver them. Two recent publications, one directed more at the social care sector *Improving the Life Chances of Disabled People* (Department for Work and Pensions, Department of Health, Department for Education and Skills, Office of the Deputy Prime Minister, 2005), and the other at primary care and community-based health services, *Our health, our care, our say: A new direction for community services* (Department of Health, 2006), both give mention to the importance of work for people with disabilities and health problems respectively, but give little indication of how this ideal is to be achieved or moved forwards.

Meeting the health needs of workers needs collaboration across traditional government departments, and one such initiative resulted in the publication of *Health, Work and Well-being – Caring for our future* (Department for Work and Pensions, Department of Health, Health and Safety Executive, 2005), which set out a strategy to improve the working lives and health of working-age people. Perhaps the most sweeping changes are, however, yet to come. The Green Paper, *A New Deal for Welfare: Empowering people to work* (Department for Work and Pensions, 2006a) launched plans for a radical reform of the benefits system, as part of a wider Welfare Reform Bill, set to come into effect in 2008.

Since a number of the policies which are touched on here have had a direct result on OT in VR, we will return to discuss the practical application and implications of a number of them at various points throughout this book. We have, however, for the meantime, brought ourselves up to date, and therefore it is time to move on from this historical text to consider other aspects of OT and work.

3 The Meaning and Value of Work

Without giving it too much thought, we all assume that we know what work is. It may be the time you spend in the office or at the hospital, doing your job. Or the place you have to be from 9am – 5pm, in order to get paid. You may define it as the opposite of your leisure or free time. However, if we delve a little deeper, we come up with a number of instances where the situation is not quite so clear cut. Checking your work e-mails at home in the evening, or just finishing off a report for an early morning meeting the following day, are clearly work even if they are done outside of contracted working hours. If you are a student, do you consider this to be work? It is likely that you do, even if others around you don't necessarily share your views.

Occupational therapists organise daily occupations into three categories: self-care, work and leisure. Yet there are a number of activities that don't fit very neatly into these boxes. For example, is shopping work or is it leisure, or does it depend on what you are shopping for? The purpose behind an activity is an important factor in determining whether we consider it to be work. When supermarkets first came into existence, they were widely criticised for expecting the customer to do the work. People were not accustomed to selecting their own groceries and then packing them into the bags; this had previously been the job of the shopkeeper behind the counter. Let me illustrate this point with another example. How would you classify preparing a meal – as work, leisure or even an activity of daily living? Is your answer dependent on the time, place, meaning and purpose attached to the task? A hastily prepared sandwich at lunchtime, purely directed towards addressing your hunger, may well be seen as an activity of daily living. If you have to prepare an evening meal for your family after returning home from a long day at work, you may well consider this to be just a different form of work. While a carefully planned and prepared special meal for friends at the weekend could perhaps fall into your definition of leisure. However, if you were a trained chef preparing meals in your restaurant, then this activity clearly would be work.

You will notice from both of the examples above that our judgement about whether an activity is, in fact, work is significantly influenced by the personal meaning and value which we attach to it (Noon and Blyton, 1997). These meanings have been extensively researched (Castillo, 1997; Tausky, 1995; Montgomery *et al.*, 2005) and are shaped by the culture in which we live, as well as our own attitudes and beliefs. We all have feelings about our work. We may consider it to be stimulating, challenging and enjoyable, or monotonous, tedious and uninspiring. We will be examining more ideas about the meanings of work, later in this chapter.

What the above examples also serve to illustrate, is that 'work' is perhaps not quite as clear cut as we may have at first thought. In order to understand work, it is necessary to examine it from multiple perspectives, and this is what this chapter sets out to do. Despite a strong belief in the link between work and health, there has been little debate about our collective understanding of the nature of work within the occupational therapy (OT) literature. What 'work' means, is perhaps even more complicated to get to grips with than the concept of vocational rehabilitation (VR), but it is an essential prerequisite. We need a shared understanding of what we, and our clients, mean when we use the word 'work', before we can begin to support them to achieve their aspirations in this area of their lives.

This chapter opens the debate about how we may start to define the occupation of work, classify it, and how we may gain a clearer understanding of the activities which it encompasses. This is not a discipline-specific field, and therefore we can draw on the wealth of information available from a variety of different sources. By pulling together the views of researchers, theorists, employers, health professionals, and disabled people themselves, we can begin to formulate an occupation-focused perspective of work and VR. Through achieving this understanding, occupational therapists will be able to articulate successfully their unique perspective and be equipped to defend their contribution to this field of practice in the future.

WHAT IS WORK?

The meaning of 'work' as a social construct, is shaped by wider societal events and the attitudes of the time. From a historical perspective, as noted in an earlier chapter, work has had different meanings at different points in history. Geography, too, plays a role, as the tasks, expectations and experiences associated with work vary, depending on which part of world you are in. Even within Britain itself, you will find that the meaning and value attached to work varies across communities. Understanding what work is, and what it means, is further complicated by the broad range of uses of the word 'work', being both a noun and a verb, in the English language. The Oxford English Dictionary lists an impressive 39 different meanings, and only one of these has to do with a job and making a living (Jahoda, 1982). Examples of definitions of 'work' include:

> *1. physical or mental effort directed towards doing or making something. 2. paid employment at a job or a trade, occupation or profession. 3. a duty, task, or undertaking. 4. something done, made, etc., as a result of effort or exertion.*
>
> (Summers and Holmes, 2004, p.1395).

Not surprisingly, then, there is no accepted universal definition of 'work'. It is generally assumed that work is an adult occupation, which takes place somewhere between the ages of 16 or 18 and 65 years. However, even making this distinction on the basis of age is simplistic, as the following discussion will illustrate.

Many occupational therapists work with children under the age of 18, yet they have tended to focus more on the nature of their play, than on their work activities (Larson, 2004). Despite this apparent lack of regard by therapists, children as young as six years of age have been shown to have clear ideas about what activities may be classified as work (Chapparo and Hooper, 2002). Even less attention has been given to the fact that, in Britain, children and teenagers are estimated to account for up to a quarter of all child workers in Europe (ChildRIGHT, 1998). Further research suggests that this figure may be conservative, and that the majority of school-age children, at some point, take on some form of part-time, paid employment (Penrose *et al.*, 2002). On the positive side, work can build the self-esteem, occupational competence and social skills of young people. On a negative note, however, child workers in the UK have less protection under the law than adults. A significant number also work illegally, and some even truant school to do so (Trades Union Congress, 2001).

For the older person beyond retirement age, leisure activities and interests, or perhaps voluntary work, may replace employment. However, since the population as a whole is living longer, in years to come individuals may well be expected to extend their working life. Not all western countries have a fixed retirement age, and the Government in Britain has ambitions to increase the existing limit, possibly up to 70 years. The recent introduction of anti-age discrimination laws will help protect the rights of older workers, however, little is currently known about the effects of work on the health of this group, and a recent study found that over a third of workers were concerned about still being able to do their job when they were 60 (O'Neill, 2006). We will return to the implications for occupational therapists of age-discrimination legislation in a later chapter.

The plethora of definitions of the word 'work' was mentioned earlier. This situation is further complicated by the fact that we use the words 'employment', 'jobs' and 'work', interchangeably in our culture. For example:

- a person who is workless is someone without a job
- people who hold demonstrations about 'the right to work' are really protesting because they want a job (Jahoda, 1982)
- at the heart of the current British Government's modernisation agenda, Welfare to Work is aimed at getting more people into employment
- the condition known as work-related stress is actually a negative response to employment, rather than to work itself.

This text makes no attempt to untangle these complexities, even were it possible to do so. It is important that you, the reader, are aware that these inconsistencies exist within the wider literature. Furthermore, these confusions in terminology may be a barrier to gaining a better understanding of what work is. Therefore, the next section divides work activities into four main categories. Collectively, these groups describe the different types of work which may be found in our society today.

THE CLASSIFICATION OF WORK

While there is no consensus within the OT literature as to what work is, occupational therapists do recognise work to be an important form of human occupation. It is for this reason that we need to be thinking and debating more about how we may quantify and define it. As a starting point for this discussion, we will conceptualise work in a broad and inclusive way. To this end, we may identify four different forms of work:

1. paid work
2. unpaid work
3. hidden work
4. substitute work.

PAID WORK

This first category is the most common form of activity to be associated with work. Paid work may include some form of employment or a job, but can also extend to those who are self-employed (Brown, 1997). This type of work takes place mainly under contractual obligations in return for a specified material reward, which is usually financial. Within western capitalist economies, paid work has the highest status of the four categories of work that we have identified. As Bassett and Lloyd (2000, p.480) rather cynically point out: 'we live in an industrialized and technologically driven world where people are defined not by who they are but by what they do to get paid.' Paid work can be sub-divided according to the functions of the work undertaken; for example, professional, managerial, skilled manual, unskilled and so on. There have been immeasurable changes to the form and nature of employment and, consequently, to the demands which are placed on employees.

People have widely different experiences of paid work. Some, but by no means all, are fortunate to have work which they consider to be meaningful, and have career opportunities to retain their interest and commitment. For others, it is a struggle to find a work–life balance which allows them to manage the various commitments in their lives. Most people in paid employment find that there are elements of their job which they find satisfying and rewarding, and other elements which do not provide the same emotional reward. Job satisfaction will be considered in more detail later in this chapter and we will also examine a number of other aspects of employment in subsequent chapters.

The current British Government's Welfare to Work Programme is targeted primarily at reducing the number of welfare claimants by assisting them into paid work. While the economic need to have people in employment is clear, the drive toward full employment risks further undermining, and devaluing, other forms of work, in particular unpaid work. At the same time, this campaign has the undesirable effect of narrowing the range of valued work roles which are available to people, so depriving them of alternative options to participate and make a worthwhile contribution to society in other meaningful ways.

UNPAID WORK

Much of the work carried out in our society does not attract financial remuneration. Yet despite this lack of tangible acknowledgement, unpaid work plays an important supporting role to paid work. For this reason, some argue that the contribution made by unpaid workers, particularly towards sustaining capitalism within our society, should attract some form of payment (Smith, 2003). With or without payment, however, it is clear that in order to maintain society's infrastructure it is necessary 'to see all occupations as generating, not just a market price but also a social product' (Toulmin, 1995, p.49).

Examples of unpaid work activities include volunteer work, housework or household work as it has also been called, and caring for dependents. These activities are most commonly undertaken by women. The value attached to both household work and volunteering is often highly personal in nature. For example, the successful high-powered executive who unexpectedly gives up her well-paid job to raise her children, or the father who campaigns tirelessly on behalf of a charity concerned with improving road safety, following his child's death in a road traffic accident.

The meanings and significance that individuals attach to participation in this form of work may differ from their perceptions of participation in paid work, in that they are more likely to describe it in terms of 'love' (Primeau, 1996). The significance attached to these occupations is aptly illustrated by the flow and rhythm of the traditional homemaking activities of women, observed by researchers within a rural culture in a developing nation. The patterns and routines of their daily work occupations are seen to blend into one another to help create a sense of well-being (Ekelman et al., 2003).

Many of the activities involved in housework and care-giving recur throughout the day. They also have a repetitive element; for example, washing dishes and tidying up. Yet many other work tasks in the home are unseen, even though considerable behind the scenes effort is required to create and maintain a satisfying family life. Despite an acknowledgement of the valuable contribution unpaid work makes towards maintaining and enriching our society, it is, on the whole, less highly valued than paid work. The effects of this low value may be reflected in the attitudes which people may show towards these occupations. It is not uncommon for a woman, caring full-time for young children, to apologetically state 'I'm just a housewife,' when asked what she does. Increasing numbers of adults are now also taking on caring responsibilities for older family members. It is estimated that around seven and a half per cent of the adult population provide some form of informal care for the elderly, and the economic cost of this care, should it need to be met by the state, would be substantial.

In contrast to household work and caring for dependents, volunteering usually takes place outside of the home. This is an advantage, as it can reduce the risk of the social isolation which may be experienced during home-based work (Primeau, 1996). For some individuals, volunteering can be a valued, meaningful and purposeful occupation which contributes towards developing a positive social identity (Rebeiro and Allen,

1998). Despite this, it is important to acknowledge that not all clients or potential workers may view volunteering as a constructive occupational choice for them. For those who do, this form of work may provide opportunities for increased confidence and self-esteem, social support, a feeling of active participation and inclusion in the life of the community, and replacing lost roles. As such, it can have a positive influence on the participants' health and well-being (Black and Living, 2004). It may also, for some, provide a stepping stone into paid employment. Within our society, the role of volunteers is a crucial, yet undervalued, form of work. In financial terms, it is estimated that over one million full-time workers would be needed to replace formal volunteers, at an estimated cost of more than £25 billion, based on the national average wage (Wilding *et al.*, 2006).

The final category of unpaid work encompasses education and training. Some may not define these to be work activities, yet we would not necessarily consider them to be leisure or activities of daily living. If we continue to think about work in a more expanded way, we will see that there are many similarities between education and training, and other work activities. They may help provide a formal structure to time through regular routines. What is expected of the student, in common with more traditional forms of work, is largely dictated by others. As with volunteering, these pursuits may bring with them certain benefits, particularly in social contact and personal development. Some participants take the adjustment to becoming a student in their stride, and consequently may experience feelings of enjoyment, satisfaction, involvement, and a sense of commitment to the student role. For others, however, the student role may prove a considerable challenge, or even have a negative effect on their well-being, and potentially their health.

Education and learning are no longer considered the exclusive domain of the young. There is now an expectation that learning activities will be undertaken throughout life. There are many benefits to this lifelong learning agenda, but there is also the danger that it may lead to role overload. Sometimes, education or training is taken on in addition to employment commitments or, perhaps, on a full-time basis alongside caring responsibilities. In some instances, employees may feel compelled to engage in training activities in order to further their career. The nature of education courses, in particular, means that they invariably lack flexibility, and this means that the student often has very little control over the timing, pace and intensity of the work. In common with some forms of paid employment, this lack of flexibility may lead to role conflict. For example, the mature student who has to juggle attending lectures alongside collecting children from school, or the young student living away from home for the first time, who is forced to learn new life skills such as budgeting or cooking, in addition to making the transitions from school to college or university. These conflicts and issues may be minimised by ensuring strong social support systems are in place (Campaniello, 1988). Under the terms of the Special Educational Needs and Disability Act (2001), students with disabilities entering further or higher education courses have the right not to be discriminated against and to have reasonable adjustments made to accommodate them. However, many will still be faced with attitudinal barriers and stigma.

HIDDEN WORK

Sometimes also known as the 'informal sector', hidden work generally involves activities of an illegal nature; some of which may be morally questionable as well. This type of work may include services or goods provided for cash, which are then not formally declared as income for taxation purposes. Two possible examples of hidden work include: a mum at home who buys clothing and footwear at car boot fairs and then re-sells the goods through an internet auction house for profit; or perhaps the day tripper to France who comes back with his van stocked up with cheap alcohol and tobacco for re-sale in Britain, where the prices are much higher. Although there is no status attached to these forms of work in society at large, within certain communities they may become a normal and accepted part of life.

In some instances, employers use a 'cash in hand' strategy to avoid paying tax and national insurance contributions, and meeting their legal responsibilities, such as paying the minimum wage, and ensuring health and safety regulations are observed. It has been estimated that this grey economy is worth around £75 billion each year. Many low-paid homeworkers, doing tasks such as data entry, assembly work and packing, will also fit into this category (Trades Union Congress, 2006).

On an even more sinister level, hidden work also includes activities with an exploitative element, for example, forced labour. It is estimated that more than 12 million people worldwide are the victims of forced labour. This includes drug trafficking and supply, women and girls forced into prostitution, and migrants who are unable to escape debt bondage. Many sweatshop workers and farm labourers are forced to work for little or no money. Child labour is on the decline around the world, but there are still more than 200 million children who do work and many are exposed to dangerous types of work, often on a full-time basis (International Labour Organisation, 2006). Clearly these forms of work are not health-enhancing. Collectively, occupational therapists need to add their voice to those of others who advocate for decent work in safe and humane working conditions, which will allow people to flourish and thrive. Within the UK there is currently a rapidly expanding migrant labour force, mainly originating from eastern European countries. While many work legitimately in this country, and are therefore protected by legal safeguards, there are others who work illegally, and this group are therefore at greater risk because of their potential for exploitation.

Any occupational therapist who is based in an inner city community mental health team may well have encountered clients with a dual diagnosis of mental illness and substance misuse, who undertake hidden work as drug dealers or couriers. The challenge in this situation is to work collaboratively with the client to try and identify alternative, acceptable, valued occupations to replace this form of work.

SUBSTITUTE WORK

This final type of work is one which has traditionally been reserved for disabled people. It is often contrived work, which is nearly always unpaid or provides minimal 'therapeutic earnings'. It takes place in a segregated environment, usually with other people with a similar disability. Examples of this replacement work can be found in sheltered workshops and work projects, often run by voluntary sector organisations, local authority day centres, and some out-patient OT services. This kind of work flourished with the de-institutionalisation movement in the 1980s. Its purpose was to provide a replacement daily structure for those people who had moved into community settings from former institutions and mental asylums. Since that time, attitudes have changed and the segregated nature of this form of work is now at odds with the current social inclusion agenda. A number of services which provide substitute work are re-focusing their service towards other forms of work, as a result of the withdrawal of their funding for these sorts of activities. Substitute work is not highly regarded by society, or indeed by many disabled people themselves (Drake, 1999). The variable quality of the services provided also means that while some may provide meaningful and enjoyable diversional activities, others are exploitative and afford their trainees or workers less rights than they would otherwise have if they were in paid employment.

Now that we have grouped work activities into the four broad categories of paid, unpaid, hidden and substitute work, we will move on to look in more depth at a selection of other ways in which work has been construed. This will also provide us with some insights into the reasons and motives which we, as individuals, may have for working, as well as help us define those activities which come under the work umbrella.

WORK VERSUS LEISURE

Making a distinction between work and leisure activities is common practice, although, as we have discussed previously, this division is often somewhat arbitrary. Many people impose physical and mental barriers around work and home. For some, commuting to and from a workplace is experienced as the bridge between the two (Nippert-Eng, 1996). Leisure may be understood as an occupation with subjective experiences and meanings attached to it (Suto, 1998), and concepts which have been linked with leisure include 'time, activity, attitudes, space, freedom and experience' (Neumayer and Wilding, 2005, p.319). Leisure activities are frequently directed towards enhancing health and well-being, such as going to the gym or taking a bike ride. It is qualities such as a greater freedom of choice and more discretionary elements which often distinguishes leisure activities from work ones (Deem, 1988).

Within OT, work and leisure have historically been viewed as key occupational performance areas. Leisure, in particular, is routinely used as an activity directed towards achieving clients goals (Suto, 1998). However, there remains a need to build a solid understanding of these concepts from an OT perspective (Suto, 1998; Kumar, 2000). Occupational therapists recognise that there is a strong and binding link between work and leisure activities and also the need for balance between the two. So, individuals often experience them as symbiotic – with each deriving meaning from the other. When someone loses their job and becomes unemployed, for example, their leisure interests invariably suffer as well. It is clear, then, that leisure should be viewed as complementary to employment, rather than as an alternative to it (Glyptis, 1989; Jahoda, 1982).

Nowadays, paid work is seen as a form of social inclusion and a way out of poverty for disadvantaged people, whereas leisure is viewed as a commodity. Popular forms of leisure outside of the home include holidays, cinemas, sports and shopping (Neumayer and Wilding, 2005; Deem, 1988). Participation in these interests is influenced by the work–leisure relationship, since they require money in order to pursue them. It follows, therefore, that both the quality, and quantity, of leisure activities may be reduced by unemployment or financial hardship (Lobo, 1999).

Many modern day leisure pursuits have been criticised as being unhealthy, unsatisfying, purposeless and unfulfilling (Smigel, 1963; Di Bona, 2000). Consumerism drives an increasing desire to purchase ever more goods, products and services. This, in turn, means that more money needs to be earned to fund these pastimes, so significant increases in hours spent working have resulted. This culture of working ever longer hours in Britain now means that one in nine employees work more than a sixty hour week; and this tendency is reflected elsewhere in the developed world (Watson, 2003).

The ratio of time spent in leisure activities to that spent in work activities varies from person to person. It follows that the amount of time a person has for leisure is often inversely proportional to the time they spend in work activities, since there are only 24 hours in each day. Therefore, for example, a factory worker who works a 12-hour shift, and spends an hour travelling each way, has little remaining time for leisure. Some higher-paid workers may find that they have more money available to spend on leisure, but that they have less time during which to spend it (Neumayer and Wilding, 2005).

In addition to a time component, there is also an age dimension to the leisure–work continuum. Those who have investigated this subject have found that younger people tend to be more attracted to work activities – although leisure has been found to be of benefit, since it allows this age group to experiment, take risks and face challenges and also provides an opportunity for relaxation and personal development (Lobo, 1999), in ways that work may not afford. It has also been suggested that the relative value attached to leisure activities appears to increase with advancing age (Morgan and Yongbloed, 1990). This is most likely because age and life stage influence leisure participation in particular types of activity (Deem, 1988). Consider for a moment how your own leisure interests have evolved over the years.

The status attached to both work and leisure is culturally bound and has changed over time. For example, the ancient Greeks viewed work as undignified – not fit for the free man. Instead, the free man took part in worthy leisure activities such as politics, debate, art and sport. The meaning of leisure was 'freedom from the necessity of being occupied' (De Grazia, 1962, p.14 cited in Smigel, 1963, p.ii). Protestant views held in later times could not have been more different. Calvinism emphasised that work was all important; leisure or spare time was to be used purely for prayer, in order to recover to be able to perform more work. The concept of 'work ethic' originated in this era.

WORK AS STATUS

Over half a century ago it was asserted that work was 'an essential part of a man's life, since it is that aspect of his life which gives him status and binds him to society' (Brown, 1954 cited in Hutchinson, 1982, p.1). This statement makes plain the perceived link between an individual's status or position in society and his or her work. Modern western society continues to place great esteem on the occupational status of individuals. The existence of this relationship between work and status may help explain the high value attached to being able to acquire a worker role by people who are excluded from the workforce, possibly because of a health condition or a disability (Ross, 1998).

However, while status is attached to being in work, not all forms of work are valued equally. This point is of particular relevance to occupational therapists, since disabled people are disproportionately found in low-paid, low-status, low-skilled jobs (Christie and Mensah-Coker, 1999). For example, an analysis from the Labour Force Survey found that, on average, disabled people are less represented in managerial, professional and technical occupations, and are more likely to be in administrative, secretarial, personal service or elementary jobs (Smith and Twomey, 2002).

A SOCIO-ECONOMIC PERSPECTIVE OF WORK

Recognising and appreciating the socio-economic perspective of work is important, as it is widely acknowledged that countries with higher levels of employment generally enjoy greater prosperity. Communities and families with no form of employment are often in a state of poverty (Towner, 2005), with all the negative consequences attached to this situation. With this in mind, it is easy to see how work becomes synonymous with paid employment. There are currently just over 28 million people in employment in the UK, and almost a further one and a half million seeking it. However, nearly a third of people of working age are not in employment (Office for National Statistics, 2005). Of this group, a significant majority have health or disability problems. Even where people are actively participating in the labour force, the estimated cost of sickness absence to the economy is nearly £11 billion (Confederation of British Industry, 2001). Furthermore, the population as a whole is growing older, so the size of the potential workforce is decreasing exponentially. As Britain is one of the wealthier countries in the world, these trends and figures represent a significant challenge to policy-makers and business leaders alike, if national prosperity and economic competitiveness are to be maintained, or improved, in the future.

WORKING TO MAKE A LIVING

As mentioned previously, work is most commonly associated with paid employment. For the majority of the world's people, even painful, degrading or dangerous work is a necessary evil, just in order to survive. There seems little reason to doubt that for many, money is one of the main motives for working. The tangible rewards which may come from employment, such as good benefits, pay and a secure job, may be more highly valued by workers than a sense of contributing to society or the opportunity for personal growth and achievement in some sectors (Baker *et al.*, 2003). This reality may, perhaps, be seen to be in conflict with the OT philosophy which tends to place stronger value on an intrinsic value to occupational performance, as we shall see later in the section on occupation and work.

In western society, however, the protection afforded by social security systems means that work is not linked to survival. Those who are unable to support themselves financially are assisted by the state. There is no clear evidence, however, that employment is valued any less because this safety net exists. This is evident when considering the position of many disabled people, the majority of whom, despite receiving assistance in the form of disability benefits, frequently express a desire to work and have a job (Department for Work and Pensions, 2002).

Although there is a firm association between work and some form of payment, the traditions and customs which influence the ways in which the financial rewards for work are distributed, are often irrational, unfair and unjust. Equal opportunities legislation has failed to address the pay discrepancies which still remain between men and women, different ethnic groups, and non-disabled and disabled people. A recent global report by the International Labour Organisation shows that significant forms of workplace discrimination still remain a real cause of concern. For example, the gross hourly earnings for women in Europe are 15 per cent lower than for men (International Labour Organisation, 2007). In addition, some types of work attract far higher rates of pay than others, regardless of how well that job is executed or its perceived societal value. Examples illustrating these inconsistencies can be seen in the media on an almost daily basis.

In some sectors, high performance and outputs earn bonuses as a form of additional reward. There are often difficulties in achieving fairness and equity within these systems, and the factors which are measured are not necessarily linked to the quality of the work performance of the actual individual (Doyle, 2003). For example, a bus company may offer its bus drivers a weekly bonus for ensuring that they keep to scheduled times on their route. If they are late arriving at their destination more than a couple of times during the week, they do not receive the additional payment. On the one hand, this may be seen as a positive incentive, because it helps ensure that buses keep to time and passengers are not inconvenienced by late running buses. On the other hand, however, it could also result in the driver being less concerned with the safety of the passengers than with making sure he or she sticks to the timetable. It is not difficult to imagine how this form of incentive may encourage risk-taking and less careful, or even reckless, driving, as the driver tries to make up time lost in a traffic jam rather than lose his pay. How often have you seen an elderly person stumble, or even fall, on the bus because the driver takes off in haste before all the passengers are seated? The labour market is rife with examples of these perverse types of incentives.

The value of money in motivating the individual to work, or indeed to work as efficiently as the employer would like, has attracted much attention from work psychologists and sociologists alike. These two large professional groups have approached the subject from different angles, however both have shown interest in the association between work and rewards for work. We will turn, for a moment, to some of the main ideas which have emanated from these disciplines, as they can help to explain the rationale behind some modern-day work practices.

SOCIOLOGICAL AND PSYCHOLOGICAL PERSPECTIVES OF WORK

Sociologists, in particular, have made an enormous contribution to our knowledge and understanding of work. So much so, that in a number of undergraduate OT programmes, a sociological perspective currently dominates key aspects of the curriculum which are concerned with work (Ross, 2006). In common with others, sociologists have varying viewpoints as to what activities constitute work. Despite the fact that some have limited their discussions of work to employment, others recognise that work dates back to times far earlier than the notion of employment came into existence (Allen, 1997). Elements of sociological and psychological theory are of value to occupational therapists for two main reasons. Firstly, some theories and ideas are compatible with an occupational perspective of work and, as such, can enhance our own knowledge base and understanding. Secondly, key theories may assist the occupational therapist to gain a better understanding of the workplace culture within a particular organisation. Current managerial thinking and working practises may well be based on evidence drawn from such theories. While these viewpoints may at times come into conflict with a more occupation-focused philosophy, it is important to recognise the contribution that they may make to the organisation of the workplace as a whole.

Taylorism (after F.W. Taylor 1856–1917), which follows Taylor's principles of scientific management, has had a large impact on job design. Introduced at a time of increasing mechanisation, workers were reduced to little more than machines, as the planning and execution of work were separated out. Workers were de-skilled as the total job was broken down into fragmented parts. Taylor also believed that it was man's natural instinct to try and get the maximum reward for minimum amount of effort and therefore strong management practices were needed to prevent this. Workers were intensely monitored to ensure the various elements of the total job were co-ordinated and the managers who undertook this scrutiny kept their distance, having as little interaction with workers as possible. Increased worker output and effort was reinforced by using incentive payment systems.

Elements of these principles can still often be found in the labour market of today, particularly within the manufacturing sector and in situations where work activities can be easily routinised (Watson, 2003). Other sociological theories, brought about by differing world views, have also contributed to existing understandings of work and the workplace. More well-known examples include Marx's theory of capital,

Durkheim's informal and formal organisations, and Weber's theory of bureaucracy (Hatch and Cunliffe, 2006).

The field of work or occupational psychology, as it is also known, has put forward numerous theories, particularly to do with individual's experiences of work and the relationship between the workplace and the worker. Warr (1987), for example, identified key factors which influence an individual's well-being in the workplace.

An area of common interest for psychology and OT is that of job satisfaction and its relationship to health. Occupational therapists will find much of interest within the extensive psychological literature on this subject (Faragher *et al.*, 2005). Job satisfaction may be influenced by factors such as perception of significance, financial rewards, continuity, intrinsic interest, achievement, social status, security, advancement, self-improvement and social interaction (Hutchinson, 1982). It has been suggested that:

> *the most satisfied employee is one who is in a secure job, with a high level of individual discretion and participation in decision-making, but not requiring highly intensive work effort. They will be well-matched to their job in terms of both qualifications and hours of work, be well-paid but have relatively low pay expectations.*

> (Green, 2005, p.1)

If this is indeed an accurate representation of a satisfied worker, then perhaps it is unsurprising that levels of job satisfaction have fallen, since modern work trends mean that fewer and fewer jobs fit this description. However, this may be a somewhat narrow definition, since others argue that work motivation and job satisfaction are linked more to the meaning that the individual person attaches to working. These contrasting viewpoints reinforce the need for occupational therapists to begin to understand some of these determinants, so as to better puzzle out the complex association between work and health (Baker *et al.*, 2003).

WORK AS OCCUPATION

Key socio-economic, sociological and psychological perspectives of work have been touched upon briefly. However, each of these perspectives fails to address adequately the intrinsic need for, and value of, work. Work is an essential form of human activity which may provide meaning within the broader context of an individual's life. Since the early 1990s, research by occupational scientists has led to increased understanding of the concept of human 'occupation' and this subject has received much attention and discussion in the professional literature in recent years (Christiansen and Townsend, 2004; Molineux, 2004).

Occupational science, which is increasingly contributing to the OT knowledge base, has drawn strongly on a humanist perspective by emphasising the potential of each individual to control their life and make their own choices about their life. An occupational perspective also takes the view that humans are, inherently, productive beings. They choose to pursue, and attach value to, different occupations across the lifespan. They experience, and express, personal meanings through their participation in their daily occupations (Hocking, 2001) and their use of time. OT is underpinned by a firm belief in the relationship between occupation and health and well-being (Christiansen, 1999; Wilcock, 1998). The concept of occupation, therefore, extends beyond work alone. These occupations may take place, for example, in the home, community, workplace or school.

The dynamic balance and relationship between different occupations creates complex patterns of occupational performance which are unique to each individual. Participation in meaningful occupations provides a sense of satisfaction and purpose. A balance of occupations, which includes productive activities, is considered to be an essential pre-requisite of health (Farnworth, 1995), and it is this very personal, very individual, balance which needs to be stressed. The centrality, or importance, of work will vary between individuals. It may also change across a person's lifespan and the onset of a disability later in life may act as a catalyst for a re-evaluation of an individual's occupational priorities. We also know that the meanings which individuals find in work can have an effect on their perceived levels of job satisfaction. But, even though the role of worker is a primary occupational role, we cannot separate it from an individual's wider identity. Nor should we try. A sense of accomplishment and independence, or perhaps achieving a valued lifestyle, may all contribute to a particular individual's identity (Spencer *et al.*, 1998). In addition, factors outside of the workplace, such as social and family supports, and a work–life balance, can also impact on meaning and job satisfaction at work (Brown *et al.*, 2001). We need to regularly remind ourselves of the necessity, first and foremost, to retain a broader understanding of the worker as an occupational being.

At a service level, it is suggested that 'occupation focused services within the health and disability sectors are typically aimed at enabling people or groups to increase participation in, and gain control over, their everyday lives when their usual occupations are interrupted' (Brown *et al.*, 2005, p.274). In order to achieve this, systems need to be directed towards overcoming, or minimising, the barriers which are preventing people from participating in their day-to-day occupations (Law and Baum, 2001). Sometimes, this may require change at a societal level. An empowering stance towards groups and communities is needed, for 'occupational justice' to be achieved. In this way, individuals will be enabled to take part in a diverse range of meaningful, satisfying occupations in daily life (Townsend and Wilcock, 2004). There is a degree of compatibility, despite some differences in jargon, between the viewpoints of occupational scientists and the social inclusion agenda, which we will continue to explore in more detail.

WORK AS SOCIAL INCLUSION: DISABLED PEOPLE'S PERSPECTIVES

The current political stance towards tackling social exclusion is directed towards increasing participation in paid employment (Levitas, 1998). Creating more opportunities for disabled people to join the labour force is viewed as a way of assisting them out of poverty. It is also seen as a way of integrating those people who are deemed to be socially excluded, into society. While there are clear advantages to enabling more people to enter paid work, there are also some inherent dangers in making the assumption that securing a job will automatically lead to social inclusion for people with disabilities (Abberley, 2002).

The figures show that paid employment is no panacea. The majority of disabled people report wanting a job (Meager *et al.*, 1998), yet it is often more difficult for this group to hold onto a new job. One in three of those who do manage to secure employment become unemployed again within the year. Of those who become disabled while they are in work, about 17 per cent lose their job within12 months (Burchardt, 2000). The average take-home pay of disabled employees is lower than that of non-disabled employees and they are more likely to work in manual or lower paid jobs. Those who have a disability and are from an ethic minority background are also more likely to be unemployed (Meager *et al.*, 1998). Despite changes to the law, disabled people continue to face stigma, discrimination and less favourable treatment in the workplace (Office of the Deputy Prime Minister, 2004).

These findings suggest that securing entry to paid work cannot be seen as an end in itself. The social inclusion agenda is unlikely to be delivered in this way alone. The need is rather to enable people to lead meaningful and fulfilling lives through participation in a range of valued occupations. This viewpoint is supported in the OT literature on occupational justice and argues for a society where people can develop their potential to participate fully in life, not just fit pre-established work roles (Wilcock, 1998; Jakobsen, 2004). This point is also aptly illustrated by Nagle *et al.* (2002), who describe how people with mental illness – unable to sustain competitive employment – make occupational choices which enabled them to stay well and socially engaged. They found that the demands imposed by traditional forms of employment, and its inherent inflexibility, meant that the participants felt unable to maintain the occupational balance that they needed to stay well when engaging in this activity. These viewpoints raise important considerations for OT practitioners and we will continue to explore them further in subsequent chapters.

ILLNESS AND DISABILITY: EMPLOYERS' PERSPECTIVES

Social and legislative changes have had a positive influence on the opportunities for disabled people in the workforce. Employers have become increasingly mindful of ensuring that their recruitment and selection procedures do not discriminate against people with disabilities which, in turn, has meant that there are now more people with disabilities who are working in a wider variety of jobs. Employers have consistently claimed that they consider competitive skills and job readiness to be essential characteristics of any potential recruit (Greenwood and Johnson, 1987). While the Disability Discrimination Act (DDA) makes it unlawful for employers to discriminate against people with disabilities, either when they are applying for work or when they are in employment, they do not, however, have a legal duty to ensure that disabled people are represented in their workforce (Drake, 1999).

A study which surveyed businesses about their responses to the DDA (1995) found that around 37 per cent of employers reported having previously employed disabled people. This was more likely to be in larger businesses and in the public, rather than the private, sector. Small employers were found to lack knowledge of disability, and it was more commonplace for them to associate disability with visible, physical impairments rather than, for example, mental health problems or other forms of disability covered by the DDA (Roberts *et al.*, 2004). This perception amongst employers is longstanding, as several studies from over 20 years ago reported that employers were influenced by the nature of the potential employees' disability (Burton *et al.*, 1987), and that they considered physical disabilities easier to accommodate than mental health problems (Combs and Omvig, 1986).

From an employer's perspective, absence from work may result in lost production, disruption, a decrease in efficiency, missed opportunities and reduced quality of the goods or services; all of which have a negative effect on the competitiveness and profitability of any business (Bevan and Hayday, 1998). Yet in the UK, only a quarter of employers offer any sort of rehabilitation to their employees (Employee Health Bulletin, 2001 cited in Tehrani, 2004). Different legal requirements in different countries mean that the extent of participation by employers, in making provision for disabled employees, varies enormously. In Sweden, for example, employers are, by law, responsible for the work environment. In this capacity they must identify situations where rehabilitation is needed, develop a rehabilitation plan, and then take the necessary action to ensure that it is implemented (Larsson and Gard, 2003). This stance may encourage more of a preventative approach, with the need for earlier intervention and in-service training about the workplace environment emerging as themes from this research. We will return to the role of employers in the rehabilitation to work process, in later chapters.

REHABILITATION FOR WORK: HEALTH PROFESSIONALS' PERSPECTIVES

Health professionals have a key role to play in facilitating a safe, effective and timely return to work, particularly since returning to work is now being hailed as an important part of an individual's recovery. However, concerns have been raised that practitioners in the health service (British Society of Rehabilitation Medicine, 2000), occupational health (Wynn *et al.*, 2003), and the employment services (Floyd and Landymore, 2000), do not necessarily have the knowledge and skills required to practice effectively within this field. In addition, poor communication between health professionals has been found to act as a key barrier to effective rehabilitation for work (Sawney and Challoner, 2003), particularly between general practitioners and occupational health professionals (Beaumont, 2003).

Health professionals and rehabilitation services have been criticised as being slow and unresponsive (British Society of Rehabilitation Medicine, 2000), inappropriate to today's needs (Waddell *et al.*, 2004), incorrectly deployed (Joss, 2002), and failing to recognise the needs of disabled people (Swain *et al.*, 2003). It is unsurprising in the light of these criticisms that the individual with a disability or a health condition is often faced with innumerable barriers, including contradictory or conflicting advice about their ability to return to work. In the case of OT, only a small minority of occupational therapists working in statutory services offer work rehabilitation to their clients (Wright *et al.*, 2005).

Not wishing to be pessimistic, the importance of work has been pushed up the political agenda and this is a positive move. It is important, however, to make the point that effective systems which support and deliver this agenda still need to be advanced. Clear routes into good quality, sustainable work roles for people with health problems and disabilities are still poorly signposted. Pro-active, preventative measures to help individuals maintain a valued worker role are also under-developed. Gaining an increased understanding of the meaning and value of work, to the health and well-being of individuals and to our society as a whole, has a significant role to play in taking this specialty forward. We will return to our exploration of some of the issues which have been raised in this chapter, later in the book.

4 Theoretical Frameworks in Vocational Rehabilitation

This chapter introduces theoretical frameworks which can be drawn upon to guide and underpin vocational rehabilitation (VR). For the therapist beginning to introduce VR into his or her practice, this is a good place to start. There may be a temptation to pass over this theoretical knowledge in favour of the more applied knowledge to be found in later chapters. To do so, however, would be misguided for a number of good reasons.

Theoretical frameworks provide an important structure for our practice. In the same way that scaffolding within the construction industry helps to support and shape a new building, the theoretical framework provides similar help to form, hold up, and define, our interventions. Frameworks assist clinical judgment and decision-making. The concepts within a framework help us to understand, and explain, an event or situation. They can therefore provide important justification for a particular intervention or approach. This, in itself, is all the more essential in a field where there is a wide range of practitioners, both with and without professional qualifications, who claim to **do** VR. Without the support of a framework to guide reasoning, and defend decision-making, there is a risk that occupational therapy (OT) may be viewed as just a disparate assortment of unconnected interventions.

A theoretical framework must be selected for the perspective it can provide as well as for its relevance to the particular context or situation. A brief search of the literature identifies models of motivation for work (Hackman and Oldham, 1980; Shamir, 1996), theories about the meaning of work (Jahoda, 1982), job satisfaction models (Locke, 1976) and models of work functioning (Sandqvist and Henriksson, 2004), to name but a few. Despite the numerous options available, OT models, already familiar to many practitioners, offer a good starting point for an increased understanding of the occupation of work. The Canadian Model of Occupational Performance (CMOP) (Townsend, 2002) and the Model of Human Occupation (MOHO) (Kielhofner, 2002) are two such models, both of which have successfully been applied within the work context.

It is important to emphasise at the outset that there is no 'one size fits all' framework. In some cases, therefore, it may be desirable to use a combination of models or approaches. Choosing the most appropriate framework for the particular situation which faces you is part of your therapeutic reasoning skill, as a therapist. As you move from competent to expert practice, you may develop the ability to move outside of the constraints of any particular model of practice, while still being able to ground your practice in theory. This is a skill to aspire to, since it will enable you to clearly articulate your knowledge base as well as your rationale for treatment (Kelly, 2004). In order to achieve this aptitude, you will first need to develop an understanding of, and familiarity with, key models within your area of developing expertise. For this reason, the frameworks included in this chapter have been drawn both from sources within, and outside of, OT. Each one may usefully add to your understanding of work and VR and case studies are included to demonstrate their application. There are many other models and frameworks which could potentially have been included and the interested reader will find a wealth of material on this subject, particularly within the psychological literature.

The main purpose of this chapter is to provide some useful scaffolding, as a starting point, to help support your awareness, reasoning and practice in the context of work and the workplace. No attempt has been made to disentangle models from approaches from theories. There is no consensus on terminology in this area and it is outside the scope of this book to delve into these issues. Rather, the term 'theoretical framework' is used as an all-encompassing phrase for the different conceptual perspectives that have been selected.

We will begin by relating two well-known OT models of practice, the CMOP and the MOHO, to the work context. In order to apply these models to the workplace setting, the work of occupational scientists has been drawn on to illustrate some of the key elements of each model.

THE CANADIAN MODEL OF OCCUPATIONAL PERFORMANCE (CMOP)

The CMOP is perhaps the most well-known of a collection of models which may be grouped around three main components:

- the person
- the occupation
- the environment.

CMOP postulates that these three components work together, and interact (Law *et al.*, 1996 cited in Townsend, 2002), and in doing so they produce occupational performance. Occupational performance is dynamic and responds to changes in the person–environment–occupation relationship. Changes may also occur throughout each day and across the course of the lifespan.

Key underpinning elements of the model may be summarised as follows:

- The main purpose of OT is to enable occupation
- Occupation is health-giving
- An individual's choice and performance of occupations is influenced by the environment
- A client-centred approach will assist individuals to select, organise and perform occupations which are important and meaningful to them

- Occupation is defined as:

  groups of activities and tasks of everyday life, named, organized and given value and meaning by individuals and a culture. Occupation is everything people do to occupy themselves, including looking after themselves (self-care), enjoying life (leisure) and contributing to the social and economic fabric of their communities (productivity).
  (Townsend, 2002, p.34)

For our purposes, we are particularly interested in productivity, which, as the above definition illustrates, has a meaning beyond that of paid employment. Productivity is an occupation which is undertaken throughout the lifespan, from the play and schoolwork of the child to employment, home maintenance and parenting occupations of adulthood through to, perhaps, voluntary work undertaken by older people.

The words 'productivity' and 'work' are often used interchangeably by occupational therapists in the UK. Outside of the OT profession however, productivity has a totally different meaning which is often linked more with increased business efficiency and profitability. To avoid this confusion, we will continue to use the term 'work', throughout this text, as well as for the sake of clarity and consistency.

> If you are interested in reading more about CMOP you might like to read: Townsend, E. (editor.) (2002) *Enabling Occupation: An occupational therapy perspective*, Ottawa: Canadian Association of Occupational Therapists.

THE PERSON

The remainder of this section illustrates how the CMOP framework may be applied to the work situation. At this point, let us remind ourselves that we are focusing first and foremost on the person as a worker, or potential worker, rather than a patient with a particular disability or health condition. This is important since, the person will need to take an active decision to resume their daily occupations, rather than remaining in a passive patient role. This 'worker identity' is an important notion which we will return to in a later chapter.

Person = Worker

Using CMOP, we can begin understand that the person, as a worker, has affective, cognitive and physical components. Some examples are provided in the box below.

> Ted is a long-distance lorry driver (worker) who develops back pain (physical component).
> Lynda is a secondary school teacher (worker) who begins experiencing very high levels of anxiety (affective component) at the start of the school day.
> John is a window cleaner (worker) who, having recovered from a fall from a ladder, now has difficulty remembering his customers' address details (cognitive component).

Of course, the person may experience difficulties with more than one performance component. Let's return to Ted, the lorry driver. After several weeks off work with his back pain, Ted is suffering financial hardship. With no signs of improvement in his condition, this is placing a growing strain on his family role and relationships. He starts to believe that he will never get better or be able to return to work. Ted begins to show signs of depression (affective component) in response to these additional pressures. This example illustrates how an individual's illness beliefs and attitudes, and also perhaps feelings of fear about going back to work, can present significant barriers to actually returning to work (Frank and Thurgood, 2006). Any difficulties which a person experiences in their affective, cognitive or physical functioning may impact on their performance of their work occupations.

There is one further element of the person which we need to attend to within the CMOP. It is not a component of function, rather a central core. This is the person's spirituality. Occupational therapists have widely differing views and understandings of spirituality and its importance, place and relevance within OT (Unruh et al., 2002). Within CMOP, however, spirituality means 'the essence of self', and it is this which makes us individual and unique human beings. In other words, it is our spirituality that determines what is important and meaningful to each of us – what we value and believe in – and how we express this through our actions. Our drive and motivation to be a particular type of person, or engage in particular activities or occupations, are expressions of our spirituality. Our spirituality may also influence our career preferences, since it guides us in how we express our choice. It may affect the value that we attach to our work and the meaning we draw from it, since spirituality is a source of self determination and personal control (Townsend, 2002).

> Shannon had always wanted to be a primary school teacher. She enjoyed the company of young children and had fond memories of her own school days. She believed that positive early educational experiences were crucial to the development of happy, well-adjusted children. Shannon worked in a small village primary school for five years after qualifying. Although there was a lot more paperwork than she had anticipated, she gained much personal satisfaction and enjoyment from her job, which she did well. Shannon then had a child of her own. She had not anticipated the difficulties she would encounter trying to find suitable childcare, or the feelings of guilt she would experience at leaving her baby in the care of others. This conflicted with her deeply held views and values on her role as a good mother to her child. Shannon returned to work but could not bring the enthusiasm to her job which she had done previously. She began to neglect the paperwork as she attempted to juggle her roles as a teacher and a mother. Her sleep patterns became disturbed, as she lay awake worrying about the tasks she wasn't completing. She began to lose weight and felt tearful and unable to cope. The final straw came when an angry parent demanded to know why her daughter had not brought home a new reading book for two weeks. Shannon burst into tears and was sent home from school. Her doctor signed her off sick with anxiety and depression.

This example demonstrates how spirituality – what Shannon thought was important and meaningful, and what she valued and believed in – was expressed through her actions. Shannon experienced feelings of conflict between her occupations as mother and teacher. This conflict had a profoundly negative impact on her occupational performance.

Listening to an individual's occupational and life stories can provide the occupational therapist with insights into those occupations which are of significance and importance to an individual. Although not addressed directly by CMOP, additional personal factors, such as self confidence, self esteem, assertiveness, motivation, personality and emotional vulnerability, need to be considered by the therapist during the VR process (Frank and Thurgood, 2006).

THE OCCUPATION

Having examined the person in terms of their physical, affective, cognitive and spiritual components, let us now move on to the second core element of CMOP: occupation. Occupation is a powerful force within the lives of each of us. It encompasses just about everything we do. It is also apparent that the more knowledge we gain about the complexities of occupation, the more we realise how much we still have to learn.

There are many different ways to examine the subjective meanings and values that we attach to all of our activities, and the processes and patterns through which we engage in them. In reality, we cannot hope to gain more than a fleeting insight into the gamut of occupations of any person at any particular point in time. Our efforts to understand another person's occupational identity are constrained by a number of factors. These may include internal factors, such as our own values and judgements, and external factors, for example a limit on the prescribed number of treatment sessions we are able to provide.

In our attempts to aid understanding, we tend to dissect occupations and occupational performance. We separate them, compartmentalise them, classify them, order or rank them. The inherent difficulties in trying to simplify occupations in this way have been discussed in earlier chapters. Remember, for example, the difficulty in separating work from leisure, or classifying the activity of cooking a meal, which we discussed earlier? CMOP divides occupations into self-care, productivity and leisure, but we must not lose sight of the fact that this is an oversimplification of occupation – the boundaries around each of these domains are not clear cut. Equally, our focus within this text is on the occupation of productivity/work but we recognise that this must be considered within the wider context of an individual's life.

Occupation = Work

CMOP emphasises the link which can exist between occupational performance and health, just as we know that positive health benefits may be achieved through participation in work (Waddell and Burton, 2006). Let us briefly refresh our memory about what we already understand about the occupation of work. Earlier, we classified the different forms of work as paid, unpaid, hidden or substitute work. We also examined the value and meaning which may be attached to work by an individual and by society and these are certainly important dimensions of this occupation. Understanding a person's feelings towards their work is an important element in assisting a person into, or back to, work.

In addition to the more subjective dimensions of the person's own perceptions of their work, there are also the more tangible qualities of the work itself to consider. The occupational therapist needs to gain an understanding of the nature of the work and the work tasks which the person performs, since the components and requirements of any given type of work will differ. As you seek to learn about a particular job you will need to ask such questions as:

• What are the main work tasks?
• What are the demands of the work?
• Where, when and for how long are they performed?
• What is the skill level of the tasks?

The occupational therapist's ability to undertake task and activity analysis, which can be transferred to the work setting, will give an indication of the requirements of the work, or job. Job descriptions and person specifications, if available, may provide an initial starting point. It is important to reflect on how well an individual's skills, abilities and interests match the needs and demands of the work they need to perform. This fit, between the worker and the work, is a critical element in the success or failure of a return to work or an initial engagement in work activity. We will come back to these points when we look at the assessment in the VR process later on in the text.

THE ENVIRONMENT

The third, and final, component in the person–occupation–environment framework of CMOP is the environment. Occupational performance takes place in an environment which consists of physical, institutional, cultural and social elements (Townsend, 2002). The particular environment in which we are interested is that of the workplace, but this extends beyond just the physical location in which the work takes place.

Environment = Workplace

The workplace may be seen as having different 'levels'. Firstly, at the level of the individual worker, there is his or her immediate workplace environment. There is probably greater diversity in this work environment than in, say, the home environment, which may be more familiar territory to many therapists. The characteristics of each workplace will differ according to the nature and purpose of the business.

The physical environment of the workplace may include the person's workstation, their office, the staff restroom and the car park, amongst others. The workplace may be indoors or outdoors, or a combination of the two. It may be a noisy factory or a quiet office. There may be a large number of employees or just a handful. As previously mentioned, each form of work, and workplace, puts forward its own set of barriers and facilitators to occupational performance in work, particularly for the person with a disability or health condition. We will return to consider the physical characteristics of work environments in far greater detail in later chapters.

Many people report that social interaction with colleagues is an important aspect of work. This social environment may be a positive or a negative feature of a particular individual's workplace. For many people with disabilities or health conditions, the attitudes of co-workers, management and wider society are significant obstacles to work. The social model of disability, discussed later in this chapter, expands on this point further.

The environment extends far beyond the immediacy of the physical and social elements of the workspace alone. The institutional environment includes political, legal and economic aspects too. These are of particular relevance in the area of VR. The economic component of the environment dictates the availability of jobs within the labour market. As Britain's economy is currently strong, there are more job opportunities for people with disabilities than there have been during periods of recession. This point was illustrated in the earlier historical account of work and VR.

The introduction of legislation such as the Disability Discrimination Act in 1995, for example, is a political element of the institutional environment. As such, it requires employers to make goods and services more accessible to people with disabilities and makes it unlawful to discriminate against them. The institutional environment may also affect housing provision, transport accessibility, the availability of affordable childcare and benefit entitlements. Any combination of these factors may impact on an individual's ability to engage in work.

The cultural environment may be viewed at two levels: that of society at large, and that of the specific workplace or employing organisation. Our capitalist society influences the types of jobs which are available, as well as attitudes to work and to the workforce. At an organisational level, the policies and procedures, and terms and conditions which govern the employment contract, reflect the value that the organisation places on their employees. The size of an organisation, how it manages sickness absence, and the ethos within the organisation are also important factors (Frank and Thurgood, 2006). We will return to these aspects of the environment later in this chapter.

In summary, the CMOP framework can usefully be applied to assist our understanding of the individual and their environment when their condition or disability is negatively affecting their occupational performance of their work. We will continue examining frameworks which may usefully guide our practice, by moving on to another well-known OT theoretical model, the MOHO.

THE MODEL OF HUMAN OCCUPATION (MOHO)

A second OT model which may help us to understand an individual's work performance, or work dysfunction, is the MOHO. In common with the CMOP, discussed in the previous section, the MOHO, which originated in America, can be applied to any individual, regardless of their age or disability. This text assumes that the reader has some familiarity with the central tenets of MOHO. The MOHO has a number of assessment tools which can be used by the occupational therapist in work-focused practice. These are discussed further in the later chapter on assessment in the VR process.

If you are interested in reading more about the MOHO you might like to read: Kielhofner, G. (2002) *The Model of Human Occupation: Theory and application* (3rd edition), Philadelphia: Lippincott, Williams & Wilkins.

THE PERSON

Within the framework of the MOHO, we understand work behaviour by recognising that each person is made up of:

- volition
- habituation
- performance capacity.

The person's volition influences their experiences and choices. The habituation component identifies how a person's occupation is organised into habits and routines. The final component of the person, performance capacity, refers to an individual's innate physical and mental abilities in carrying out an occupation. Since we do not exist in a vacuum, the environment is a further core element of the MOHO, since this is where an occupation takes place (Kielhofner *et al.*, 1999).

Each of these four components is interrelated, and each can also be further subdivided as follows. Our volition, or motivation for occupation, is determined by how we view our capabilities and how effective we see ourselves as being (personal causation), what we consider to be important (values) and what we enjoy or get satisfaction from doing (interests). Others have illustrated how individual's values and views of work may differ, and how this may impact on their occupational life when they have to adapt to a disability (Mentrup *et al.*, 1999). The following two examples illustrate this point further.

Bill works as a fundraising manager for a small wildlife charity. Last year his efforts brought in enough money from sponsorship to allow the charity to expand its work in protecting the habitat of endangered wildlife. Bill believes himself to be an effective fundraiser and this view is reinforced by the praise he receives from his co-workers (personal causation). Bill enjoys his work. He has a strong belief in the charity's mission as he is an avid birdwatcher himself (values). He gets tremendous satisfaction from raising money for this cause (interest).

This example demonstrates the positive relationship which Bill has with his work. It shows a high level of compatibility between Bill's personal values and interests and his work. Contrast this scenario with the following one.

Ben has worked for a multinational insurance company for the past six years. He is based in a large open plan office with 60 or so other insurance salesmen. There is a high staff turnover and a number of people, including Ben, are currently job hunting. He finds his work day passes slowly, and the time he spends there is boring and unsatisfying (lack of interest). His division has performed poorly over the last 18 months and this has resulted in a reduced volume of work. Ben knows that many of his co-workers spend a lot of time looking busy, while surfing the internet or sending personal e-mails. Ben does not like the insurance sector and wants a career change (lack of value). There are strong rumours that his division will soon be shut down (this uncertainty contributes to his reduced personal causation). Ben is worried about being made redundant as he has a family to support and high financial commitments.

It is clear from this second example that there is a poor match between Ben and his job. Ben experiences little pleasure in his work; he feels trapped yet he cannot leave for financial reasons. The job insecurity will add to his feelings of not being in control. Occupational choice and work satisfaction are key functions of volition (Kielhofner *et al.*, 1999).

The second component of the person in MOHO is habituation; the semi-automatic patterns of behaviour which allow us go about our daily routines in an almost effortless way. Think about your routine when you arrive at work in the morning. Do you hang up your coat and make yourself a hot drink, or do you immediately sit at your desk and turn on your computer? Do you stop and chat to colleagues, or launch yourself immediately into the tasks of the day? Each of us has our own particular pattern of activities which we build up to form habits and roles.

For the person with a health problem or disability, well-established habits can be disrupted.

Sue works for the local authority as a housing advisor. She has been in this position for ten years and has always prided herself on her punctuality. Of late, she is finding it difficult to get to work for her 9am start. Sue has rheumatoid arthritis and this has disrupted her previous early morning routine of getting herself ready and prepared for the day ahead. This is now taking far longer than it did previously. It also requires far more effort, because of the early morning pain and stiffness she is experiencing. Although no one at work has commented on her lateness, Sue feels increasingly uncomfortable and concerned about it.

The MOHO has usefully added to occupational therapists' understanding of occupational roles. The worker role is currently attracting widespread attention, because of its potential in assisting to reduce social exclusion and poverty within our society (Organisation for Economic Co-operation and Development, 2003). At an individual level, roles can also help provide a personal identity, meaning and satisfaction in life (Brown *et al.*, 2001), so that for some of us, the type of work we do forms an important part of who we are. Our participation in work occupations is not static, but rather responds and changes to the opportunities and challenges which present to us during our lifetimes.

These experiences gained during our occupational career shape, and are shaped by, us as occupational beings. Some people commit to a particular form of work occupation over a number of years. We have all come across, or read about, occupational therapists who have dedicated their entire working life to the profession. For others, work occupations and roles are more varied, and sometimes more colourful, as people explore and develop their occupational identity over time by engaging in different types of work activities. In some instances this is out of personal choice, but, increasingly, the labour market is dictating these changes. Maintaining employability has become an important element of successfully maintaining a worker role throughout a working life (Furnham, 2005).

The concept of an occupational career was introduced into the OT literature some 30 years ago. This early interest focused on how roles were acquired, and changed, across the lifespan (Heard, 1977; Black, 1976). It was suggested that the role career was usually an orderly progression from player, to student, to worker, to volunteer or homemaker, and then to retiree. These early concepts continue to be of relevance to the occupational therapist today, although this developmental sequence no longer exists with the same degree of certainty as it used to. For many, there are no longer easily definable career paths as global shifts from production-based economies to knowledge-based ones continue unabated (Vierling, 1999). In an earlier chapter we examined some of the effects of the changing nature of work.

Roles organise use of time, and, as mentioned previously, place an individual within the social structure (Oakley *et al.*, 1986). Therefore, each particular worker role has social expectations attached to it. We also make our own individual interpretations of what these expectations might be. The person who identifies strongly with the worker role, and considers it a central component of their personal identity, for example, is more likely to put a great degree of effort and time into their job. Role strain may occur when there is a poor match between an individual's capabilities and the demands of their job, or between other roles and their worker role (Kielhofner *et al.*, 1999). This point was illustrated earlier in the chapter, in the case of Shannon, the teacher.

Following a serious traumatic injury or sudden severe illness, therapists are frequently called upon to support individuals through the significant role disruption which these events may accompany. Throughout this book we encounter case studies of individuals who have had to make significant adjustments in the face of injury, illness and disability. You may have come across these situations in your own personal or professional life. You will know, therefore, that some clients in these circumstances need considerable assistance, and often creativity, to help them re-establish their worker role (Hammel, 1999).

The third component of the person in MOHO, performance capacity, may be affected by changes in either an individual's volitional or habituation systems, or by their own subjective views of their capabilities.

> Karen is a data input clerk for a local shipping firm. She has been off work for four months following a whiplash injury sustained while travelling to work. An MRI scan after the incident did not reveal any structural damage to her neck. Karen is however, still experiencing sharp pains on head movement. She believes, erroneously, that these pains are evidence of further ongoing injury occurring to her neck. She thinks that she must therefore avoid all head movement so as to not worsen her condition. She refuses to take analgesia or anti-inflammatory medication as she thinks this will just mask the damage that is taking place. Her fears are preventing her from returning to her normal daily activities, including work. She spends much of her day sitting in a high-backed chair, supported by cushions, watching television.

It is evident from this example that Karen's subjective views of her performance capacity are hindering her recovery. However, her volitional and habituation systems are also clearly influencing her behaviour as well.

THE ENVIRONMENT

The final component of the MOHO is the environment, which has both physical and social dimensions. For the worker with a disability or injury, the environment can pose significant barriers to work. Disabled people have fewer opportunities to enter employment and even those who are successful in this regard are often faced with negative or patronising attitudes from co-workers or management (Kielhofner *et al.*, 1999). The stigma attached to disability, in particular to mental illness, is a critical element of the social environment, and, as such, has a profound influence on the disabled person's experience of work. Education and awareness-raising of these sorts of issues are important components of the occupational therapist's role in the workplace.

As far as the physical environment is concerned, greater strides are being made. The introduction of the Disability Discrimination Act means that some of the physical barriers which existed previously, such as building inaccessibility, now need to be addressed by employers. Similarly, schemes such as Access to Work, part of the Jobcentre Plus service, may also help address these physical obstacles to work. This is also an important domain of concern for occupational therapists and we will be referring back to these issues in successive chapters. However, having now examined the application of two OT models within VR, we will move on to examine other theoretical frameworks which may assist our understanding. The first of these is the bio-psychosocial model.

THE BIO-PSYCHOSOCIAL MODEL

The bio-psychosocial model was originally put forward in the mid-1970s by an American OT educator. At this time, theoretical perspectives specifically to do with OT practice were still in their infancy. Practice was driven by the medical model and was largely concerned with signs, symptoms and pathology (Mosey, 1974). Mosey argued that the use of a bio-psychosocial model would help the occupational therapist focus on the body, the mind and the environment of a given client. The model encompassed a biological component, such as muscle strength and co-ordination, and a psychological component, including human development and psychodynamic theories. The sociological element of the model was located in an understanding of group dynamics, socialisation and the development of role patterns. By viewing the client in this way, without a disease-specific focus, Mosey believed that OT would be better placed to work with clients in community settings. The major assumption of the model was that 'man has a right to a meaningful and productive existence. This includes not only the right to be free of disease but to participate in the life of the community' (1974, p.139).

Ironically, the potential of the bio-psychosocial model over a medical model approach appears to have been recognised more by other professional groups (Silcox, 2006), than it has within the OT profession itself. However, a number of the applications presented in the literature fail to reflect Mosey's original vision of the philosophy of the model. Since its inception, the model has been applied to a variety of conditions, such as cardiac arrest (Engel, 1980) and chronic pain (Nielson and Weir, 2001). It has been adopted by a number of different professional groups including nurses (Julliard *et al.*, 2006), GPs (Horton-Salway, 2002) and psychologists (Hoffman, 2000). Settings where the model has been used include primary care (Mårtensson, 2001), the hospice (Cassileith, 1984) and community mental health (Vasile *et al.*, 1987). Mistakenly, it has been referred to as the bio-psychosocial model of illness (Taggart *et al.*, 2003) and of disease (Huyse *et al.*, 2001). The model has been applied to the practice of VR (Waddell and Burton, 2004), disability and worklessness (Schulman, 1994) and to work hardening (Fisher, 1999).

The observant reader will recognise that this model is based upon an understanding of the inter-relationship between the person and his or her environment. This may partly explain why, anecdotally, occupational therapists who work in VR feel able to identify with the model. This concept has, however, been expanded upon and developed further as it has been incorporated into more recent OT theory, such as the MOHO and the CMOP, discussed earlier in this section.

THE INTERNATIONAL CLASSIFICATION OF FUNCTIONING, DISABILITY AND HEALTH (ICF)

The ICF provides a common framework and language for health professionals and service users. It is intended to create a shared understanding of the determinants of health and barriers to participation for people with disabilities, across multi-professional and cultural boundaries. The ICF has four main sections (World Health Organization, 2001):

1. body structure and function
2. activity

3. participation
4. environment.

There is a strong resonance between the values and beliefs which underpin OT and those of the ICF.

Occupational therapists have been encouraged to 'address the barriers to participation in occupation by creating home, work and community environments that facilitate engagement in occupation' (Canadian Association of Occupational Therapists, 2003, p.1). Others have advocated that occupational therapists need to align themselves more strongly with the ICF definitions and terminology. Terms such as 'participation' and 'activity', should, it is suggested, be used to describe outcomes of interventions (the end product), and the term 'occupation' should be reserved for the process involved in getting there (the means) (Royeen, 2002). This simplification, Royeen has argued, may reduce confusion around the OT role and allow others, such as service commissioners and the general public, to better understand its contribution.

While it is beyond the scope of this book to debate the best use of language in this regard, it is clear that the ICF may act as a useful tool to help justify and explain, in a manner which others understand, the OT role and contribution to assisting people to participate or remain in the activity of work.

THE IMPORTANCE OF THE ENVIRONMENT

Now that we have examined some possible applications of some commonly used frameworks, we will move on to a selection of concepts and ideas from other disciplines, which may usefully assist our understanding of the context in which VR takes place. Each of the frameworks explored thus far include the environment as a key component of work performance and behaviour. Since this is such a central theme, we will continue to expand on this concept in this next section.

THE SOCIAL MODEL OF DISABILITY

The social model originates from within the disabled community. It describes disability as a socio-political issue rather than an individual one (Bricher, 2000). From this perspective, disability arises out of the oppression which is experienced through societies' failure to adequately address the needs of people with an impairment (Craddock, 1996). It asserts that people with impairments are unable to participate in education, work and the social aspects of life, because of barriers that are erected by the non-disabled majority. These barriers may be either physical or attitudinal in nature. The social and environmental barriers which are faced by disabled people continue to contribute to their exclusion from the labour market (Barnes and Mercer, 2005).

Strong voices within the disability movement argue that a job is a fundamental human right, and the central issue is the amount of control the person has over their everyday routine, rather than how many tasks they can perform (Brisenden, 1986).

The social model therefore makes an important contribution to highlighting social barriers which are faced by disabled people in society. As such, it is an important reminder of the need to address a wide range of environmental factors which may be preventing the person with a health condition or disability from participating in work.

THE HEALTHY WORKPLACE

For work to bring about positive benefits to health, this occupation needs to take place in a healthy environment. Our discussions about the workplace environment will therefore centre on the notion of a healthy workplace. As our starting point, we will consider the benefits of a preventative approach, aimed at minimising the risks of acquiring an illness or disability, through placing a stronger emphasis on both health and well-being at work. Firstly, the potential of health promotion to achieve this objective will be explored. We will then briefly touch on Warr's (1987) Vitamin Model to help us understand how individuals may respond differently to stressors in the workplace and, finally, we will examine the disability management model. This is another Canadian model, which enables us to better understand how to re-integrate the worker, who has sustained some form of injury or illness, back into the workplace.

Health promotion

In the field of health promotion, there are plenty of opinions, but little consensus, about what constitutes health and well being, and how these can best be evaluated. Constraints within the existing health service in the UK mean that promoting and maintaining health has not tended to be a primary role of occupational therapists. Other western countries have long since recognised the potential for occupational therapists in this field (Canadian Association of Occupational Therapists, 2001). Despite this, many of the core beliefs underpinning both health education and health promotion will be familiar to occupational therapists, since they are often targeted at changing people's attitudes, beliefs and behaviour in some way (Calman *et al.*, 1990). Allen (1986) describes two employee health promotion programmes carried out by an occupational therapist and Unsworth (1999) uses a health promotion framework to reduce the risk of injuries, at home and at work, for people who have epilepsy.

The Ottawa Charter for Health Promotion (World Health Organization, 1986, p.1), which is based on a social model of health, defines health promotion as:

> *... the process of enabling people to increase control over, and to improve, their health. To reach a state of complete physical, mental and social well-being, an individual or group must be able to identify and to realize aspirations, to satisfy needs, and to change or cope with the environment. Health is, therefore, seen as a resource for everyday life, not the objective of living. Health is a positive concept emphasizing social and personal resources, as well as physical capacities. Therefore, health promotion is not just the responsibility of the health sector, but goes beyond healthy life-styles to well-being.*

This influential charter has broadened the focus of health promotion, to include the wider determinants of health and health inequalities. Its agenda has helped to inform both national and international policy in the area of health promotion. The key objectives include building public health policy, creating supportive environments, strengthening community action, developing personal skills and reorienting health services to include the promotion of health (Scriven, 2005). The World Health Organization (WHO) has since extended the principles of the Ottawa Charter to the workplace. We will examine this influential strategy further when we discuss the links between work and health, and ill-health, in a later chapter on employment in the open labour market.

Traditionally, there has been a strong medical focus to health promotion, and many existing strategies reflect this perspective. Interventions continue to be directed at an individual level, rather than an organisational or societal one (Perkins *et al.*, 1999). More recently, however, there has been greater recognition of the need to also address the cultural and social environment, for health promotion to be more effective. To take an example from the young person's workplace, namely the school, extensive interest in the concept of the 'health promoting school' has led to health education messages being reflected in the types of food served from the school canteen.

Increasingly, the concept of health in the workplace (Hayday *et al.*, 2004) is attracting similar interest. There are three main stands to health promotion in the workplace. These are:

1. raising awareness of health issues
2. interventions to help people to make changes to their lifestyles
3. creating and sustaining a healthy work environment.

Examples of these may include larger companies who have corporate membership of fitness centres or gyms. In some settings, anti-smoking policies have been introduced. Yet others employ a variety of complementary therapists to help reduce stress and muscular tension. These sorts of initiatives are important because they recognise that healthy workers in healthy workplaces are good for both the individual and the business.

This is a positive beginning since, traditionally, health at work has been viewed in a much narrower way. For many years it has been measured in terms of occupational accidents, injuries and diseases. The dominance of the biomedical model in this area has restricted understanding of workplace health and well-being. It has reduced ill-health at work to just those causative factors which it is possible to measure and control. Furthermore, the tendency has been to focus only on those conditions which research has proved are caused directly by the workplace itself. This has resulted in a lack of recognition of a much broader number of conditions which may be aggravated by work, or by poor quality work.

Symptoms of an unhealthy workplace may include:

- reduced performance and an increase in work-related errors and work-related accidents – this can be a particular problem for people with irregular shift patterns involving night working (Doyle, 2003)

- reduced productivity and wasting time during working hours (Bolchover, 2005)
- high levels of conflict at work and poor interpersonal communication
- job dissatisfaction, low morale and poor motivation
- high turn-over of staff and reduced employee commitment to work (Furnham, 2005)
- frequent short absences for illnesses
- poor customer satisfaction and complaints by customers and staff
- poor organisational image and reputation
- strike action may result if the issues are not resolved.

Let us illustrate some of these points through the use of a case study.

Rosemary is employed on a part-time basis by a local supermarket. Her job involves working on the customer services desk and occasionally operating the tills at the check-out. Rosemary has been struggling with depression for the past three months. Her family doctor has prescribed medication, which has not had much impact. Rosemary is the main carer for her mother who has dementia and lives with the family. Her mother's condition is deteriorating and she now needs a lot of personal care assistance. The situation at home has been made worse since Rosemary's husband Dave has been made redundant. The car manufacturing plant he worked for closed down unexpectedly at the end of last month. The family now has financial worries as well.

Rosemary makes an appointment to see her line manager to discuss her problems. She requests a swap from the customer services desk to check-out duties as she is finding it difficult to deal with customer's complaints, particularly as some can be quite hostile in their attitudes. She often finds herself going home in tears. The manager reminds her of the store's zero tolerance policy to harassment of staff and that she should be reporting any incidents. As none have been recorded in the incident book, the manager decides that this must be a training issue and recommends Rosemary attends a half-day training course in her own time so she is able deal with customers more effectively.

This example highlights how social and personal difficulties can impact on a person's ability to perform their work tasks. Rosemary was finding certain elements of her job were aggravating her depression. She was able to recognise that this was lowering her work quality. Her manager was unsympathetic to her problems since they were not directly related to the workplace, or caused by it.

Warr's Vitamin Model

We have seen that it is possible to identify the features of an unhealthy workplace, so can we then determine what makes a healthy one? Warr (1987) identifies nine key elements which can positively contribute to our sense of mental well-being, and can suitably be applied to the workplace situation (Doyle, 2003; Hodson, 2001). These elements act in a similar way to vitamins – we need a certain amount of each to maintain our health. Too much or too little of any particular 'vitamin' may have a detrimental effect on our health. They are:

- opportunity for control
- opportunity for skill use
- externally generated goals (negative effect)
- variety
- environmental clarity
- availability of money
- physical security
- opportunity for interpersonal contact
- valued social position.

However, unlike vitamins, there is no recommended daily dose. Warr did, however, examine the fit between the person and their work, by linking each of these elements to particular personality characteristics (Furnham, 2005). The degree of variety in an individual's work, and the right amount of social contact are largely determined by our specific needs according to our particular personality. As a general rule, each of us strives to find the right amount of 'vitamins' for ourselves. For the occupational therapist, these concepts may help explain why jobs with certain characteristics may be perceived as stressful by a particular individual, but not by another. We are able to recognise the application of Warr's model if we look back at a couple of the earlier case studies. Ben's job, for example, lacked variety, security and clarity. Rosemary's job, on the other hand, lacked opportunity for control, and she was also subject to goals which were generated externally, by her manager.

THE DISABILITY MANAGEMENT MODEL

In addition to advocating for healthy workplaces, the occupational therapist needs a good understanding of how to assist the worker with a health condition or acquired disability back to work. We can draw knowledge from the disability management literature to help us in this task. Disability management is an approach aimed at finding timely solutions, including rehabilitation, to address functional limitations which may arise in the workplace. In this way it aims to prevent further disability from taking place. The goal is to enable people to keep their job, or return to work, after a disability. It has been defined as

> ... a workplace prevention and remediation strategy that seeks to prevent disability from occurring or, lacking that, to intervene early following the onset of disability, using a coordinated, cost-conscious, quality rehabilitation service that reflects an organizational commitment to continued employment of those experiencing functional work limitations. The remediation goal of disability management is successful job maintenance, or optimum timing for return-to-work...

> (Akabas et al., 1992, p.2)

In support of this positive approach, the International Labour Organisation has produced guidelines to assist employers in managing disability-related issues in the workplace (International Labour Organisation, 2001).

Disability management is an expanding area of practice in North America, Canada, Australia and parts of Europe (Shrey and Hursh, 1999), and is slowly emerging in areas of the UK as well. It is not discipline specific and is practiced by occupational therapists, kinesiologists, nurses, insurance specialists and others in the field. It has its own code of practice (National Institute of Disability Management and Research, 2000), and some have called for disability management to be recognised as a profession in its own right (Harder and Scott, 2005). Disability management is a successful approach to work injury prevention (Isernhagen, 2000), and to reducing work disability for those with musculoskeletal conditions (Williams and Westmorland, 2002). It has, however, been less widely used for people with mental health conditions (Olsheski *et al.*, 2002).

A model of disability management, which illustrates key factors to take into account, when supporting the individual with a disability to return to work, has recently been put forward (Harder and Scott, 2005) (see Figure 4.1). This model highlights

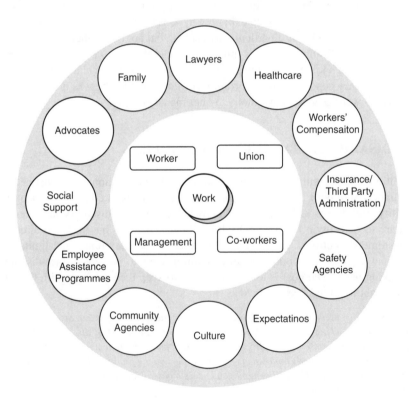

Figure 4.1. The disability management model. Reprinted from Harder, H.G. and Scott, L.R. (2005) *Comprehensive Disability Management,* p.27, with permission from Elsevier

the range of environmental factors, both within the workplace itself and beyond, which may impact on the outcome of the rehabilitation for work programme. Any combination of the identified factors may influence the return to work process, either in a positive or a negative way. Although this model is based on practice within a Canadian context, there are common elements which are compatible with practice in the UK. The model has been designed with a return to paid employment in mind, however aspects may also be useful when an individual is entering an unpaid work environment, such as in voluntary work participation.

The disability management model identifies that each workplace has its own unique characteristics. The philosophy of the workplace, together with the policies and procedures which operate within it, will have an impact on the workers' experience of working. Within the workplace, represented inside the circle, in Figure 4.1 there is a complex interplay between five central elements which are the:

1. work
2. worker
3. co-workers
4. management
5. union (if one is present).

Within this model, work is conceptualised in a way which will be familiar to many occupational therapists. It is placed at the centre as it forms a central component of life, bringing with it a sense of meaning and well-being, confidence and self-worth. The personal characteristics of the worker, such as personality, capabilities, beliefs and values, will influence both the reaction to the disability or condition, and the attitude towards returning to or remaining in work. Research within OT has shown the importance of these personal dimensions in the return to work process (Kemp and Kleinplatz, 1985; Tse and Walsh, 2001).

The attitudes and responses of co-workers may either be positive or negative. In these circumstances they present a very real barrier to the return of the disabled person to work. Co-workers may resent what they see as having to carry the disabled person, particularly in instances where they are expected to take on additional duties as a result. In contrast, where there is support from co-workers, and genuine concern for the well-being of the employee, combined with understanding, believing and good communication, then this environment will be far more enabling as a result (Shaw et al., 2003).

The management component of the workplace will be influenced by the objectives and strategies of the company itself. These will, in turn, influence attitudes towards disability. A tension is always likely to exist between the employers' drive towards increased productivity and the capabilities and effort expended by employees. Attitudes of the immediate manager and human resources departments will have a significant impact on the success or failure of the return to work. The employer–employee relationship will be returned to later, when we will further examine concepts such as absence management policies and job retention.

The union is far less of a force within modern workplaces in the UK than in the industries of the past. The nature of the relationship between the union and the management in a given company will influence the part played by the union within the disability management process. As with any of the other factors in the model, this influence may, or may not, be constructive in nature. Unions have the potential to be a powerful supporter of the disabled worker and therefore, where they exist, the role they may play will be an important consideration (Trades Union Congress, 2002).

Having considered the inter-relationships between the key components within the workplace, there are a further 12 factors outside of the workplace itself which may potentially play an important role in the return to work process. These external elements make up the outer circle of Figure 4.1 and include:

1. family
2. lawyers
3. healthcare
4. compensation
5. insurance
6. safety agencies
7. expectations
8. culture
9. community agencies (voluntary sector organisations)
10. employee assistance programmes
11. social and family support
12. advocates.

It is beyond the scope of this section to do more than touch on these key factors. Some will be covered in later sections of the book.

CULTURE AND EXPECTATIONS

Attitudes towards health, disability and work are shaped by values and beliefs of the wider culture. Even the culture within an organisation and attitudes towards expected behaviours, such as what you do when you are unwell, will impact on the worker's expectations of when, or if, it is appropriate to go back to work.

> Ed works in the print room of a leading national newspaper. He is 56 years old, and has held a similar job with the company since he left school aged 15. Ed was recently diagnosed with diabetes. Since he is over 55, he assumes that this diagnosis signals the end of his working life. He expects that he will now take early retirement, on medical grounds. Many of his former colleagues have already gone down this route. Ed makes these assumptions in spite of the fact that, if properly controlled, his diabetes is unlikely to markedly affect his ability to do his job.

The expectations of the worker may be affected by many other factors. For example, if the person has a strong work identity and expects to return to work, this can positively reinforce their return. In Britain however, existing policies do not always support this approach. There has traditionally been an expectation that the worker must be fully fit before resuming work activities. This assumption negatively impacts on the likelihood of a person returning to work because the longer someone is off work, perhaps waiting for symptoms such as back pain to disappear, the less likely it is that they will successfully return to work (Department for Work and Pensions, 2002).

In a similar vein, where a lawyer becomes involved because a claim for compensation is being pursued, an employee may focus their energy more on the case and possibly on maximising any potential financial settlement, than on actively participating in their recovery. This perverse incentive is a real barrier, and may clearly have implications for the outcome of the client's return to work programme. Health professionals, including occupational therapists, have expressed their frustration with clients' reluctance to engage in the return to work process because they have effectively put their life on hold while their case is being pursued. Since the legal process can be drawn out over several years, this contradicts the evidence which shows that early intervention in return to work has the best chance of success.

The International Underwriting Association of London, which is the world's largest representative organisation for insurance and reinsurance companies, formed a Rehabilitation Working Party in 1998 to encourage greater use of rehabilitation in the claims process in cases of injury. The working party included representatives of bodies such as the Association of British Insurers, primary insurers, legal groups, care providers and NHS representatives. This resulted in the publication of a voluntary Rehabilitation Code in 1999. The main aim of the code is to promote the use of rehabilitation and early intervention in the claims process, so that an injured person is enabled to make a speedy medical, social and psychological recovery. More recently, the Association of Personal Injury Lawyers has produced a best practice guide on rehabilitation (Association of Personal Injury Lawyers, 2004) which provides additional guidance and support for their members.

SUPPORT NETWORKS

The role fulfilled by the worker within the family, and attitudes and responses to the worker's disability from family members, may also influence the outcome of the disability management process. Similarly, social support networks may contribute to an individual's perceptions about their ability to return to work. An advocate, either within the workplace, or from extended social or family networks, may also feed into these perceptions. Consider the following two contrasting scenarios.

Elaine works full-time, which includes shift work, as a midwife. In the last six months she has had nearly seven weeks off work – usually three to four days at a time – because of recurrent migraines. She is awaiting further tests to try and establish the cause of the migraines. Elaine lives with her husband and has two grown up children. Both children live locally and have recently started families of their own. Elaine's family feel that work is taking too much out of her and are encouraging her to give up her job to allow her to spend more time with her grandchildren. Three months later, Elaine decides to resign from her job.

Don is a 26–year-old firefighter who loves his job and is well respected for his skills in combating fires. Recently, he was seriously injured by falling debris while attending a fire. He is making a good recovery, and is working hard during rehabilitation sessions. He has frequent visits in hospital from his parents, friends and from his co-workers, all of whom reinforce his talents in his chosen vocation. They are supportive of his eventual return to work. Nine months later, after a phased return to work, Don resumes full duties as a firefighter.

These two examples illustrate how the views and attitudes of family and friends may potentially influence an individual's return to work, in very different ways.

THE ROLE OF OTHER ORGANISATIONS IN DISABILITY MANAGEMENT

There is an extensive network of voluntary sector organisations (community agencies) in the UK which may play an important contributory role in the return to work process. Some provide training, or retraining, others offer practical and emotional support. The role of these organisations and government safety agencies, such as the Health and Safety Executive and the Health and Safety Commission, will be discussed in later chapters.

The majority of healthcare in the UK is provided by the state-funded National Health Service (NHS). However, the modern-day NHS remains largely unconcerned with the health of the workforce. Lengthy waits for investigations and treatment are often a significant barrier and delay return to work (British Society of Rehabilitation Medicine, 2000). Some larger companies provide their employees with private medical insurance so as to avoid these holdups. They may also provide in-house employee assistance programmes, such as workplace counselling or alternative therapies. The attitudes of the healthcare professionals who are involved in a person's medical treatment may also impact on whether an individual perceives that they are capable of returning to work (Department for Work and Pensions, 2004).

By law, all employers have to take out compulsory employers' liability (EL) insurance to cover them in the event of workplace-related illness or injury. The Association of British Insurers has identified that the current system of EL is not sustainable because claims are becoming increasingly difficult to predict, the costs of claims have risen dramatically, and policies are therefore becoming unaffordable to employers. A reform has been called for, in the system, to allow more widespread use of rehabilitation of injured workers and greater emphasis to be placed on good health and safety practice (Association of British Insurers, 2005). In addition to EL insurance, a percentage of mainly larger companies extend their insurance to cover sickness absence or injuries which are not caused by work itself, often though the purchase of income protection policies.

If you are interested in reading more about disability management you might like to read: Harder, H.G. and Scott, L.R. (2005) *Comprehensive Disability Management*, Edinburgh: Elsevier Churchill Livingstone.

A CONCEPTUAL FRAMEWORK OF THE CYCLES
OF VULNERABILITY

Another theoretical framework which can guide the occupational therapist's understanding of return to work, and the risk of job loss associated with illness or disability, is that of the cycles of vulnerability framework (James *et al.*, 2003), which is illustrated in Figure 4.2. This framework is primarily targeted at the job retention of the ill or disabled worker. It illustrates the increasing risk of job loss which the person may face, either on a voluntary or compulsory basis. It also suggests how VR may help to reduce this risk and facilitate continued employment.

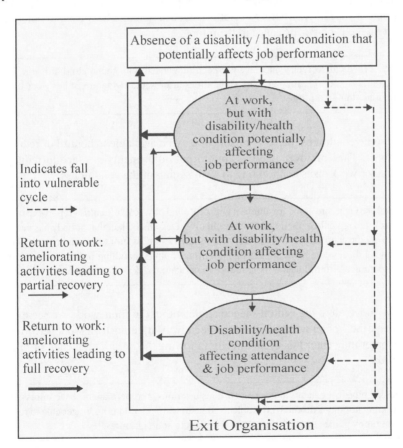

Figure 4.2. Cycles of vulnerability conceptual framework. Reprinted from Health and Safety Executive (2003) *Job Retention and Vocational Rehabilitation: The development and evaluation of a conceptual framework*, p.63. Crown copyright material is reproduced with the permission of the controller of HMSO and the Queen's printer for Scotland

Let us now consider this framework in more detail, using examples to demonstrate its application.

The box at the top of the diagram represents those workers whose work performance is not affected by a disability or health condition. The worker may have an illness or a disability, but this does not have a negative impact on their work ability.

> Mike, a plasterer, is partially blind in one eye following an assault in a pub a number of years ago. He has continued working and his work has not suffered as a result of his visual deficit. Mike does, however, have his vision checked regularly, particularly to ensure he remains fit to drive.

The top shaded circle is the first cycle and represents workers who develop a health condition or disability, whether or not it is work-related, which has the potential to impact on their job performance in the future.

> Kirsty, a medical secretary, has recently been diagnosed with rheumatoid arthritis. Even though this is not affecting her work capabilities at present, the nature of her work means that it may do in the future.

For some conditions, medical treatment may be available to control or reduce the symptoms. The employer may be able to put adjustments in place to reduce the potential of work tasks contributing to a worsening of the condition.

> Several staff in a care home for children with profound physical difficulties report experiencing back and leg pain to their union representative. Despite the fact that nobody has been off work with these problems, there is very real concern amongst staff that their health is at risk. Following discussions with management, hoists, a manual handling policy, and additional staff training are introduced to help reduce the potential risk of a work-related injury.

If we move on to the central shaded circle within the framework, we see that this represents the worker whose condition is negatively affecting their work performance. The worker may enter this cycle directly following the onset of a mental of physical condition.

> Gerald, a physical education teacher, sustains a serious, and permanent, knee injury while on a skiing holiday. Although he is able to come to work, Gerald is no longer able to referee school rugby games or drive the school mini-bus to sports fixtures.

Alternatively, the worker may enter this second cycle of vulnerability from the first cycle. This may be due to a worsening of their condition or disability, or a failure of the employer to make adjustments to the nature of the work or the workplace.

The third cycle represents the worker whose condition is affecting both their performance and their attendance. Again, the worker may move directly into this cycle.

Hadiya develops a chronic depressive illness following the death of her spouse. She has difficulty concentrating on work tasks while at work as a library assistant, and frequently fails to arrive at work in the morning, leading to high levels of work absence.

Alternatively, a worker may move into this third cycle from cycle two.

Returning to the example of the PE teacher above. Gerald has developed chronic pain in his injured knee, which is being aggravated by the amount of physical exertion his job entails. This pain is resulting in increasingly extended periods of absence from work.

On the left-hand side of the diagram, the two lines of varying thickness suggest how VR interventions may help reduce the impact of the health condition or disability. Appropriate forms of intervention may contribute to increased job stability, thereby helping to reduce the risk of the individual losing his or her job. Clearly the ideal outcome is reflected by the thick black line, which represents a return from any of the vulnerable cycles to a health state where performance is not negatively affected. The thinner line represents a reduction in the impact of the disability on job performance, however the employee within any of the cycles remains at greater risk of job loss.

You will see that this framework is useful for displaying how rehabilitation may, potentially, help prevent job loss. Assisting the individual to retain their job in this way may reduce the health risks, and other negative consequences, which have been associated with unemployment.

In this chapter we have discussed a range of theoretical frameworks, both from within and outside of OT, which may usefully enhance our understanding of VR, as well as helping to guide our practice. We will now move on from these theoretical models, to examine an array of different service models intended to meet the rehabilitation needs of workers across the spectrum of VR.

5 Service Models in Vocational Rehabilitation

THE CONTINUUM OF VOCATIONAL REHABILITATION

In the previous chapter we examined the profession-specific and generic theoretical frameworks that occupational therapists may use to guide their reasoning and practice within Vocational Rehabilitation (VR). In this chapter we will move on to look at the types of service models that exist to help disabled people participate in work occupations. There is, unfortunately, no getting around the fact that the range of services to be found under the banner of VR is complex; with a number of different stakeholders involved. This complexity has been compounded by the fragmentation and piecemeal approach to the development of services in the past. The diverse array of service models in VR can sometimes make it difficult for the novice practitioner to gain an understanding of what is available, and to whom. The number of occupational therapists working within this sector, outside of the confines of traditional health and social care delivery, is still relatively small. Yet the scope and contribution that they may make are clearly demonstrated by those who have moved into this area of practice. The over-arching aim of this chapter, therefore, is to outline a broad range of different service models and initiatives. Exploring these wider dimensions will provide occupational therapists with a greater familiarity of a broader range of possible work opportunities which may be available to their clients, as well as increasing their knowledge and understanding of practice within commercial settings.

In an ideal world, there would be a comprehensive range of services which enabled people to access, maintain and return to a valued work occupation. These services would be contained under the broad umbrella of one integrated system. Unfortunately, however, this is not the case. Services can only exist where finances are available to fund them, and so the configuration of available services is almost wholly dictated by socio-economic objectives and priorities.

Conventionally, VR services have been divided into two distinct categories. The first deals with the collection of services that are directed towards those people who have a disability and are unemployed. They may never have secured a job, or they may have been out of any form of employment for a long time. The severity of their condition may mean that competing for work in the open labour market is unrealistic. Traditionally, services for this group of individuals has been funded by the public purse, though provision from healthcare organisations, local authorities and government employment services. The voluntary sector is also, increasingly, playing a significant role in this area.

The second category are the VR services available to people who are already in employment. The person may not be attending work at present, because of an illness or injury, but they have a job to return to. In a nutshell, these services are funded by employers, either directly or indirectly. Directly, through the provision of occupational health services, or indirectly through purchasing insurance cover. At this level, a further division is, most commonly, made between conditions suffered as a result of work, in which case the employer may perhaps be held to be responsible in some way, and those where the condition was not work-related, in which case the person is not entitled to assistance through this route. A simplified outline of this principle is outlined in Figure 5.1.

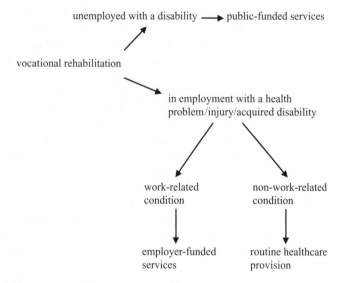

Figure 5.1. A simplified outline of the traditional organisation of vocational rehabilitation provision

In our modern world, these rather rigid delineations can be unhelpful. This is particularly so, if our purpose is to enable each person to acquire and retain a meaningful and valued worker role, as an important dimension of their individual occupational profile. With this aspirational intention, there is a need to re-examine and re-design existing service provision in quite a different way. However, before thinking about how things might be, we first need to be able to understand how existing systems operate.

Chapter 2 included some observations of developments in different countries. Around the world, countries such as Canada, the United States of America, Australia, New Zealand, South Africa and some European countries, such as Sweden and Finland, have had established programmes for many years to assist people into, and back into, work. There is no plan to describe these services, nor indeed to undertake a comparison between them, since this task has already been admirably performed by others (Pratt and Jacobs, 1997; Floyd, 1996; Koch and Rumrill, 2003; Curtis, 2003; O'Halloran, 2002).

As mentioned in the Introduction of this book, the terminological differences across these different countries makes it difficult for us to gain a sense of the strengths and weaknesses of the different programmes available. If you are interested in exploring this area further, you will find that the configuration of the majority of these service models is based, at least to some degree, on the funding streams outlined above.

As mentioned previously, a key element of the present UK Government's welfare reform programme includes a drive towards increasing the numbers of people in paid employment. This Welfare to Work policy promotes employment as a fundamental way of addressing social exclusion, reducing poverty and as a means of improving health. The need to tackle this on different fronts, by reducing the risks of employees becoming ill, improving the retention of employees, and supporting rehabilitation for people who experience illness or disability, has been recognised as crucial to the success of these endeavours (Department for Work and Pensions *et al.*, 2005). Throughout this chapter we will be exploring some of the ways in which this agenda is being implemented, and the practical initiatives which have stemmed from it.

Many services in the UK are still largely in a fledgling state, but despite this, there has been a shared recognition amongst the different stakeholders of the need for VR (British Society of Rehabilitation Medicine, 2000). This spirit of collaboration is leading to a blurring of some of the more conventional service boundaries, resulting in more innovative service delivery approaches. In order to address the problems of work, ill-health and disability, further developments will be necessary. Consequently, this chapter has not been structured around the traditional model of service delivery outlined above. Rather, a person-centred perspective has been used to examine this problem. Services have been grouped on the basis of a continuum, where an individual may move along or between three distinct phases, as seen in Figure 5.2.

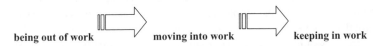

being out of work   moving into work   keeping in work

Figure 5.2. The three phases of a person-centred continuum of vocational rehabilitation services

This continuum begins with the notion of being out of work, and what this means to individuals and society at large. This first section aims to help the reader understand the nature and extent of unemployment, as well as the policies and agendas that are directed towards addressing the situation. Following on, the second section is based around the theme of moving into work. It outlines the range of services available, which may assist individuals to gain a worker role. There is a need for different service models in order to enable as many people as possible, with a wide range of disabilities, health conditions and other disadvantages, to access meaningful work.

Working in the open labour market is an aspiration of many people with a disability, yet statistics demonstrate that only the minority are successful in this regard. This section therefore focuses on exploring access routes into paid employment. It examines the role of the employment services in helping people into work and the advantages for the occupational therapist, and his or her clients, in establishing collaborative working relationships with them. Supporting people in the transition from being out of work to establishing a worker role, is an area with considerable scope for an occupational therapy (OT) contribution.

The third element of the VR continuum identifies the current range of services which may help people to keep in work and preventing them from losing their worker role. Initiatives aimed at preventing job loss for people who acquire health problems or disabilities during their adult life are currently still few and far between. In contrast to other countries, such as Canada and Australia, there is a lack of robust legislation in this field in the UK. As a result, the complexity of developing effective strategies means that sound, evidence-based pathways are still in their infancy.

SERVICE MODELS ACROSS THE CONTINUUM

Of course, it goes without saying that unfortunately services are not neatly organised into a client-centred continuum of VR services as has been described here. However, by organising them in this way, it allows us to consider what is currently available and what may be needed to fill the gaps in the future.

This chapter attempts to provide a balanced overview of different forms of work. You will recall from an earlier chapter, that our broad understanding of valued work occupations extends beyond just paid, competitive employment. Supporting a client to make the work choices which are right for them at a particular stage in their recovery, as well as respecting their decision, should always be an occupational therapist's first priority. This viewpoint may contrast somewhat with current political drives, which are very strongly directed towards increasing participation in open labour market employment. Similarly, insurers and employers will no doubt be motivated, at least to some extent, by their interest in cutting their overheads. We should not ignore these pressures, indeed it would be foolishly unrealistic to do so. Equally, however, as professionals who believe that a relationship exists between occupation and health, we do not have to blindly follow the agenda set by others. There is clearly a balance to be struck between these two, sometimes opposing, perspectives and we will continue to debate this tension as this chapter progresses. Let us explore, at this point, what it means to be out of work; the problems which contribute to it, and the problems which it creates.

BEING OUT OF WORK

Since we commonly link work with employment, it is unsurprising that we take the connection further to make the assumption that being out of work means being unemployed. As you read on through this section you will, however, see that unemployment is just one dimension of the problem. For the purpose of this book 'being out of work' has been defined as currently not fulfilling, or participating in, a valued worker role. Being unemployed does not necessarily mean that a person does not have a worker role. Deciding what constitutes a meaningful worker role is a very individual viewpoint, although this perception will be shaped by the person's wider community network as well as by the views of society at large.

Being out of work may be short-term and temporary, or it may be long-term in nature. There are several reasons for both. Short-term interruptions may result when someone sustains an injury or illness, and is consequently off work on sick leave. They still have a job, but they are not performing their usual worker role. They may well, however, plan to resume this role when they are recovered. For others, the loss of their worker role may be due to redundancy. While for many this is a temporary stoppage, their return will depend on factors such as the person's employability and existing local labour market conditions. Another good example is child-rearing. This involves the temporary loss of a paid worker role, in order to take up an unpaid work role as a parent and home maintainer.

In other instances, the loss, or failure to gain, a worker role may be chronic, long-term or permanent. There are disadvantaged groups in our society who find it difficult to enter work. Disabled school leavers are a good example. Another example may be found in certain communities, where several generations of families have been out of work – being workless has become the accepted norm. Sometimes, the systems which are in place actively discourage people from seeking a return to the worker role. Elements of the healthcare, benefits and legal systems are particularly at fault in this regard.

We will learn throughout this chapter about some of the initiatives which have been introduced to attempt to address some of these issues, such as the current incapacity benefit (IB) reforms. Let us move on to examine the nature and extent of the most widely recognised form of being out of work: unemployment.

Unemployment

Unemployment, for most people, is a negative experience. There are few who are able to replace work with leisure activities in a meaningful way (Glyptis, 1989). An examination of the health status of unemployed people suggests that being out of work is an important determinant of health inequalities, particularly in the effects it has on people's behaviours and their habits. For example, those who become unemployed are more likely to increase their smoking and alcohol consumption, reduce their physical activity, gain weight, and have reduced psychological well-being (Department of Health, 2004). It is not uncommon for people who lose their job to develop secondary mental health problems in addition to their presenting ailment (Waddell and Burton, 2004). This is particularly the case when they have been unemployed for a prolonged period of time, following, say, an injury (Banks, 1995). Families also suffer and bear much of the burden in these situations (Dale *et al.*, 2003).

Some have linked long-term unemployment to social exclusion (Danson, 2005), as well as higher levels of mortality from lung cancer, suicide, heart disease and mental illnesses, such as anxiety and reactive clinical depression. It is for these reasons, amongst others, that Douthwaite (1994) challenges occupational therapists to become more involved in addressing the employment needs of their clients, rather than just dealing with the consequences of their unemployment.

In early 2005, the unemployment rate in the UK was 4.8 per cent (Dewson, 2005). However, measuring the actual number of unemployed people is not a straightforward task. The definition of what constitutes unemployment varies over time, as well as between countries. Factors such as the welfare provision within a particular country and the level of family support, will impact on the experience of unemployment for the individual (Paugam and Duncan, 2004). There tends to be a reliance on citing the numbers claiming unemployment benefits, but this is an inaccurate indicator since it doesn't represent the full picture. In order to receive benefits you must be eligible for them in the first place, so this excludes some groups, for example refugees, some homeless people and traveller communities. Frequent administrative changes also affect the accuracy of the figures, as people are moved between different types of benefits, often to meet political ends.

There is no single cause of unemployment, however, it is possible to identify certain groups who are most at risk of losing their job. These include:

- the poorly qualified
- the unskilled
- the young and inexperienced
- the older worker, particularly ten to 15 years before retirement age
- those in poor health or with a disability
- those from an ethnic minority.
(Convery, 1997)

In addition to these demographic variables, the availability and supply of local work is also a factor which influences the likelihood of being in employment. For people with a health problem or disability, the more severe their impairment, the poorer their prospects of securing a job in the first place (Berthoud, 2006). There is also a clear link between qualifications, previous experience and employment. Those people without qualifications have the highest levels of unemployment and a greater likelihood of experiencing job instability with regular periods of unemployment. Conversely, people with a degree, particularly a vocational qualification such as nursing or teaching, have the lowest levels of unemployment (Convery, 1997).

This is reflective of the UK labour market's fastest growing industries being in the services sector. As well as jobs within health, education, and welfare, this sector also includes transport, communications, government, administration, financial services, leisure, personal services, retail and so on. In contrast, less than two per cent of the population are now employed in agriculture, forestry and fishing. Manufacturing, once the largest sector, now only accounts for less than a fifth of jobs (Brown, 1997).

Not only are the types of job changing, but so too are the ways in which work duties are performed. For some years now there has been a move towards more flexible working, restructuring, demands for more transferable skills, along with increased expectations to hold an educational qualification. This has meant that large numbers of people skilled in traditional occupations, men in particular, now have problems with employability (Danson, 2005; Brown, 1997). In the same vein, changes to the nature of work means that the 'job for life' culture of industrial times has largely come to an end. A significant number of people are therefore likely to need to cope with periods of unemployment during their working lives (Walker and Walker, 1997; Noon and Blyton, 1997).

Fortunately, many people who lose their job through redundancy will successfully find another job. For example, during the early 1990s there were particularly high numbers of redundancies and 1.2 million people lost their jobs. Six months later, nearly half had secured alternative employment, despite the less than favourable economic conditions of the time (Convery, 1997). However, the current social geography of the UK reflects that there are some deprived areas of the country with continued high levels of worklessness. These are evident in inner city areas, the old industrial areas, and those areas which depended on mining, as well as some costal towns and rural areas.

A series of Government initiatives, including designated employment zones and action teams, has been put in place to attempt to tackle the identified problems in these specific areas. A more recent initiative, the Working Neighbourhoods Pilot, was set up to address what has become known as the 'culture of worklessness', which is found in some of the worst affected areas. Demographics show that this is not a straight-forward task, as people in these neighbourhoods experience multiple barriers to employment. The remit of the Working Neighbourhoods Pilot is to provide intensive support for people, to help them secure jobs within their local areas. Early evaluations found the project to be successful in helping more people into employment, as well as achieving softer outcomes, such as improvements in self-confidence and motivation (Dewson, 2005).

Under-employment and economic inactivity

At this point, it is important to make the distinction between unemployment, under-employment and economic inactivity. People who are unemployed do not have a paid job, and, as we have learned, there are a number of reasons why this group of people may not be participating in the labour market. Others do not want, or need, to be in employment. Furthermore, as the education process has lengthened over time, many more young people are now entering paid work at a later age.

Some people are under-employed. That is, they are prevented in some way from working more hours, despite perhaps a desire or willingness to do so. A good example of this is the restriction placed on disabled people's working hours. If they exceed their allowable working hours, their benefit entitlements are put at risk. Yet other job-seekers are only able to obtain part-time work, despite perhaps wanting to do more.

Economic inactivity applies in instances where people drop out of the labour market, but do not move onto state benefits, preferring instead to live on their savings. The largest group of economically inactive people are men over the age of 50. This number has been steadily rising since the early 1990s. When these figures are combined with those of unemployment, as many as a quarter of men of working age are not in employment (Convery, 1997). Earlier we discussed the socio-economic role of work, and highlighted Government concerns about the dwindling number of people who are actively participating in the workforce.

It is interesting to digress a little at this point, to consider that much of what we currently understand about the meaning of work (Brief *et al.*, 1995) and the health benefits of being in employment (Waddell and Burton, 2006), have been inferred through studying the effects of unemployment. The danger in making these inferences is the assumption that it is being in employment which provides these benefits. This conjecture fails to recognise that these benefits are probably conditional on that employment being of good quality. Work which is of poor quality does not necessarily confer health benefits – quite the opposite, in fact. Other work-related factors, besides unemployment, which have been identified as having a potentially negative effect on the health or well-being of individuals include:

- under-employment
- poor quality and unproductive jobs
- unsafe work and insecure income
- rights which are denied
- gender inequality
- migrant workers who are exploited
- lack of representation and voice
- inadequate protection and support for those facing disease, disability or old age.
(International Labour Organisation, 2005)

It has been well-documented that tiring, mindless, mundane, stressful or unchallenging work also has negative effects on well-being (Farnworth, 1995), and, in the longer term, potentially on health.

Work imbalance and role conflict

For some, work occupations conflict with each other. This is often the experience of parents, particularly mothers, who are also in paid employment. Although there have been some improvements in the entitlement to parental leave, parenthood, particularly motherhood, is an undervalued role within our society. The current drive, therefore, is towards getting mothers re-engaged in the paid workforce as soon as possible. This emphasis means that parents are often faced with role conflict and role overload, as we witnessed in the earlier case study of Shannon.

The need for an improved work–life balance, as it has become known, has been recognised, but for many workers this remains elusive. A culture of long work hours means that about 840, 000 people do more than ten hours of unpaid overtime a week, with teachers and lecturers being the worst affected (Trades Union Congress, 2007). Combined with other factors, such as increased job intensity and office politics, this means that the incidence of work-related stress continues to rise (Health and Safety Commission, 2006a). In this next section we will continue to examine some more negative consequences of poor-quality work.

Work-related ill-health, injury and death

Illness or injury may strike anywhere, yet when it is in some way linked to the workplace it has traditionally been singled out for particular attention. And for good reason. The number of fatal accidents which take place at work, for instance, is a key indicator of the conditions and the nature of the work environment in which that work is carried out. Keeping records of these incidents helps identify risk factors which may be present in particular industries. This, in turn, assists with the development of strategies to minimise and reduce these risks (Takala, 1995).

Obviously there are enormous variations in the safety of work across different countries. Taking a global perspective illustrates this point. An annual estimate ranges from 100 to 270 million occupational accidents and injuries, resulting in 200,000 deaths. In addition, conservative estimates suggest there are 68 million–157 million new cases of occupational disease caused by hazardous exposures or workloads (World Health Organization, 2004). In total, it is believed that more than two million men and women around the world die from accidents at work or occupational diseases each year (International Labour Organisation, 2005).

If we consider the UK picture, we find that the number of fatalities and work-related injuries continues to fall in response to improvements in working practises designed to help make workplaces safer places. The risk of being fatally injured at work has shown a general downward trend since the early 1990s. In 2005/2006, 212 workers were killed – a rate of 0.7 fatal injuries per 100,000 employed. Higher-risk industries include construction and agriculture, forestry and fishing which, when combined, accounted for nearly half of the recorded deaths (Health and Safety Commission, 2006b). If we look at the picture more closely, according to the Royal Society for the Prevention of Accidents (1998–2007) the rate of fatal and major injuries in small firms (<50 employees) is over twice the rate in firms employing more than 1,000 people. The most common kinds of accident which result in fatal injuries are: falling from a height; being struck by a moving vehicle; and being struck by a moving or falling object.

Work-related driving is one of the biggest single causes of all reportable accidents, with car and van drivers who cover 25,000 miles a year as part of their job having the same risk of being killed at work as coal miners. These are therefore important factors to be incorporated into any occupational risk assessment. A further 150,559 non-fatal injuries to employees were reported; a rate of 587 per 100,000 employees. In addition to these recorded deaths and major injuries, the Labour Force Survey suggests that 363,000 unreported injuries occurred, which is a rate of 1,330 per 100,000 workers, based on 2003/2004 figures. The combined cost to industry of workplace injuries is up to seven million working days.

In contrast to injuries and deaths, work-related ill-health is more difficult to measure. There are relatively few conditions which may be directly attributed to particular forms of work, and in many instances these are only discovered, or confirmed, many years after the exposure took place. While recognising these complexities, it is known that as many as two million people in the UK have reported suffering from an illness which they believe was caused, or made worse, by either their current or past work. More than half a million of these were new cases reported in the last year. Of these cases, over 20,000 were severe enough to warrant being seen by a specialist doctor. (Health and Safety Executive, 2006). Each year there are about 40,000 new assessments for the Department for Work and Pensions' Industrial Injuries Disablement Benefit Scheme, of which about 6,500 receive compensation under this scheme (Wright *et al.*, 2005). We will learn more about the Industrial Injuries Disability Benefits in a later chapter.

The Health and Safety Executive statistics also indicate that 27,000 people leave employment permanently each year after becoming ill or sustaining an injury at work (Trades Union Congress, 2002). Work-related ill-health was responsible for a total of 28 million days of sickness absence. When work-related injury and illness are combined, 35 million working days were lost (averaging 1.5 days per worker) over the past year. These findings clearly have significant implications for the long-term health and well-being of the working population as well as for industry.

Fatal illnesses, resulting from past exposure to toxins at work, are still affecting significant numbers of people. These conditions include cancers, such as mesothelioma and asbestos-related lung cancer. It is estimated that they account for four per cent of cancer deaths. Smaller numbers of people have died from asbestosis and other types of pneumoconiosis, mostly associated with inhaling coal dust and silica. Past exposure to fumes, chemicals and dusts at work are also likely to be responsible for up to 15 per cent of chronic obstructive pulmonary disease, including bronchitis and emphysema. This is estimated to cause around a further 4,000 deaths each year (Health and Safety Executive, 2006).

Common work-related illnesses

Over the years, the nature of work-related conditions has changed. In recent years, the most common ailments experienced by workers in the UK have been musculoskeletal disorders, particularly back and upper limb disorders, stress and other types of mental health problems. These now account for 75 per cent of self-reported non-fatal work-related illnesses. Other commonly reported forms of ill-health related to work include respiratory diseases, such as asthma, and skin diseases, such as dermatitis. Deafness and infections also account for a percentage of reported cases.

As well as informing us about the conditions which are most commonly associated with work, statistics can also help us identify particular groups of workers, or certain occupations, which put people at greater risk of developing those conditions.

For example, it is known that nurses, care assistants and home carers, construction workers and drivers self report higher than average numbers of musculo-skeletal disorders. The occupational groups who most frequently consult specialist doctors because of musculo-skeletal problems included typists, people who assemble vehicles and other metal products, and road construction workers. Not surprisingly, the actual job tasks which are most likely to be linked with work-related musculo-skeletal conditions are working with tools, and heavy lifting, carrying, or pushing and pulling activities (Health and Safety Executive, 2006a).

Mental health problems such as stress, depression and anxiety can be found across a wide range of occupational groups. Teaching professionals, health and social welfare associate professionals, such as nurses and social workers, and corporate managers, have reported higher than average rates. Army personnel, medical practitioners, police and prison officers, have been identified by consultant psychiatrists as experiencing the highest rates of work-related mental ill-health. Work pressures and inter-personal difficulties were singled out as common precipitating factors in these conditions. Workers who have stressful jobs are more than twice as likely to die from heart disease than those who do not (Kivimakäki et al., 2002).

Jobs which hold the greatest risk for developing respiratory conditions are those where workers are exposed to particular substances. So, vehicle spray painters and bakers, for example, are amongst the groups of workers who are most at risk of developing occupational asthma. While hairdressers, barbers, beauticians and those who work with chemicals or glass and ceramic production, have the highest rates of contact dermatitis. Care assistants and home carers have very high levels of work-related infections.

Industries which involve the use of noisy equipment, such as mining, manufacturing and construction, have the highest rates of noise-induced deafness. Workers who use hand-held power tools extensively, for example miners and builders, may also be at greater risk of developing conditions like carpal tunnel syndrome and hand–arm vibration syndrome. Both of these conditions affect the circulation, sensation, co-ordination and strength in a worker's hands and can have an impact on a person's functional abilities. There may be associated pain, and sustained exposure may lead to permanent damage (Health and Safety Executive, 2005).

Understanding the risks of work to health

The occupational therapist involved in helping workers return to work needs an understanding of the potential risks and hazards which may face the worker in the workplace. Obviously, these dangers will vary according to the type of job which a person performs. For instance, a construction worker is at greater risk of falling from a height than a data-entry clerk. While rehabilitation may not be indicated for some work-related conditions mentioned, such as contact dermatitis, any effective programme designed to promote workplace wellness and well-being will need to acknowledge these risks. This point highlights the benefits of working within the context of a multi-disciplinary team, and we will return to this issue in later chapters.

As you will no doubt have realised from the discussions so far, not everyone is fortunate enough to experience a positive relationship between employment and health and work can have a negative impact on the health and well-being of a particular individual, or group of individuals. It is, however, important to keep in mind that work **can** provide health benefits, given the right environment. In this next section, we will learn about some of the conditions which may help to create a positive, health-giving work environment.

Improving working conditions and the quality of work

We should bear in mind that just because a person is in paid work doesn't necessarily mean that they gain satisfaction or a sense of value from holding that position. The overall conditions of work shape and define people's experiences of work. Each country has its own minimum standards for working conditions, however, a sizeable majority of workers are not included within these protection measures. The United Nations agency, the International Labour Organisation (ILO), advocates for both health and safety at work, as well as for decent quality work. They argue, not unreasonably, that all workers should be entitled to opportunities for productive work that pays a fair income.

Furthermore, workers should have better prospects for personal development and social integration as well as the freedom to express any concerns. They should be able to organise and take part in those decisions that affect their lives, and finally, there should be equal opportunities and treatment for both men and women. The notion of decent work needs to be a central feature of global, national and local strategies so as to encourage economic and social progress. This in turn will have a positive effect on efforts to reduce poverty, and a means for achieving sustainable development (International Labour Organisation, 2006).

The World Health Organization (WHO) has also contributed to the agenda of improving health at work. It has done so by building upon the principles of the Ottawa Charter – which we came across in an earlier chapter – and extending them to the workplace. WHO argues that the highest attainable standards of health are a fundamental right of each worker. WHO's global strategy of 'Occupational health for all' (World Health Organization, 1994; 2006) advocates for access to occupational health services for all workers regardless of age, sex, nationality, occupation, type of employment, or the size or location of the workplace. We will return to look specifically at occupational health provision in the UK in a later section of this chapter, but first we will touch on some of the measures introduced by the Government to address these international agendas.

Ambitious targets have been set by the Health and Safety Commission to reduce health and safety failures in the workplace. Through the *Revitalising Health and Safety Strategy* (2000) they aim to significantly reduce work-related illness and accidents by the year 2010. These targets include:

- reducing the number of working days lost per 100,000 workers from work-related injury and ill-health by 30 per cent

- reducing the incidence rate of fatal and major injury accidents by 10 per cent
- reducing the incidence rate of cases of work-related ill-health by 20 per cent.

This has been followed up by further strategies directed towards the workplace, including creating effective partnerships (Health and Safety Commission, 2005) as well as practical campaigns to encourage wider participation in the strategy. For example, 'Backs!' was a national campaign aimed at raising the awareness and profile of back pain so as to reduce the incidence of work-related back pain. The construction industry accounts for 15 per cent of all major accidents at work, therefore a national campaign to reduce the incidence of slips, trips and falls in this sector was also launched recently (Health and Safety Commission, 2006c). We will return to this agenda in the final part of this chapter, when we examine initiatives to help people keep in work. But first, we will turn our attention to strategies, service models and initiatives to help people move into work.

MOVING INTO WORK

There are well-established benefits to being in work, for both the individual and for our society as a whole. As discussed previously, there is the promise of financial gain, as well as positive influences on self identity, health and well-being. It is recognised that people who are in employment visit their GP less often, and have generally fewer health problems than those who are unemployed (Department for Work and Pensions, 2002). As a group, however, disabled people face some of the greatest difficulties when moving into employment, as they often experience multiple disadvantages. Not only are they less likely to secure work because of their disability, but those who have been disabled as children often also leave school with no, or few, educational qualifications. Despite a number of different approaches and policy initiatives, including quota schemes and the provision of special aids and equipment, a realistic long-term solution is yet to be discovered (Hutchinson, 1982; Burchardt, 2000).

Service providers who support people into work

Services which aim to support people to move into work are mostly provided by the state employment services and the voluntary sector. Less frequently, these services may be available within independent, NHS or local authority organisations, in certain parts of the country. This section briefly introduces the role of public sector employment services, such as Jobcentre Plus. We will also discuss the part played by the voluntary sector, since they are also an expanding provider of employment and vocational services for people with disabilities.

Jobcentre Plus

Jobcentre Plus comes under the remit of the Department for Work and Pensions. There has been a roll-out programme of new Jobcentre Plus offices across the country over the past few years. This process began in 2002, following the amalgamation of Jobcentres and the Benefits Agency, which used to distribute benefits through social security offices. The primary role of these services is to assist people who are unemployed to seek and gain paid employment within the open labour market. They are mainly targeted towards people who are having difficulty securing a job through their own endeavours. The employment services also play a lesser role in helping people with disabilities to remain in their existing jobs, and we will be touching on these schemes in the later section, 'Keeping in work'. As well as assisting more people into paid work, the Jobcentre Plus role is also to help employers to fill their vacancies. We will return, in some detail, to the range of services which are available through the Jobcentre Plus later in this section.

The Voluntary Sector

We will start this section by examining what the voluntary sector is. It is also called the not-for-profit sector, the voluntary and community sector, the third sector and the charity sector. The definition of a charity is narrower than, for example, a sports and recreation club, and charities are required to be registered. There are nearly 200,000 registered charities in the UK with a combined annual income of £ 40 billion. They employ 600,000 staff and have between them a further 13.2 million unpaid volunteers and over 900,000 trustees (Charity Commission, 2005). Charities receive their funding from five main sources. These include:

1. donations and gifts from individuals
2. grants from charitable trusts and companies
3. fees for delivering services, such as government contracts
4. income from their investments
5. profits from charity shops and other retail sources.

Government policy to diversify service provision has meant the transfer of resources from the statutory to the voluntary sector. As a result, this sector has seen enormous recent growth. New European funding streams have also added to the opportunities available. In 1991 there were 98,000 charities increasing to 169,000 in 2004. Over half of this number were small charities which had an annual income of less than £ 10,000, but there are nearly 3,000 large charities with earnings in excess of £ 1 million. Fourteen organisations, which have become well-known household names, each have a turnover of over £ 100 million. Much of this growth in the charitable sector has been as a result of their increasing role in delivering public services. This has meant that a larger percentage of their income now comes from earned income, particularly for services which they provide to the state, rather than from traditional voluntary income, such as grants and donations from the public (Wilding et al., 2006).

The voluntary sector has also taken on an increasing role in the field of vocational and employment services, particularly through service contracts with Jobcentre Plus and local authorities. A project which was designed to quantify employment-focussed services, surveyed 2,500 work projects around the country. They found that:

- less than ten per cent provided services for both disabled and non-disabled people
- over eighty per cent were targeted at people with a specific disability, most commonly mental health problems and learning disabilities
- services provided included vocational training, work placement, supported employment and sheltered employment, with most focus being on the pre-employment stage
- there were wide variations in geographical distribution of services, with some areas being over-represented by certain types of services for particular groups of clients
- there were very few job retention services.

(Arksey *et al.*, 2002)

The findings from this survey suggest that there remains a need to work towards more integrated, mainstream employment services which are focused on common barriers to employment, rather than creating artificial boundaries based on medical diagnosis.

Service models to assist people to move into work

The purpose of this next section is to briefly outline some of the services which are available to people who have work- or employment-related difficulties. The literature identifies a number of service models for people who are not, at this point in their recovery, in a position to pursue competitive, paid employment. We will consider a broad range of these service alternatives, which may be available to people who have a disability or health condition, and are without work. Some are intended specifically for particular client groups, for example, clubhouses set up for people with mental health problems. Others have been designed for people whose productivity level is below that which would be required in the open labour market.

For some people, their aspiration will be a job in the open labour market. Others may prefer to be involved in a social enterprise or employee mutual (EM) scheme. Some may choose a place in sheltered employment. Then, there are other options such as supported employment, individual placement and support (IPS), social firms, volunteering and clubhouses. The features of these different service models, and their similarities and differences, are highlighted in this next section.

In Figure 5.3 these different service models have been arranged to demonstrate their relative proximity to paid employment in the open labour market, although, of course, there will be inevitable blurring and overlaps between these different models.

Occupational therapists may be found in many of these different types of service models, or they may be working collaboratively with staff in them. We will continue by exploring aspects of each in turn.

Vocational day services

These traditional services were mainly set up as part of social care provision in the community, for people who left long-term institutional care. They offer segregated

- Vocational day services
- Sheltered workshops and industrial therapy units
- Volunteer programmes
- Supported training and education
- Clubhouses
- Sheltered employment
- Local exchange trading systems
- Self-employment/user-run enterprises
- Social firms/co-operatives
- Supported employment/IPS model
- Employment services (Jobcentre Plus)

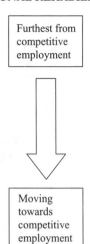

Furthest from competitive employment

Moving towards competitive employment

Figure 5.3. Proximity of service models to paid employment

provision, and any work which is undertaken would come under the definition of substitute work (see Chapter 3). No income is generated from the work activity, and no payment is attached to it. The ethos of these services is not compatible with the current social inclusion agenda, therefore, many of the services based on this model are currently undergoing review and modernisation.

Sheltered workshops and industrial therapy units

The 1944 Disabled Persons Act, which we read about in Chapter 2, required local authorities and voluntary organisations to set up and operate sheltered workshops for disabled people. These services were based on humanitarian objectives underpinned by a belief that some disabled people needed an artificially-created work environment to accommodate their lower levels of productivity (Hyde, 1996).

Industrial therapy units were a core part of the fabric of the old, long-stay asylums. Patients attended this form of work as part of an overall therapy programme including recreational and social activities. A survey of psychiatric hospitals in 1962 found that these units were most commonly managed by a head occupational therapist. They took on contract work from local businesses involved in box making, cosmetic packaging and assembling plastic flowers, for example. Sometimes they also undertook work for the hospital, such as making store bags and waste paper bins. For this work, the patients received small sums of pocket money, although the unit charged normal union rates of pay for the work (Hill, 1967). So, in some cases, they produced a valuable source of income for the old asylums.

The industrial therapy units were a product of their era, and their demise took place alongside that of the asylums to which they were attached. Technological advances have meant that the type of low-skilled repetitive work which they offered is also mostly a thing of the past. Few, if any, industrial therapy units now remain in the UK.

Volunteer programmes

Volunteering, as mentioned in an earlier chapter, can be a meaningful and valued occupation. Where there is a good fit between the worker and the volunteer work, within a supportive working environment, the perceived benefits may be similar to those which an individual experiences when they are in open labour market employment (Rebeiro and Allen, 1998). Occupational therapists, particularly those who work in mental health, continue to develop partnerships with community organisations to help create volunteering opportunities to assist clients to attain a worker role.

Occupational therapists may find further information about voluntary groups within their local area either through the council website or by visiting http://www.guidestar .org.uk (accessed 02/04/07). To find out about national charities concerned with people who have a particular form of disability, visit: http://www.directgov.gov.uk/en/ Dl1/Directories/UsefulContactsByCategory/DisabledPeopleContacts/index.htm (accessed 02/04/07).

Supported training and education

For people who are unemployed and perhaps with few skills or other disadvantages, supported training or education may provide useful alternatives. In contrast to volunteering, participation in these types of activities should generally be viewed as a stepping stone to other work options; that is, a means to an end, rather than the end.

A range of supported local training opportunities can be accessed through the Jobcentre Plus services. The service also funds residential training at 11 centres around the UK for some adults with disabilities and health conditions. Some centres cater specifically to the needs of certain client groups, while others do not discriminate on the basis of the nature of the disability. These centres are:

1. St Loyes Foundation, Devon
2. The Enham Trust, Hampshire
3. Dorton College of Further Education, Royal London Society for the Blind, Kent
4. Queen Elizabeth's Foundation Training College, Surrey
5. Royal National Institute of the Blind, Surrey
6. Queen Alexandra College, West Midlands
7. Royal National College for the Blind, Hereford
8. Royal National Institute of the Blind College, Leicestershire
9. Portland College, Nottingham
10. Doncaster College for the Deaf, South Yorkshire
11. Finchale Training College.

Each college provides a range of training opportunities and qualifications, often using work-based learning, in subjects such as electrical engineering, construction, horticulture, business administration and accounting, and information and communication technology. The contact details and websites for each of these centres can be obtained from http://www.directgov.gov.uk (accessed 07/02/07). It is important to bear in mind that residential training is not the right option for everyone. Since it is also very costly, there may be a limited number of funded places available each year. Further information may be obtained from the disability employment advisor at your local Jobcentre Plus.

Within education settings, particularly in further education, the social inclusion agenda is resulting in a shift away from segregated course provision, towards participation in mainstream courses. Legislation requires colleges and universities to improve the accessibility of their buildings and to make reasonable adjustments, so as not to discriminate against people on the grounds of their disability. This may therefore allow more individuals to engage in training or education, with the necessary supports, in a similar way to the practice of supported employment, described later in this section. Occupational therapists may work collaboratively with local colleges to help develop a pathway into education for clients who have chosen this route. Alternatively, they may work in partnership with training organisations in order to achieve accreditation, such as National Vocational Qualification recognition, of specific training programmes. Garner (1995) describes how this was achieved in a regional secure unit for offenders with mental health problems.

Clubhouses

The first clubhouse, Fountain House, emerged from a self-help organisation of a small group of people who had been discharged from a psychiatric hospital in New York. With the help of volunteers it was established in 1948 as a therapeutic environment. Its aim was to help people with serious mental illnesses re-establish their lives within the community. The clubhouse aimed to provide members with satisfying work and social lives, despite their mental illness (Angers, 1995). There was a requirement that staff and clubhouse members ran all aspects of the clubhouse operations together, in partnership. The Fountain House programme became a template for the clubhouse model of rehabilitation. A national training programme on the model was set up in 1977 and this has resulted in the development of more than 400 similar programmes in 32 countries around the world. For further information see http://www.fountainhouse.org (accessed 25/10/06). All clubhouses throughout the world aim to help members lead their lives productively and in a way which is meaningful at both a social and vocational level (McKay et al., 2006).

The UK was slow to adopt this model and the first UK clubhouse, Hillside House, was only established in 1991. There was initially a rapid spread of the clubhouse approach, but few new clubhouses have been established in recent years. The clubhouse acts as a half-way house, filling the gap of social isolation and exclusion which is experienced by many people with serious mental illness. Lifelong membership to clubhouses allows individuals to work towards their recovery at their own pace. It also fosters a sense of ownership by encouraging active participation in the affairs and running of the club. A criticism of this permissive approach may be that it has the potential to foster dependency which is counter-productive to the mission of the organisation (Di Masso *et al.*, 2001).

There are three underpinning beliefs to the clubhouse model:

1. each person, regardless of the severity of their mental illness, has potential competencies
2. housing should be pleasant, affordable and provide opportunities for friendship, companionship and mutual support
3. there is considerable restorative value of meaningful work, especially where it offers the opportunity to achieve gainful employment.

(Beard *et al.*, 1982 cited in Di Masso *et al.*, 2001, p.24)

Literature is limited regarding the effectiveness of the clubhouse model in treating mental illness in comparison to more traditional programmes. However, research does suggest that the clubhouse model is effective in both supporting people back to work (Schonebaum *et al.*, 2006) and reducing hospital re-admissions (Di Masso *et al.*, 2001).

There are three core elements to the programme provided within the clubhouse model:

1. the work-ordered day
2. the social programme
3. the employment programme.

The work-ordered day Each clubhouse revolves around meaningful work, through what is known as the 'work-ordered day'. The work-ordered day is formed by having various work units within the clubhouse. The units are generated by the development and operation of the clubhouse community and therefore differ from clubhouse to clubhouse. For example, there may be a kitchen unit where members prepare the lunchtime meal for the members. There may be a clerical unit which answers telephones and produces a monthly newsletter. A low-cost clothing shop unit may offer reasonably priced goods for sale to other members. An Outreach unit may be responsible for contacting and supporting members who have not attended for a while. Membership and education units may also be available.

Each unit is divided up into specific tasks and supervised by a member of staff. As each new member joins the clubhouse they choose a unit to work in, and the tasks they will perform within that unit, according to their interests and abilities. Through participation in the necessary work of the clubhouse, an important goal is to achieve better work habits and improved social skills. Participation is voluntary and each member's right to choose to join in is respected. However, inactivity is discouraged and a milieu which encourages people to take part is fostered (Di Masso *et al.*, 2001).

Staff numbers are deliberately kept low within clubhouses and there are no separate staff areas such as those found within traditional, more hierarchical services. The staff are also club members, and as such are expected to work alongside others to ensure that each unit completes its designated task.

The social programme A social programme takes place outside of office hours and members are encouraged to participate to enhance their social communication skills, confidence and self-esteem. A wide range of other member services, such as housing support and benefit advice, are also often provided.

The employment programme This is one of the most successful aspects of the clubhouse approach. The emphasis on the inclusive and healing nature of work is a key feature of the clubhouse model. Clubhouses offer transitions through three levels of employment (McKay *et al.*, 2006). Namely:

1. transitional employment (TE)
2. supported employment (SE)
3. independent employment (IE).

The clubhouse may support members to return to paid work in the community, rather than through segregated clubhouse enterprises or sheltered workshops. Each clubhouse is expected to offer TE and IE programmes away from the clubhouse itself. The strength of the TE rehabilitation programme is that it provides a more normal work experience, and is therefore consistent with the clubhouse objective of getting people back to work in the community. The TE programme gives members who express a desire to work, opportunities from a diverse range of job placements in business, industry and the public sector. The clubhouse programme should, ideally, be able to offer a variety of placements to reflect the current interests and skills of members. TE programmes are intended to help members overcome vocational problems in real work situations. An important feature of the TE programme is that the individual does not have to go through a competitive interviewing process to secure the placement. To help members at work, support is provided through the relationships and understanding previously established with other members and staff while working in the work units.

Transitional employment placements are part-time and time-limited, and seldom last beyond nine months. Members work at the employer's workplace and are paid directly by the employer. They are paid preferably at the prevailing rate for the job, but at least the minimum wage is required. These important factors add to a sense of having a normal job within the community. TE placements are managed by clubhouse staff and members. The clubhouse has the responsibility for selecting and training members. It also guarantees to cover placements should a member be absent for any reason. In this way the employer is assured that the job will get done.

Members who want to upgrade to better jobs are supported to do so. If they move into full-time work they continue to be supported and entitled to participate in the social programme outside of work hours or to access any of the other services the clubhouse provides. We will return to supported, independent and competitive employment later in the chapter.

The International Center for Clubhouse Development is an organisation which was set up in 1994 to serve and represent the clubhouse community. Part of its role is to support and co-ordinate the development and training of clubhouse staff and members. It also maintains international standards for clubhouse programmes and has an international certification process. More information about this organisation and a list of accredited clubhouses can be found at http://www.iccd.org (accessed 02/02/07).

Sheltered employment

Sheltered employment differs from sheltered work, in that it enables some disabled people to earn a living under open labour market conditions, while at the same time affording them some concessions for below-average productivity (Ekdawi and Conning, 1994). It may also be a useful option for those who may be preparing to move on to supported employment or open employment later in their recovery (Oxley, 1995). Workers wages are subsidised and this form of work generally takes place in sheltered factories. Traditionally, this model has catered more to the employment needs of those with moderate physical or developmental disabilities and is perhaps less well-suited to those people who have fluctuating health conditions, or perhaps poor basic work habits, such as punctuality. The Remploy organisation is a good example of a sheltered employment model.

Remploy was set up in 1946 as part of the provision under the 1944 Disabled Persons (Employment) Act. Its first factory in Bridgend, South Wales, produced furniture and violins made by disabled ex-miners. Since that time, it has expanded to employ more than 5,700 people in 83 factories located around England, Scotland and Wales. This makes Remploy the largest employer of disabled people in the UK. Remploy businesses are mainly targeted at the manufacturing and service sector. In manufacturing, the organisation produces goods such as school furniture, protective clothing for civilian and military use, and electronic components for a variety of customers. In the service sector, Remploy undertakes a diverse range of activities from recycling computers and white goods, to providing packaging, printing and data management (Blackhurst, 2005).

In addition to its role in providing sheltered employment opportunities for people with disabilities, Remploy has also taken on a job broker role. Through this initiative, Remploy Interwork, which is based on a supported employment model, supports about 3,500 people in mainstream employment. We will learn more about the supported employment model later in this section. This shift to expand the services offered is important, since it helps to create more opportunities for social integration for those who may benefit from this opportunity. Further information about Remploy can be found at: http://www.remploy.co.uk (accessed 23/02/07).

Local exchange trading systems or schemes (LETS)

LETS originated in Canada and can now be found in the UK, Ireland, the USA, Canada, Australia and New Zealand, making this probably the most widely-used model for community currency systems in the world. The system allows people within a local community LETS network to exchange a variety of goods and services with each other, without any financial transaction taking place. Participating members earn credits by providing goods and services and then are able to spend their credits on different goods and services offered by other people in the scheme. The types of things which may be exchanged include: childcare, transport, groceries, home maintenance or hiring tools and equipment.

LETS schemes are open to any individual, and they may also be used by local clubs, voluntary groups, charities, community groups and small businesses. Although the popularity of the scheme may have decreased a little in recent years, an average scheme currently has around 100 members, and there are about 300 LETS across the UK. Newer models of the traditional LETS system include timebanks, commercial barter, fairtrade campaigns, and other forms of community networks. The Government's Green Paper *Independence Well-being and Choice: Our vision for the future of social care for adults in England* (Department of Health, 2005b) suggests that timebanks provide ways to reduce inequalities in health and encourage social inclusion. Giving time can be empowering to individuals and create feelings of self-worth.

These initiatives also create opportunities for those who have traditionally been in receipt of care or services and enable them to offer something back to the community, thereby increasing their sense of inclusion. Being enabled to participate in this way can have positive benefits. Timebanks are also positive for communities because they provide a means of trading services which they may not be able to do within a conventional economy. They enable more support to be offered to those people who are the most socially disadvantaged and who often experience poor health. Some LETS may have also developed into more formal organisations, such as social firms, which you will read about later in this section. Further information about LETS in the UK can be found at: http://www.letslinkuk.net (accessed 04/02/07).

Self-employment and user-run services

The literature provides examples of user-run enterprises, such as home cleaning services (Bertram and Linnett, 1995), particularly for those clients with mental health problems. Self-employment may be an alternative for the disabled person who has learned, and understands, the principles of successful business. For some people who have gained the skills and expertise to do so, this can be a viable option to achieving financial independence. Self-employment can, however, be a stressful, socially-isolating form of work, which therefore makes it unsuitable for those who may find these work characteristics hard to cope with.

For those clients who may be interested in setting up their own business, information, advice and training can be obtained through the Learning and Skills Councils in England and Wales, and Local Enterprise Companies in Scotland. In England, Business Link also offers support to small businesses. More details can be found at: http://www.businesslink.gov.uk (accessed 15/01/07). Business Eye (Wales) and Business Gateway (Scotland) offer similar services.

Social enterprises, social firms and co-operatives

A social enterprise is a business that has a social objective. While social enterprises trade goods and/or services and follow approved business processes, such as having a business plan in place, they differ to mainstream businesses by investing any trading profit back into the business or the community, rather than passing it on to the owners or shareholders. In this way, social enterprises combine business objectives with the provision of positive benefits to the community. Companies set up as social enterprises are founded on a variety of legal models, from limited companies to provident societies and registered charities. They also include development trusts, intermediate labour markets, community businesses and credit unions. The trade or services they provide are also diverse. For example, they may offer social or environmental goods and services, such as recycling or childcare. In order to be viewed as a social enterprise, the business needs to earn at least 50 per cent of its turnover through sales of goods and/or services, and it must not be motivated by individual profit.

Social enterprises often aim to provide employment, support and training opportunities to groups who are excluded from social and economic participation within society. The benefits of social enterprises are that they:

• help increase productivity and competitiveness
• contribute to social inclusion
• help in the regeneration of local neighbourhoods
• bring new ways of delivering and reforming public services
• help create an inclusive society.

The concept of social enterprise organisations has spread throughout the world. Most are established to address a specific local or community need. In North America, for example, the sector began some 40 years ago. It was directed towards addressing some of the issues raised by inner-city riots and cuts in public services. Social enterprises in the USA are often highly successful with large turnovers, in some cases up to $55 million per year. US-based social enterprises have several advantages over those in the UK, as they benefit from a range of tax exemptions and receive widespread support from mainstream businesses. This support may be in the form of goods to assist with the start up of an enterprise or placing orders with them.

Social enterprises may start out as voluntary sector organisations, where they are dependent on grants and volunteers for their continued existence. Becoming a social enterprise puts them in a position to be able to increase their traded income. There are at least 55,000 social enterprises in the UK with a turnover of about £ 27 billion. They account for five per cent of businesses which have employees (Department of Trade and Industry, 2006).

A good example of a successful social enterprise is The Eden Project. This £ 86 million centre consists of two enormous greenhouse-type structures which house more than one million plants from around the world. The centre has a mainly educational purpose, which is to inform about environmental issues and the dependent relationship which man has with plants. The Eden Project is located in Cornwall, which is one of the poorest regions of the European Union. It has attracted more than eight million visitors, produced an operating surplus of nearly £2 million and generated around £650 million of additional income to the region. The project is administered by a charitable trust, which ensures that any profits are re-invested into the project to ensure its sustainability. For further information about The Eden Project, visit: http://www.edenproject.com (accessed 10/03/07).

Another successful example is The Big Issue – a scheme which allows homeless people to earn a living by selling newspapers on street corners. Further information can be found at: http://www.bigissue.com (accessed 10/03/07). New types of social enterprise, such as community interest companies, continue to emerge and there is likely to be further expansion of these kinds of organisations in the future. More information about social enterprises can be found on the Social Enterprise Coalition (http://www.socialenterprise.org.uk) and the Social Enterprise London (http://www.sel.org.uk) websites (both accessed 10/03/07).

The British Government recently produced the *Social Enterprise Action Plan* (Office of the Third Sector, 2006) which aims to foster a culture of social enterprise, while ensuring that advice and finance are available to support social entrepreneurs to develop the sector. This commitment extends into the health and social care market as well. The Department of Health set up their own social enterprise unit in 2006. Funding has been made available to enable a number of health and social care programmes and services around the country to re-structure themselves as social enterprises (White, 2006). This trend towards a more mixed economy of provision is likely to continue. Some occupational therapists, particularly those based in community services, may become part of social enterprises in the future.

Social firms and co-operatives are types of social enterprises. The purpose of a social firm is specifically to create employment for people with a disability and/or mental health problems. The social firm model began in Italy in the 1960s. Ten years ago, Italy further expanded the concept of the social firm by introducing new regulations aimed at increasing the number of social co-operatives in the country. This has successfully helped the sector focus beyond delivering benefits solely to members to contributing wider benefits to the local community as well. There are clear guidelines as to what constitutes a social firm and the constitution needs to reflect the stated objective of employing disabled people. Social firms pay market wages within a supportive workplace environment. In 1997 there were just six known social firms in the UK. A recent mapping exercise found that there are now 46 social firms and 70 emerging ones. They have high levels of retention and employ over 1,500 people. Of these, 55 per cent have a disability. Most employees do, however, work less than 16 hours per week. There are a further 1,000 trainees in the sector, the majority of whom are expected to go on to be employed within it. The small business model has been found to successfully offer a sustainable, long-term option for the social firm. Examples of businesses set up as social firms include guesthouses, catering businesses and IT businesses.

Social firms offer a very real alternative to competitive employment for people with a health condition or disability to engage in meaningful paid work. Further information about social firms, and examples of organisations which trade as social firms, can be obtained from the Social Firms UK website: http://www.socialfirms.co.uk (accessed 10/03/07).

A co-operative is a business owned by its members. This means the members own the wealth of the business together, not as individuals. Co-operatives are international and take many forms. There are worker co-operatives and housing co-operatives, for example. Although they may be organised in different ways, they all have common principles, values and ethics which provide guidance as to how they should function. The six values on which co-operatives are based include:

1. self help
2. self-responsibility
3. democracy
4. equality
5. equity
6. solidarity.

These, in turn, reflect the ethical values of honesty, openness, social responsibility and caring for others. Co-operatives are community-focused, autonomous, democratic organisations. They are controlled by their members and any surplus funds generated are re-invested into the organisation. Further information on co-operatives is available at http://www.cooperatives-uk.coop/ (accessed 10/03/07).

Supported employment/the individual placement and support model (IPS)

The supported employment model originated in America over 20 years ago. It is a model which has been used extensively to assist people with learning disabilities and chronic mental health problems into competitive open labour market employment, and then provide intensive on-going support to help them remain there.

There are various spin-offs of the supported employment model, with a host of different titles, including the choose–get–keep model, the place-then-train model, and the direct entry approach, to name but a few (Auerbach, 2001). Out of these various approaches, the IPS model is perhaps the most widely acknowledged and researched in the UK. It has been suggested that supported employment may offer greater promise as a social model of recovery for people with mental health problems than existing clinical models do (Secker *et al.*, 2002).

The core principles of the IPS model are:

• a goal of competitive employment
• a rapid job search, rather than a lengthy pre-vocational programme
• an integrated approach to rehabilitation and mental health treatment
• choices based on the client's preferences, rather than those of the provider
• on-going and thorough assessment of progress, barriers and possible pitfalls
• support for as long as it is needed, either on- or off-site.
(Becker and Drake, 1993 cited in Bond, 1998)

Occupational therapists familiar with the model have commented on the compatibility of its values and philosophy with those of OT (Moll *et al.*, 2003; Auerbach, 2001). The evidence base has demonstrated that this approach can successfully assist a percentage of people with mental illness into open labour market employment. It has also been successfully used with people with learning disabilities, and other forms of disability as well. The British Association for Supported Employment, a membership organisation, provides further information on the processes involved in successfully developing this type of access into employment (http://www.afse.org.uk, accessed 15/04/07).

However, since people are individuals, it is important to recognise that it is not possible (Ekdawi and Conning, 1994), or indeed necessarily desirable (Nagle *et al.*, 2002), for all people with a health problem or disability to follow this particular route. This recognition means that new models continue to emerge. One such concept is that of the employee mutual (EM). It has been suggested that EMs offer disabled people a supportive, integrated environment, with some level of financial security, while at the same time meeting the needs of modern businesses for flexible labour. The EM 'is a new form of labour market body, a blend of recruitment agency, training provider, trade union, mutual aid association and co-operative enterprise' (Christie and Mensah-Coker, 1999, p.37). This innovative service concept is illustrative of the need to create integrated, joined-up services which are flexible enough to meet the work needs of people with health conditions and disabilities.

Employment services

We have looked at service models for people who need work alternatives to competitive employment, and for those individuals who need significant levels of support to allow them to secure and hold down a job. We will now move onto our final category of services for people who want to move into work. These are the services provided through the state employment services.

Jobcentre Plus services

As mentioned earlier in this section, Jobcentre Plus has the dual role of assisting jobseekers into paid employment in the open labour market, as well as helping employers fill their vacancies. A brief outline of a selection of useful schemes which may be available to jobseekers through the Jobcentre Plus is given here, but since these schemes are regularly updated, and some are better established in some areas of the country than others, the interested reader is advised to find out about the current range of services on offer at their local Jobcentre Plus. It is also highly recommended that this section is read in conjunction with the later chapter on the multi-disciplinary team. This will help you familiarise yourself with the roles and responsibilities of the various Jobcentre Plus team members you may come across. Each of the services described below is accessed through one of these team members.

The **Job Introduction Scheme** allows an individual the opportunity to try out a job to see if it is suitable for them. It also allows the employer to decide if the person is right for the job. The scheme offers the participating employer help towards the person's wages and any other employment costs for the first couple of weeks, to allow both parties time to determine the person's suitability for the job. The scheme can apply to any full-time or part-time job lasting at least 26 weeks. The rationale behind this scheme is that it provides reassurance for both the person and the employer, thereby providing a route into permanent employment for those who may otherwise find this difficult.

The **WorkPath** programmes are intended to help remove any barriers which may face a disabled person and prevent them from gaining a job. Two examples of Work-Path programmes are WORKSTEP and Access to Work.

WORKSTEP provides individualised support for disabled people with more complex needs, who may experience the greatest barriers in getting and keeping a job. Opportunities available through WORKSTEP include supported jobs with mainstream employers, or work in supported factories and businesses. This programme also aims to help people develop and improve their job skills, thereby providing the opportunity to move into employment in the future. Long-term support may be provided in some cases. The scheme is also intended to encourage employers to support the development of their disabled employees.

Access to Work assistance is available for people with a long-term disability just about to start a new job and for those who are already in work but who are facing difficulties performing their job tasks because of a disability. This scheme can provide advice and practical support to help overcome any obstacles which face the disabled person at work. For example, a grant for specialist equipment, such as ergonomic seating, may be provided under a joint funding arrangement with the employer. Fares to work may be paid for people who are not able to use public transport. Access to Work can provide funds to assist employers make modifications to improve the physical access to their premises under the terms of the Disability Discrimination Act. Unfortunately, the level of awareness and knowledge of the Access to Work scheme amongst employers remains low (Taylor, 2003), and the value of the service is sometimes undermined by lengthy delays in providing the necessary support packages (Roulstone *et al.*, 2003).

More information about Jobcentre Plus services can be found on their website: http://www.jobcentreplus.gov.uk/JCP/index.html (accessed 26/02/07).

Connexions

The Connexions services, also part of the Department of Work and Pensions provision, are for young people between the ages of 13 and 19, or 25 for people with a disability. The service offers careers and learning support and advice on jobs, training, housing, money, relationships and health, and may refer onto other services as appropriate. Personal advisers may also provide information about volunteering opportunities, community projects and other local leisure activities which are available for young people. Occupational therapists working with young people may find it helpful to spend some time developing a collaborative partnership with their local Connexions service. Connexions offers a range of on-line services. More information can be found at http://www.connexions-direct.com (accessed 22/04/07).

GOVERNMENT INITIATIVES TO HELP DISABLED JOBSEEKERS

Having discovered a little about the sorts of packages that are commonly available through the employment services, we will move on to look at some of the key strategies which have been put in place by the present Government to support and assist disabled jobseekers into employment. Some of these initiatives, such as Pathways to Work, were initially introduced as pilot schemes to test out their effectiveness, before rolling them out on a wider scale. We will discuss the Pathways to Work programme a little later in this section. However, we will begin by examining an initiative which was introduced in 1998, called New Deal.

New Deal For Disabled People

A number of the services provided by the Jobcentre Plus are delivered through a scheme called the New Deal programme. This has been aimed at specific sectors of the population, known to have high levels of unemployment. They therefore included those groups commonly disadvantaged in gaining employment, such as young people, single mothers, ex-prisoners and older workers. Some schemes were voluntary, others mandatory.

One of the New Deal programmes was targeted at people in receipt of benefits because of their disabilities or long-term health problems. The New Deal for Disabled People (NDDP) is a voluntary scheme that has been in place since 2001, which provides individualised support to each customer from a network of employment specialists (sometimes also called job brokers). Job brokers are often small, local organisations who are under contract with the Department of Work and Pensions to offer a range of job-seeking and employability services. These services are accessed through a personal adviser, or other job centre staff. Broadly, the types of services which are provided may include advice on how to get a job, help to match existing skills and abilities to those employers are seeking, and support for the individual when they first start a job. They can also assist with benefits calculations to ensure the person will not be worse off when they enter paid work. More specifically, the sorts of activities that job brokers undertake include help with filling in application forms and writing CVs, interview preparation and self-presentation skills.

Job brokers are often in a good position to provide advice on local job vacancies. However, as with any other type of organisation, the range, standard and quality of the services provided varies across the country. Since many job brokers are paid by results, the service quality and accessibility to people with particular disabilities or health problems may also be influenced by the nature of the targets set and the outcomes that they are expected to achieve.

In the early years of implementation, the New Deal programme achieved significant successes, and the numbers of unemployed people across many of the target groups declined. However, this scheme did not sufficiently address the diverse needs of people with disabilities. This was evident from the rising levels of IB claimants: those people who were considered to be too ill or disabled to work any longer, as well as the small numbers of claimants from this group who engaged with the NDDP programme (Loumidis *et al.*, 2001). In the light of these shortcomings, the Government has since introduced additional measures, and trialed different types of service provision, which we will explore next.

Pathways to Work pilots

The introduction of the Pathways to Work pilots was outlined in the Green Paper *Pathways to Work: Helping people into employment* (Department for Work and Pensions, 2002). The rationale behind these pilots was that, despite improvements to the overall health of the population, the number of people receiving incapacity benefit (IB) – the main benefit for those who can no longer work due to ill-health – had trebled since 1979.

IBs are accessed through general practitioner (GP) sickness certification procedures, although few GPs would wish to be viewed as the gatekeepers to social security entitlements. Jobcentre Plus is responsible for administering this benefit to those who are entitled to receive it. To stem the in-flow of claimants they have put in place additional measures to actively encourage people back into the workforce, in preference to becoming permanently reliant on welfare payments. For example, there are now mandatory work-focused interviews for the majority of new IB claimants.

Although these measures have helped to slow the tide, there are still over two and a half million people who receive IBs. Each year, there are more than half a million new claimants, of whom 90 per cent expect to return to work at some point in the future. In reality, however, after a year spent on this benefit, the likelihood is that the person will remain on it until they retire. It is thought that nearly half of those on IB would like to get back into work again. An examination of the types of health complaints experienced by IB claimants has shown that the most common ones are mild to moderate mental health conditions (42 per cent), musculoskeletal conditions (21 per cent) and cardio-respiratory conditions (11 per cent) (Waddell and Aylward, 2005).

The Pathways to Work scheme is underpinned by the notion that, with the right help and support, significant numbers of people may be prevented from coming onto IB in the first place, or alternatively, they may be helped off it and back into work. Seven Pathways pilot sites were introduced across the UK in October 2003. The scheme was targeted specifically at IB claimants, and introduced a dual approach to helping individuals manage their health problems alongside providing them with employment support (Waddell and Aylward, 2005). The pilots aimed to increase the number of IB recipients who moved towards work, and ultimately entered paid employment.

This reform included three main elements:

1. a requirement to attend a series of work-focused interviews with an IB personal adviser
2. access to a range of programmes designed to boost an individual's prospects of being able to work
3. financial incentives (return to work credits) for individuals who enter paid employment.

(Adam *et al.*, 2006)

Each pilot site chose and adopted a different delivery model which included in-house, full or partly contracted out, condition-specific or generic provision. Each service extended across one or more primary care trust boundaries.

Despite these service model differences, each Pathways to Work programme is directed towards providing greater support in preparation for work for individuals claiming IBs. This includes easier access to existing programmes, such as NDDP, as well as other forms of employment support available through Jobcentre Plus. It also offers people the opportunity to take part in condition management programmes. Since these will be of particular interest to occupational therapists, we will now consider this element of the Pathways to Work programme in more depth.

Condition management programmes

Condition management programmes are the key health support component of the Pathways to Work programme and complement the employment support component supplied by the Jobcentre Plus. The existing condition management programmes are run by health professionals, including occupational therapists, who are seconded from the NHS in a partnership arrangement with the Jobcentre Plus. They provide short-term interventions which help the individual understand, take control of, and manage their health condition themselves. They have a work-focus and emphasise the positive benefits to be gained through participation in work activity (Waddell and Aylward, 2005).

A personal adviser may refer a consenting client, or customer, as they are usually known, through to a trained health professional in a local condition management programme. These health professionals are given the title of condition management practitioners and most come from an OT, nursing or physiotherapy background. They make use of many of their existing skills gained through their training and prior experience in healthcare settings. At present no additional training or qualification is required to take on this role, but this may change in the future.

Condition management programmes aim to help individuals manage their health conditions or disabilities, so as to facilitate a successful return to the labour force. Each programme is based on a self-help model underpinned by a cognitive behavioural approach. This approach supports and enables the person to develop their own strategies for taking greater control and responsibility of the self-management of their health condition (Newman *et al.*, 2004). In doing so, they are assisted to re-engage with normal, everyday occupations which they have often given up as a consequence of their health condition or disability. The programmes are targeted at people who experience the most common forms of health complaints, which includes people who experience mild to moderate mental health, musculoskeletal or circulatory problems.

Participation in the programme, which is based on a bio-psychosocial model of health and illness, is voluntary. More information about this model can be found in the earlier chapter on conceptual frameworks. The programme emphasises personal responsibility for effecting change, so as to improve personal coping mechanisms and abilities. We will return to look at the practical applications of this particular approach in a later chapter.

Condition management interventions address identified health-related barriers to work, such as anxiety, lack of confidence and low self esteem, or perhaps fatigue relating to a physical condition. Participants may also learn how to manage depression, stress and increase their assertiveness skills. Programmes have deliberately been positioned away from traditional healthcare settings so as to de-medicalise their focus (Waddell and Aylward, 2005). The individualised programmes are therefore delivered through individual or group sessions at the person's home, in community venues or in job centres. It is important for condition management practitioners to network with other agencies, for example job brokers and leisure service providers.

The Pathways to Work pilots evaluated successfully. Early results suggested that the numbers leaving IB increased by about eight per cent in the pilot areas. In light of this success, pilot status ended in spring 2006 and a phased roll-out of Pathways to Work and the condition management programmes is underway across the country. Fourteen more programmes are currently in planning and early implementation stages. However, it is important to recognise that the new programmes will be delivered within a landscape that is very different from the existing ones.

In contrast to the pilot programmes, which are being provided by professionally trained and experienced NHS staff, any new programmes will be contracted out to private and voluntary sector provision. This raises a number of unknowns, but is likely to alter their structure and focus at least to some degree, as they will need to have a greater focus on their cost-effectiveness and profitability. The skill set of the workforce within these new services is another unspecified factor. Given that VR is not yet regulated in any way, it is currently possible for anyone to call themselves a VR specialist.

It is also likely that the new posts will reflect the uncertainty of time-limited funding streams, thus making short-term staff contracts more likely. Higher expectations, including targets for numbers of participants in the programme, and for numbers successfully returned to work, are already being introduced into the current phase of the roll-out. This is not a problem in itself, since realistic targets can help give a service direction and purpose. However, planned legislative reform is likely to introduce some form of conditionality to receiving benefits payments (Department for Work and Pensions, 2006a). In other words, the majority of new IB claimants will be required to take part in some work-related activity, in order to avoid financial penalties and reduced income. This may, potentially, result in condition management programme participation being perceived as far less voluntary than at present.

The question also remains whether there are, or will be, sufficient numbers of suitable jobs for an increased number of work-ready people. Decent work is needed to improve people's well-being (International Labour Organisation, 2005). However, many IB claimants may have already suffered the damaging consequences of the poor-quality work still found in many parts of today's labour market. All of these factors suggest that the new condition management programmes may well present as very different entities from those seen in the first pilots.

KEEPING IN WORK

There are many reasons why people lose their worker role and we have already touched on a number of these reasons in earlier sections. We have also examined the extent of ill-health and injury within the working-age population. This section will be primarily concerned with people who are currently in open labour market employment. For many people who have a job, developing a chronic health complaint or acquiring a disability signals the end of their working life. In an earlier chapter on conceptual frameworks, we looked at how the cycle of vulnerability helps to explain the increasing risks of people losing their job when they have a health condition or disability. For the individual struggling to cope with health problems, the prospect of losing their job may be a frightening one.

In this final section of this chapter we will be exploring service models which may be available to help people remain in work. You will remember that the current drive is towards keeping people in work for longer, and so there is much interest in strategies and interventions which may prevent people from leaving the workforce early. A number of the initiatives to keep a person in work may come from within the person's actual workplace. Therefore, this section also explains terms commonly used in the employment sector, by human resources or personnel departments, which may be unfamiliar to health practitioners. This includes terms such as absence management, job retention and phased, or graduated, return to work programmes. It is important that occupational therapists in this field are able to use the language of business, both for effective marketing of OT and for communication around the needs of an individual client.

A greater focus on preventative occupational health services, which include the skills of suitably experienced rehabilitation professionals, may also help reduce the numbers of people who slide into unemployment and, consequently, become welfare dependent. We will therefore look briefly at occupational health services in this section. The pivotal role played by the GP and sickness certification will also be discussed, as this may often be a key issue in facilitating a safe and effective return to work.

THE ILL OR INJURED EMPLOYEE

Most of us recognise that illness is a fact of life. Even the healthiest amongst us will, periodically, succumb to an upper respiratory tract infection or an unwelcome dose of diarrhoea. Similarly, we may slip, or trip, and cause ourselves an injury in any manner of ways. For the most part, these afflictions will mean a few days off work, after which we return to our normal functional abilities, without giving it much further thought. These occurrences fall under the definition of 'short-term sickness absence'. A level of sickness absence is unavoidable, and it has been suggested that employers should anticipate this to be about 1.5 per cent, or around four days per employee per year, at its lowest (Taylor, 1998).

For a percentage of workers, however, the illness or injury may be far more serious. They may develop a life-threatening illness such as cancer, or a long-term condition like rheumatoid arthritis or multiple sclerosis. They could sustain a traumatic limb amputation while working with heavy machinery, or multiple fractures and soft tissue damage from a serious motor vehicle accident. Clearly, these sorts of events may well result in 'long-term sickness absence' from work, and possibly affect a person's ability to continue to do their job in the future. Long-term absence is usually defined as absences of four weeks and longer (Hayday et al., 2004).

While some people may return to their previous state of health and capabilities, others may need to adapt, over a period of time, to the reality of reduced functional abilities. The resultant negative consequences for individuals, families, and the wider economy, are a real cause for concern (Department for Work and Pensions, 2002). Even more so, when we realise that the UK has the second highest number of workers suffering from long-term sickness in the European Community (People Management, 2004), and significantly poorer return to work outcomes for those who experience a major injury (15 per cent), than countries such as Sweden (50 per cent) or America (30 per cent) (Trades Union Congress, 2005). Let us now examine how this problem has come about.

THE GENERAL PRACTITIONER AND SICKNESS CERTIFICATION

The decision about an individual's fitness to work remains firmly rooted within a medical tradition, and so it is GPs who have the responsibility for the certification process. The traditional route for a person who becomes unwell is to first consult their GP. In theory, the GP will then undertake a medical assessment of their condition and provide them with advice as to whether or not they are fit for work. GPs have an important role in maintaining public health in this regard – consider the case of the food handler who becomes unwell (Chambers et al., 2001). On the basis of their assessment they may issue a sick note, sometimes with advice on possible alternatives, such as 'fit for light duties'. In reality, short GP appointment times and few or no links with the workplace results in the unwell person deciding that they are unable to do their job for health reasons. Only a handful of GPs believe that it is their role, or their responsibility, to question or override their patient's decision in this regard. This is understandable, since many GPs would consider themselves to be in a supportive, therapeutic role rather than as a gatekeeper to the benefits system. The sick certificate is issued for a finite period of time, after which the individual must make the decision to either return to work, or return to their GP to request a further note to be issued.

Despite its subjectivity, the validity of the sick note has not been questioned by either the state benefits system or by employers and has been accepted as meaning that someone is currently too ill to do their job. However, the wisdom of this blind acceptance is now being challenged on several fronts. Employers are not obliged to follow the advice in the sick note (Chambers *et al.*, 2001), and some are beginning to take greater responsibility for more pro-active management of their employees' absence from work. Those who are absent on long-term sickness absence may, increasingly, be offered the opportunity of a more gradual re-introduction to the workplace. This is delivered through a graduated return to work programme, some form of which may be found within growing numbers of larger organisations. The Government has looked into the possibility of expanding the role of advising on fitness for work and issuing sickness certificates, to include other professional groups such as physiotherapists, osteopaths and nurse practitioners, but this proposal still needs to be piloted (Niven, 2004).

The entitlement to pay when on sick leave is determined by a number of factors, including length of service. As a minimum, statutory sick pay (SSP) is paid to all employees who are off work in the short term (up to 26 weeks). In the longer term, IB are also accessed through GP sickness certification, as we discussed earlier in the chapter. The majority of workers who move from SSP to IB will, again depending on the terms and conditions of their employment contract, at some point have lost their jobs due to their extended absence from work.

JOB RETENTION

There has been an identified need to more actively intervene to help prevent people from losing their jobs, by successfully returning them to work, following an injury or illness. This is known as job retention. Unfortunately, the current configuration of service provision does not support job retention interventions very effectively. Although VR takes different forms and has different meanings (O'Halloran and Innes, 2005; Kumar, 2000), international services are often better established than they are in the UK (Wright *et al.*, 2005). However, schemes to improve job retention have been introduced by both the Government and employers, and we will examine these initiatives from both sides.

The Job Recruitment and Retention Pilot (JRRP)

As part of its strategy to tackle the problem of rising numbers of disability benefit claimants, the Government recognised that more needed to be done to prevent people dropping out of the labour force in the first place. Since the evidence base did not provide answers regarding the best way to achieve this, a large-scale research project was undertaken to add to the knowledge base. As a result, the Job Recruitment and Retention Pilot (JRRP) was announced in the 2000 budget.

The JRRP was a two-year randomised controlled trial. It was aimed at identifying interventions successful in increasing the return to work rate of people who were in employment, but who were away from work because of ill-health, injury or an acquired disability – they were claiming SSP. At the time, more than 3,000 people per week were moving from SSP to IB (after 26 weeks absence). Around 80 per cent of this group remained out of work for more than five years (Department for Work and Pensions, 2001). The purpose of the trial was to see if it was possible to prevent people from moving out of work and onto IB. Three different interventions were tested across six different areas of the UK. Testing teams included occupational therapists at some of these project sites.

Participation in the study was voluntary. Those participants who expressed an interest in taking part, and met the eligibility criteria, were randomly assigned to one of four possible groups. These were:

1. a workplace intervention, where issues in the workplace were addressed
2. a heath intervention, where any health issues were addressed
3. a combined intervention of both health and workplace interventions
4. a control group.

The trial ended in spring 2005. More than 2,500 participants had taken part, each of whom had been off work for between six and 26 weeks. Evaluation of the study indicated that it had proved difficult to recruit sufficient numbers to the trial and there had been a relatively high early drop-out – possibly as high as 30 per cent – particularly from the workplace intervention group. Interestingly, findings showed that the return to work rates across each of the four groups were remarkably similar. Around 45 per cent returned to work from each group, including the control group. The conclusion drawn from this influential study was that none of the three interventions tested were successful in making an impact on return to work rates amongst people who were off sick (Purdon et al., 2006). This pilot was extensively evaluated, and a series of evaluation reports have been published by the Department for Work and Pensions (Nice and Thornton, 2004; Farrell et al., 2006; Purdon et al., 2006). Since none of the interventions demonstrated their effectiveness, this initiative has since been disbanded.

Managing sickness absence: the employer's perspective

While the vast majority of employers have a degree of concern for the welfare and well-being of their employees, ultimately this concern is balanced against the needs and requirements of the business as a whole. It is often the case that an employer's actions towards an employee with a health problem or a disability are governed more by the legislative demands placed on them than they are by more altruistic motives. The Health and Safety at Work etc Act 1974 is the main piece of legislation that covers occupational health and safety in the United Kingdom. We will examine this and other health and safety law, which employers must comply with and which is relevant to the role of the occupational therapist, in Chapter 9.

From an employer's perspective absenteeism brings legislative duties and can be associated with a high financial cost. It has been estimated that the average cost of sickness absence is in the region of between £ 465 and £ 2,261 per employee per year

(Bevan and Hayday, 2001). Other sources suggest that as many as eight working days are lost for every member of staff each year, which translates into 3.5 per cent of working time (Chartered Institute of Personnel and Development, 2006a). Clearly, these costs may have significant implications for the profitability of any company, particularly smaller companies with tighter profit margins. It may also have a negative effect on staff morale, as well as an uncertainty regarding whether the returnee will need more time off for sickness or hospital appointments in the future (Stokes, 1997).

It is important for occupational therapists considering working in this area of practice to recognise that employers need to contain these expenses in order for their business to succeed and flourish. It is not practicable for every worker to return to, or remain in, their job if they have a health condition which significantly affects their ability to perform the main tasks of their job. Larger companies may find it easier to accommodate people with a disability than smaller companies do (Combs and Omvig, 1986; Roberts *et al.*, 2004).

Most businesses are faced with an ever-increasing need to contain costs, so it is hardly surprising that employers are starting to recognise that they need to try and minimise the overheads associated with sickness absenteeism. Within the UK, this has resulted in a growing number of wellness programmes, which have a health promotion focus. These programmes often include a range of measures designed to help people give up smoking, eat a healthier diet, improve their physical fitness, and learn stress management techniques (Foot and Hook, 2005). These sorts of programmes have been found to be successful in reducing the costs associated with healthcare and absenteeism. More information about health promotion can be found in Chapter 4. In a similar vein, employers may introduce employee assistance programmes, which usually provide services such as counselling to deal with workplace stress. Employee assistance programmes and workplace counselling originated in North America in the 1960s and have been around in the UK since the 1980s. Both are directed towards coping with stress and improving quality of life at work, to provide both organisational and individual benefits. These types of services are managed and sourced through human resources departments, usually in larger companies. They are often provided by occupational psychologists or rehabilitation counsellors (Berridge *et al.*, 1997).

The absence (or attendance) management policy

It is good business practice for employers to have a policy in place for absence management (some employers refer to this as an attendance management policy). The purpose of this policy is to give the employee information about any statutory entitlement to leave, such as parental or compassionate leave. These policies usually include sickness reporting procedures and set out the roles and responsibilities of the individual, their manager, human resources or personnel, and the occupational health department, if available. The existence of a policy of this sort is important in helping to ensure fair and equitable treatment of all employees. Recording sickness absence and keeping in regular contact with the person who is off sick, are important elements of an effective absence management policy (Health and Safety Executive, 2004).

A cohesive policy should include details about contractual sick pay terms, and the relationship of these entitlements with SSP. The policy should also include the process to be followed by the employee when they are taking time off sick; who they should notify, and when a self-certificate and/or a doctor's sick note must be submitted. The policy should also advise the employee that they may be required to attend occupational health and the employer has the right to request a report from their own doctor. Increasingly, a return to work interview is also included as a requirement in these policies, as this is an effective strategy for reducing absences which are short-term in nature (Chartered Institute of Personnel and Development, 2006b).

Employers have tended to focus on short-term absence in their absence management policies, whereas an effective policy also needs to focus on ways to reduce long-term absence (Bevan and Hayday, 2001). Occasionally, occupational therapists involved in supporting someone back to work may discover that these policies contain procedures about graduated return to work programmes. The policy may include prescribed timescales, for example:

Week 1: 12 hours over 3 days
Week 2: 20 hours over 4 days
Week 3: 25 hours over 5 days
Week 4: 30 hours over 5 days
Week 5: 35 hours over 5 days
Week 6: return to full-time hours and full duties.

If you, as an occupational therapist, are involved in developing a return to work plan for an employee of a particular company, it is advisable to familiarise yourself with their existing policy, since you may well be expected to comply with its terms.

While ensuring equity amongst employees, imposed timescales of this nature may have a counter-productive effect in that they may draw out the return process more than is actually required by the individual The existence of prescribed return to work timescales may also inhibit the development of a programme which is tailored more specifically to a particular individual's needs in relation to their illness or injury. If this is the case, it is advisable to talk this over with a senior member of the human resources department. The return to work programme will be discussed in more detail in a later chapter.

Occupational health

Traditionally, occupational health doctors and nurses have been concerned with how people's work may affect their health. Chapter 2 was littered with examples of how individuals' health suffered due to the work duties they were expected to perform. In some instances this harm was caused by ignorance, for example the lack of awareness of the dangers of asbestos. In others it was due to a general lack of concern by employers for the health, safety and well-being of their workers. The modern occupational health service of today may have a far broader remit in the range of services it offers to employees. However, the availability of occupational health services varies according to the type of industry and, perhaps, also the motives of the employer (Chambers *et al.*, 2001). Where these services are available, the responsibility for managing and organising their provision often falls to the human resources or personnel department of the organisation.

The provision of an occupational health service is often related to the size of the organisation and the nature of the business they undertake. Occupational health services may be delivered by an external provider under a contractual arrangement, or sometimes they are bought-in on an ad hoc basis, as and when they are needed. Less frequently, a company has its own occupational health doctor or nurse, and larger organisations may have an in-house occupational health department. The nature of the services available through the occupational health service will depend on the background and training of the personnel involved. However, common tasks of an occupational health service include pre-employment health screening, general health surveillance and health promotion amongst the workforce, ensuring compliance with health and safety regulations, addressing sickness absence, monitoring different parts of the organisation for work-related stress and any other hazards and risks in the workplace, rehabilitation or re-deployment, and advising on ill-health retirement. The service may also extend to providing counselling and advice on ergonomic practises and workstation design and layout.

Occupational health services are recognised as being one of the most effective resources for managing sickness absence, particularly where this absence has a long-term nature (Chartered Institute of Personnel and Development, 2006c). In the light of this, it is somewhat disappointing that, since 1990, the proportion of the workforce able to access any sort of occupational health support has dropped from 50 per cent to just 30 per cent (Trades Union Congress, 2002). While there are discrepancies in these estimates, this probably depends to some extent on how they are defined. Therefore the figures vary from estimates of just three per cent of companies who provide comprehensive occupational health support for their employees (Trades Union Congress, 2002) to nearly 75 per cent of organisations who provide some form of occupational health services to deal with short- and long-term absence (Chartered Institute of Personnel and Development, 2006c). A very small minority of employers have any sort of rehabilitation policy. This state of affairs may be partly attributed to the fact that, in contrast to many other western countries, the United Kingdom does not have legislation which requires the provision of occupational health services to workers.

Workplace Health Connect

Small- and medium-sized businesses, those with between five and 250 workers, are particularly poorly served by company occupational health services. The Health and Safety Commission's *Strategy for Workplace Health and Safety to 2010 and Beyond* (2004) recognised the need to improve access to workplace health services for these smaller businesses and sought new and innovative ways to do this. As a result a free, confidential advice line, combined with a workplace specialist advice service, was established. This service, known as Workplace Health Connect, covers five regions in England and Wales. It is funded by the Health and Safety Executive and is provided by a range of public, private and voluntary sector service providers. Workplace Health Connect aims to transfer knowledge and skills to employers to enable them to address any future workplace health issues and sickness absence themselves. More information about this service can be found at: http://www.hse.gov.uk/workplacehealth/index.htm (accessed 11/12/06).

Occupational therapy in occupational health

Very occasionally, occupational therapists can be found in occupational health teams in the UK. A percentage may have secured their position by gaining an additional qualification, either in occupational health or in ergonomics. Currently, the role of OT in the workplace remains far less well-established than in countries such as Australia and New Zealand (Joss, 2002). However, the increasing Government emphasis on retaining people in the labour force, combined with employers' desire to more effectively manage long-term sickness absence and reduce their compulsory insurance costs, means that opportunities exist for suitably experienced occupational therapists that are able to market their services effectively (Joss and Pratt, 2006). A recent, influential report suggested that demands for VR for work-related injury and illness could double if trends follow those in other countries with more established provision (Wright et al., 2005).

There is a growing need to maintain people's functional abilities at work; adapting the environment of the workplace or the demands of the work tasks so as to accommodate individuals' particular needs. Legislation, such as the Disability Discrimination Act (1995), adds to employers' awareness of their responsibilities to make reasonable efforts to accommodate an individual's disabilities. Those occupational therapists who expand their existing knowledge of the impact of disability on functional performance to include an understanding of the workplace and workplace issues, may be well-placed to advise and intervene to help deliver this new agenda.

In addition, a growing number of occupational therapists who have specialised in VR are providing their services to insurance companies. This may be directly through employment with a particular insurance company, or as an independent provider or part of a provider company. It is timely, therefore to consider the growing influence of the insurance sector and how it is providing VR in the UK.

THE INSURANCE SECTOR

Insurance companies offer a range of products that are directed towards individuals and businesses who want to protect themselves from some form of risk. There are four main types of insurance products which may include cover for healthcare and/or rehabilitation:

1. personal medical insurance
2. income protection insurance
3. employers' liability compulsory insurance (ELI)
4. motor insurance.

Insurers who provide one, or more, of these schemes may be interested in what rehabilitation can offer (Waddell and Burton, 2004).

As we read earlier, ELI is compulsory for all employers and covers any workers who may be injured or become ill due to their work, whereas private medical insurance and income protection insurance schemes are voluntary. Motor insurance may be provided by the employer, if the person has a company car, or is required to drive to carry out his or her job. Alternatively, a car driver is legally required to have their own insurance policy. It is important to note that, following a road traffic accident, a private rehabilitation programme is only made available to the person who is determined to be the victim of the accident.

The UK has the third largest insurance sector in the world and operates within a very competitive market. About one fifth of the 1,100+ registered insurance companies in the UK are directed towards long-term business, such as life insurance, income protection, critical illness cover and pensions (Association of British Insurers, 2005).

Within the income protection market, payouts in 2004 were in the region of £1 billion (Association of British Insurers, 2005). A company may offer group or individual products, or both, and they are often sold through brokers. Just two per cent of households in the UK purchase this kind of protection on an individual basis (National Statistics 2003/2004), therefore the major customer group is likely to be companies purchasing group schemes. This type of insurance is taken out by companies who want to protect themselves against financial loss resulting from an employee's illness, injury or death, regardless of the origins or nature of the affliction suffered by the individual. Since it is the employer who is the policyholder, they are the recipient of any payment from a valid claim. While some employers may pass some, or all, of this payout onto their employee, they are not under any obligation to do so.

The Association of British Insurers has highlighted the need for a shift away from a culture of lengthy personal injury claims chasing large financial settlements, towards the potential benefits of VR and better occupational health services helping people return to work earlier and more effectively (Association of British Insurers, 2005).

Occupational therapy in the insurance sector

VR is not the exclusive domain of occupational therapists. Therefore, insurance companies who provide VR may employ specialists with backgrounds such as OT, physiotherapy, psychology and rehabilitation counselling. In addition, they are often employed with a different title, such as rehabilitation co-ordinator or VR consultant.

Others may be employed as functional capacity evaluators. These practitioners may be either office-based or home-based workers covering a particular geographical area.

The primary aim of VR in the insurance sector is to facilitate a timely and successful return to work for selected individuals, eligible under the terms of the insurance policy. These may be people who are absent from their job because of injury, or perhaps a health condition with a more chronic nature. For the occupational therapist using a case management approach, this may include sourcing the necessary rehabilitation providers in the individual's local area. It may also include providing support to employees and employers during the transition back to work, as well as advice and information about disability-related issues, where necessary. We will explore more about the case management and the role of the occupational therapist in these settings, in the following chapter on assessment and intervention.

In this chapter we have learned about the types of services and initiatives which may be available to people who are out of work, those who are attempting to move into work, and those who need assistance to stay in work. We have explored a range of service models which may provide a valued worker role for those who cannot, or do not wish to, secure competitive employment. In the next section we will be looking at the VR process which may be supported by the occupational therapist assisting a client into, or back to, work.

6 Occupational Therapy and the Vocational Rehabilitation Process

The aim of this chapter is to describe the process involved in assisting an individual in to, or back to, work. It takes you through each of the stages involved and touches on the main issues related to each stage. It also outlines a selection of tools and techniques which may be helpful at different stages of the process. You will notice as you read through this chapter, that there are both similarities and differences between the vocational rehabilitation (VR) process and the more traditional, perhaps more familiar, occupational therapy (OT) rehabilitation process. The focus is on the knowledge that you may need to acquire in order to apply existing OT knowledge and skills to the VR process. This chapter also attempts to illustrate that the same process may be followed, regardless of whether you are trying to help a person to gain work, return to work or maintain an existing worker role. This process can apply to any form of work, paid or unpaid. However, this is a very broad brush to use. You may find that certain discussions in this chapter will apply more closely to the stage of recovery of your particular client group than others; enabling you to draw out the aspects which are of relevance to your particular set of circumstances.

Throughout this book, a pan-disability perspective has been adopted. This is because the barriers which may be preventing a person from participating in work will most likely extend beyond purely the functional limitations which have been caused by a particular health condition or disability. This is not, of course, to suggest that these limitations be ignored, rather that, in taking an occupation-focused perspective, and in looking for effective solutions, the occupational therapist will need to take a broader perspective. An essential element of the VR process is to help the person to come to terms with their injury, disability or health condition and to understand, and manage, the ways in which it impacts on their occupational participation in work.

Let us begin with what is probably common knowledge: the core stages of the OT process which include assessment, planning, intervention and evaluation, as seen in Figure 6.1.

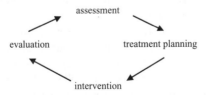

Figure 6.1. The core stages of the occupational therapy process

Although this process can be expanded to include further stages in some situations or shortened in others – for example, if we work in an assessment unit – these four basic elements still remain the essence of the OT process. Vocational rehabilitation follows a remarkably similar process, regardless of the setting in which it is practised. It does, however, have some additional stages, and, importantly, the content and focus within some of these stages may differ from what you are currently familiar with. Figure 6.2 also illustrates the main elements of the VR process.

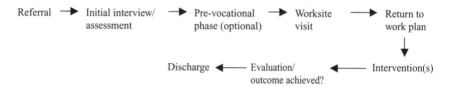

Figure 6.2. The vocational rehabilitation process

Figure 6.2 also illustrates that the VR process is stepped, thereby guiding you as you assist your client back to work. Unlike the cyclical nature of the OT process illustrated in Figure 6.1, the VR process tends to be more linear in nature. If this course of action does not result in a successful return to work, there are very few settings that have the funding to allow the practitioner to go through the process again. From beginning to end, this process may be completed in a matter of days, or it may take place across several months. The same VR process can, however, be followed regardless of whether the person is currently unemployed and seeking to move in to work, or whether they have a job which is still open for them to return to.

As we discussed in the previous chapter, it is important to remember that in countries where rehabilitation for work is far more established, the service models make a clear distinction between those people who are unemployed and seeking entry to the labour market and those who have an employer and are returning to an existing job. It is, however, primarily legislation and funding streams that have created this dichotomy. The result has been that these two groups have traditionally followed different paths, often being assisted in their rehabilitation by people from different professional backgrounds. There may also be different names for these two interventions, with the former sometimes being called VR and the latter occupational rehabilitation, although exact terminology varies from country to country. We will return to look more closely at the specific terminology and interventions used by occupational therapists later in the section.

In the emerging market in the UK, we do not have this diversity of professionals, such as vocational specialists and rehabilitation counsellors, with such clearly delineated roles. Nor is the legislation as prescriptive. Hence, at this time, services to both of these groups come under the very broad umbrella of VR. As services become more established this situation may change. Currently, however, occupational therapists and others with the necessary skills, assist people to access work or return to the workforce following the VR process outlined in Figure 6.2.

The VR process begins with the receipt of a referral and then moves through up to six further stages to discharge. Depending on the client's needs, the length of each stage will vary considerably. We will now look at each of these eight stages, to help you understand what is involved in each step of the process. We will start with the referral.

STAGE 1: THE REFERRAL

The VR process begins with the receipt of a referral. After all, without referrals there is no service to provide! This may sound a rather obvious statement to make, but there are two good reasons for emphasising this point at this initial stage in our discussion. The first reason is that within vocational practice, referrals may potentially come from a broader range of sources than occupational therapists may realise or anticipate. If you work within an NHS service which has a vocational focus, then your referrals will most likely come from familiar medical practitioner sources. However, if you are employed by an insurance company, the referral may come to you from a claims management specialist. Alternatively, if you work in an occupational health setting, it may be sent by an occupational physician or an occupational health nurse, or in some instances, directly from an employer. Then again, if you work as a condition management practitioner, your referral will come to you from a personal advisor in a jobcentre. The source of the referral is of particular importance because, in most instances, this person, or the organisation they represent, will be paying for your service and will be your customer. As a part of the organisation they are contracting with, you will therefore have certain professional responsibilities to them – for example, to provide a quality, cost-effective service.

The source of the referral will also, to some extent, determine the outcome that you will be aiming to achieve with your client. Your customer will, not unreasonably, expect demonstrable outcomes for purchasing your services. Since this notion may be an unfamiliar one to occupational therapists without a commercial background, let us illustrate this point with a few examples.

Bob is a sales representative who was the victim of a serious road traffic accident seven months ago. He sustained multiple fractures and soft tissue injuries. The insurance company has referred him to you, as an employee of a private rehabilitation provider company, to assess his medical and vocational rehabilitation needs.

Javier is a project manager for the software design company, TD Productions. He was in charge of a large project which was beset by problems and, despite working on it for over 80 hours a week, costs have begun to spiral out of control. His line manager was putting increasing pressure on him to sort things out quickly. He was also having serious relationship problems with his wife. One month ago Javier arrived at work drunk one morning. After a fierce confrontation with his boss, in front of his work colleagues, Javier stormed out. His GP subsequently signed him off sick with stress and anxiety. The human resources director for TD Productions has referred Javier to their occupational health service provider. The occupational health physician asks you to help Javier to return to work.

It is easy to identify your client as Bob and Javier in these scenarios. However, in the first case your customer is the insurance company, and in the second, it is the employer. It is important to recognise that in each of these cases you have certain responsibilities to **both** parties – to the customer, who is paying for a service to be provided, and to the individual, to whom you owe a duty of care as a registered healthcare professional. This dual responsibility places a new slant and a new complexity on the traditional client–therapist relationship for many therapists. It means that you will need to develop the ability to maintain a more neutral, considered and measured stance than perhaps you have been used to assuming in other settings. The ability to adopt an impartial perspective while taking the views and perspectives of both parties into account, may well become a crucial factor in determining the success of your intervention.

In each of the above scenarios the customer will expect you to help the referred person return to work. At this stage, the referral stage, you cannot know the likelihood of achieving this outcome. You do know, however that the earlier an intervention takes place, the greater the chances of success (Waddell and Burton, 2004). You will also be mindful of the service standards you are required to work to – the timescales by which you should have completed the initial assessment and report, for example. You will also be aware that, in the case of Javier, if your intervention is unsuccessful there is a greater likelihood this may be treated as a capability issue by the employer – this may increase the chance of Javier losing his job. You will need to recognise, and try to overcome, the strained interpersonal relationships that may exist between employer and employee in this sort of scenario.

STAGE 2: THE INTITAL ASSESSMENT

The second stage in the VR process is the initial assessment stage. There are seven key steps which will need to be attended to during this stage:

1. selecting a location for the initial assessment
2. explaining the purpose of the meeting and gaining consent
3. undertaking the initial assessment of the referred person
4. agreeing an action plan
5. completing the necessary documentation
6. assessing work readiness
7. identifying a way forward for the person who is not yet work ready.

Let us consider some of the factors that the therapist should focus on during each of these key steps.

SELECTING A LOCATION FOR THE INITIAL ASSESSMENT

Even before making arrangements to meet with the client, the first step is to decide on the most appropriate venue for the initial assessment to be undertaken. The literature, and anecdotal evidence, suggests that the environment in which the rehabilitation takes place may have an influence on the outcome of the intervention (Velozo, 1993). It is suggested that the workplace, and not the medical clinic, may be the best place to rehabilitate the majority of injured workers back to work (Innes, 1995). This environment is cost-effective and can help prevent unnecessary disability from occurring (Ganora and Wright, 1987). This will be unsurprising to many occupational therapists, who understand that the ways in which people perform and organise their occupations is determined by the relationship they have with their environment (Canadian Association of Occupational Therapists, 2002). Following on from this point, we can surmise that the environment in which the initial assessment meeting takes place may be of significance too.

This initial contact may take place at any number of venues, including the client's own home, their place of work, your place of work, a community venue, a jobcentre, a primary care centre or other NHS site, or an occupational health department. You may not have a choice in the venue selection, but do reflect for a moment on the message that each of the locations listed above may, potentially, send to the client. This point is illustrated through the following two examples.

Jean is a 54-year-old woman who is on incapacity benefit. She is a small, timid, softly-spoken woman with a nervous presentation. She has not worked for eight years, due to depression following the unexpected death of a close family member. Before that, she worked full-time as an office administrator for the local authority, where she was well-respected. She attends her local jobcentre, after being sent an appointment for a work-focused interview with a personal adviser. She expresses a cautious interest in finding out more about condition management, but does not want to commit herself at this stage. She is referred to you, as a condition management practitioner linked to this jobcentre, to discuss what the programme might entail. You make an appointment to see Jean at the same jobcentre first thing next Wednesday morning. You book a room to meet with her there.

On the day in question, Jean is very nervous. She arrives at the jobcentre ten minutes early, as she likes to be punctual. The doors have not yet opened, and a queue has formed outside. The queue, on this particular morning, includes a group of rowdy young men who are horse-playing and swearing loudly at each other. Some are wearing hooded tops and Jean feels intimidated and scared, even before she joins the queue. She decides that she has made the wrong decision and returns home, missing her appointment with you. She no longer wishes to find out about the condition management programme. With the benefit of hindsight, you realise that the choice of time and venue, on this particular occasion, was the wrong one. Where might have been a better choice?

Mike is a 55-year-old security guard at a local hospital. He is a keen sportsman and has always prided himself on his fitness and agility. His wife died about six years ago, and since that time most of his social outlets have been through his work. He is actively involved in the security department's darts team and their football team, and they have regular after-work games. Six weeks ago, he tripped and fell awkwardly while running across some uneven ground. As a result, he fractured his finger and sustained a soft tissue injury to his ankle. During his absence from work, he has been in regular telephone contact with his employer.

His finger is healing as expected, but his ankle remains painful and swollen, and he is still using his crutches. Mike worries that his ankle will never heal. He confides to his manager that he is wondering if he will ever be fit enough to come back to work again. He is very upset on the phone. Mike's manager is concerned about him, so contacts the occupational health department for advice.

An appointment is made for Mike to see the occupational health physician in the occupational health department, which is located on the hospital site. He is very keen to take part in a graduated return to work programme, and so sees you immediately after he has seen the doctor. Mike tells you how much better he feels just coming to the hospital site. 'It's silly, I know,' he laughs, 'but I've really missed the place. Just being here makes me feel like I've taken that first step towards coming back to work.'

This was an important point in Mike's recovery. It helped re-kindle some of his intrinsic coping strategies so that he could see a way forward. Visiting him at home, for example, would not have achieved the same effect. There will, however, be times when meeting the individual for the initial assessment at their workplace will not be the right choice. Some instances where the workplace may not be the best option for the initial assessment include:

- no suitable place at the worksite where you can meet on neutral territory; that is away from the person's day-to-day work environment
- there are poor relations between the person and their manager or co-workers
- the person sustained their current injury at work
- the reason for the absence is because of work-related stress
- the person has been off work for an extended period of time.

You will have your own views as to the most appropriate environment in which to meet a potential client for the initial assessment. There is no perfect venue and you will need to make your decision based on the information you receive in the referral. You will also need to be mindful of your own personal safety when coming to this decision.

EXPLAINING THE PURPOSE OF THE MEETING AND GAINING CONSENT

The initial assessment has three main purposes:

1. to develop a therapeutic relationship with the client
2. to share information
3. to agree the way forwards, which may include obtaining informed consent.

Let us examine the rationale for each of these, in turn.

Occupational therapy is based on a client-centred approach to practice (Sumsion, 1999), so establishing a trusting, collaborative, working relationship is often a particular skill of many occupational therapists working in rehabilitation settings. The value and importance of establishing this rapport cannot be over-stated, because without it, your intervention may very well stall before the first hurdle. If you are perhaps working in a case management role, and the client lives some distance from your place of work, this initial assessment meeting may also be the only opportunity you actually get meet the client face-to-face.

The second purpose of the meeting is for two-way information sharing. As you will notice, this purpose is inextricably linked with the first, since the client will only share their story, and any fears or concerns they may have about returning to work, if a trusting relationship has been established. The starting point in this information-sharing process is for you to clearly and succinctly explain your role. This is of particular importance in VR, because clients may initially, quite understandably, be somewhat suspicious of your reasons for seeing them.

If you are in any way linked with an organisation which currently provides them with some form of financial support because of their illness or disability, they may suspect that you have come to try and catch them out or check up on them, to see if they are malingering in some way. This is a natural human response. It is, therefore, important to clearly explain your role and your responsibilities. This will include making plain what you are, and are not, able to deliver, openly and honestly. If, for example, your customer is an insurance company, then they may suddenly, and without warning, withdraw funding for treatment which you have sourced for the client. This may happen if the case is due for settlement, or questions have arisen about liability, for example. Alerting the client to this possibility, right at the outset, is necessary to ensure that they understand the boundaries, and limits, of your role. In doing so, you will hopefully address, and allay, any fears the client may have about your motives and your intentions.

In some situations, the client may also need to be aware that your primary role is as a facilitator of the return to work process. In this capacity you will be helping them in their recovery, and acting as a bridge or a conduit between them and their workplace. In certain cases, you may find that the client is in some sort of dispute with their employer, or their employer may be taking some form of disciplinary action against them. It is important to ensure that you are not seen to be taking sides with the client against their employer, or vice versa. Your role is to, as far as possible, maintain a neutral stance. If relationships have broken down between an employer and an employee then you may well be trying to re-open communication channels as part of your intervention.

If the client needs an advocate, they should preferably be directed to their trade union representative, if they have one, or to their local citizen's advice bureau. You may also, of course, suggest that they may wish to seek legal advice from a solicitor if the situation they are in warrants this sort of intervention.

Having outlined your role, it is then over to the client. Allowing the person the time to tell their story should not be under-estimated. Short GP consultations do not allow an individual to discuss their difficulties beyond a very superficial level. Clients themselves have told me how much they have valued the time given by the occupational therapist to understanding their difficulties and how these were impacting on their lives. You may find that many clients have not previously had the opportunity to discuss their occupational performance limitations and their fears for their future in this way. During these discussions, you will be trying to identify the particular barriers that the client is currently facing, health related or otherwise, which may be preventing them from successfully entering or returning to work.

The third purpose of the initial interview is to agree the next step, which is usually set out in an action plan, and gain informed consent. In some settings, consent may have been obtained beforehand. Alternatively, the therapist will be expected to gain the client's written agreement to take part in the VR process. This consent may need to extend to giving you permission to contact third parties, such as the client's GP or solicitor, if one is involved. The client needs to be reassured that the information you gather will be treated confidentially. For the therapist who works in VR, maintaining confidentiality, while facilitating open and constructive dialogue with employers and others who may be involved in the client's return to work, is a delicate balancing act requiring high levels of judgment and tact. We will return to this issue in Chapter 8, when we discuss the multidisciplinary team.

UNDERTAKING THE INITIAL ASSESSMENT OF THE REFERRED PERSON

The initial assessment is most likely to take the form of a semi-structured interview. This will usually be a face-to-face meeting, although occasionally it is conducted over the telephone. The quantity of information you will need to gather during this assessment meeting will depend largely on the source of your funding and the nature of the service you are providing. For example, if you are acting as a case manager working for an insurance company, this may be the only face-to-face meeting you have with the client, who will probably live some distance away. You will, therefore, need to gather more information during this meeting than if you are working as a condition management practitioner for a local Pathways to Work programme. In this capacity, you may have the opportunity to meet with the client on a regular basis over a longer period of time. If the person is hard to engage, perhaps because of a mental health problem, for example, then you may well choose to approach the interview in a less-threatening, more informal, way. If your work setting is the NHS, you will be governed by the timescales set within your particular service.

As a general rule, there are three broad categories of information that you should gather during your initial assessment:

1. health or medical information
2. information about occupational performance
3. more detailed information about the person's work.

The following possible assessment form has been prepared in order to guide your exploration of these three areas. This assessment outlines the basic information which you would probably require from your initial interview.

Figure 6.3 illustrates that the VR assessment is not dissimilar to other client-centred OT initial assessments that you may undertake in any number of different settings.

INITIAL VOCATIONAL REHABILITATION ASSESSMENT

Health/medical information

Details of the client's illness or injury:

Treatment received by the client so far:

Any relevant past medical history:

> Contact details for the client's medical practitioner(s):
>
> Contact details for any other treating professional(s):

Client's residual symptoms:

- physical
- cognitive
- psychological.

Occupational performance information

What impact does the client think these symptoms are having on their functional abilities?

How is the client managing their activities of daily living at home?

How is the client's mobility in the community?

What are the client's leisure and recreational interests?

Are these affected by the client's condition? In what way(s)?

What are the client's main occupational roles?

Who are the client's significant others? How have they been affected?

If the client is in a relationship, or lives within a family unit, you may wish to seek the client's consent hear the views of other significant family members as well.

What is the nature of the client's work, if any? What are the client's thoughts about entering, or returning to, work?

Work information

Employment history

Current employment (if any):

- employer
- position
- hours of work
- duties
- potential barriers to returning to work (or entering work if the person is unemployed).

> Contact details for the client's employer:

Other relevant information:

Action plan/goals:

Figure 6.3. Initial vocational rehabilitation assessment

Perhaps the most significant difference is the way in which the person's work is highlighted during this information-gathering process. This is a core component of the initial assessment in VR. Since we are taking a client-centred perspective, the work section should routinely be included in the assessment, regardless of your own opinion as to the likely prospects of the person returning to work in the foreseeable future.

Obviously, you will need to obtain far more in-depth details about certain areas and we will discuss these as we work our way through this chapter. There are also other tools available to help you gather the additional information you may need. We will look briefly at a selection later in this chapter and the next. You will also want to make use of your observation skills, informally, during the interview, to add to your understanding of the client's strengths and difficulties. Experienced occupational therapists in the field report that they are often able to get a good sense of the likelihood of a person returning to work from this initial meeting.

AGREEING AN ACTION PLAN

The final part of the initial meeting with a client is to agree the next steps. Seeing a way forward, with the necessary support in place, is a crucial part of maintaining the momentum of an individual's occupational recovery. This is often achieved through the setting of goals or the creation of an action plan. The formality and the specific details of this plan will vary from individual to individual, and from setting to setting. Some will be simple, others more complex. For example, it may range from the client agreeing to keep a diary of their thoughts, feelings and/or daily activities for a week; to the person getting in touch with their employer to re-establish contact with their workplace; to setting longer-term goals based around returning to valued leisure or work activities. Regardless of these differences, goals should be client-centred and based on SMART principles. That is, goals should be specific, measurable, achievable, realistic and time-limited, since they will lay the foundations for the next stage of the VR process.

You may not be able, by yourself, to meet all the occupational performance needs that you have identified in the initial assessment. Onward referral to others may be part of the action plan agreed with the client. This may, for example, include a referral to an occupational therapist in another service, such as for home adaptations or assistive equipment, since existing service structures will dictate who may be responsible for meeting the costs of these interventions.

COMPLETING THE NECESSARY DOCUMENTATION

On completion of the initial assessment, in most instances, you will need to complete an assessment report, which outlines your findings, recommendations and any goals you may have set with your client. This is another example of the need for excellent communication skills; this time written abilities rather than verbal ones. Your report may be written for:

- the client
- the employer
- human resources department
- the claimant's solicitor
- the insurer
- the GP
- other treating health professionals
- the personal advisor (for Jobcentre Plus referrals).

Therefore, when writing your report, you will need to be mindful of your responsibility to each of these involved parties. You need to ensure that you do not breach your duty of confidentiality to your client. To this end, obtain the client's authorisation before distributing the report.

In the situation where the person has a job to return to, it is always wise to keep to factual information rather than hearsay, since you would not want to negatively influence the success of a work re-entry. The therapist is sometimes placed in a difficult situation, when it is evident from the client's account of events that the employee–employer relationship has soured. It is particularly important that the therapist is not seen to be 'taking sides' in any dispute. It is also important not to pre-judge the person's potential ability, or desire, to return to work. For example, although it may be helpful for you to know the person's feelings about returning to work, in most circumstances it is wise to hold this information in confidence at this point. You would not want to jeopardise the person's job, or the future success of their return to work, by revealing that they are not sure about returning. At this early stage, it is not uncommon for a person to have feelings of ambivalence or fear about work. It is good practice, in most settings, to have a more experienced therapist scrutinise your report before you send it out to the relevant parties.

ASSESSING WORK READINESS

By this stage in the VR process, it may be evident, in a minority of cases, to both the client and yourself, that they are not going to be able to remain in their current line of work. For example, a roofing contractor who sustains a traumatic above-knee amputation, or a paramedic who suffers a spinal fracture, will both need to re-evaluate their occupational choices. In these sorts of situations, vocational exploration will be necessary and we will learn more about this intervention later in the chapter.

The majority of clients who are returning to existing work may well be able to do elements of their current job. Assessing their work readiness is an important aspect of your formulation of the client's current situation. 'How do you decide when, or if, your client is ready to return to work?' is a question frequently asked by occupational therapists, particularly when they are still relatively new to a VR role. The answer is that there is no hard and fast rule, since it will depend on multiple factors. Safety is a paramount concern throughout the VR process, and assessing risk is an important component of determining work readiness. The occupational therapist, together with the client, will need to identify possible strengths and barriers when coming to a decision about readiness to return to work. The following list, which is by no means exhaustive and in no particular order, highlights some key factors that will influence these decisions:

- motivation to return to work
- level of job satisfaction with their job
- occupational and worker identity
- the client's values and beliefs, and those of others around them
- the client's pre-injury/illness relationships with others at work
- the nature of the client's condition and their experience of illness/injury
- the stage and pace of the client's recovery
- ongoing complications such as pain and fatigue
- the length of time the client has been away from the workplace
- the demands and requirements of the client's job
- the nature of any identified risks
- the client's age
- the client's existing financial commitments
- involvement in a legal process
- whether the client's condition is covered by the Disability Discrimination Act.

A client who is unemployed may be deemed to be work-ready, based on the above considerations, but there may be no suitable local jobs available. If the client has an existing job to return to, there are additional workplace factors that may also affect the feasibility of their return to work. These include:

- the availability of modified duties
- the employer's existing return to work policies
- the size of the company
- the willingness of the employer for the person to return
- the perceived value of the person to the company, both in financial terms and in terms of their skills, abilities and role within the company
- their pre-injury or pre-illness attendance patterns and any outstanding capability or disciplinary issues.

It is likely that you will need to gather information about these particular factors from both the client and their employer or line manager. We will shortly return to look at these aspects in more detail when we come to the worksite visit. In reaching a decision about work readiness, if the client is to return to an existing job it is helpful to have a baseline number of hours in mind. That is, the minimum number of hours that the client needs to be able to work before a return should be considered. This minimum baseline could be set at 12 hours per week, for a full-time employee. This seems to be a rough figure used by some practicing therapists.

You might like to consider whether this person is likely to have the work tolerance, at this point in time, to be able to do selected elements of their job for 12 hours, across the course of a working week. In answering this question, you will be taking into account the person's own views and priorities, their strengths, the nature of their job and work tasks, the potential ease of accommodating them back into the workplace and the barriers to be overcome, including the nature and stage of recovery of their health condition or disability.

If you think there is a good chance of achieving this, then you will be able to move swiftly onto the next stage of the VR process. Before we do this, however, we need to discuss the rationale for this 12-hour principle in a little more detail. There will, of course, be a number of exceptions to it. For example, you may be assisting a client on benefits to move into work and their benefit entitlement may limit the number of hours they are allowed to work. A.young person with a moderate learning disability, who is entering employment for the first time, perhaps through a supported employment route, may well be starting off with just one or two hours a week. Reintroduction to work for a person who has sustained a serious brain injury and needs to re-learn work tasks, will be a far more gradual and longer-term process. Alternatively, the person may have only had a part-time contract of employment in the first place.

Some occupational therapists will feel that it is beneficial for the client to ease back into the workplace for a couple of hours per week, if this is all that they can manage. However, there are two good reasons for setting a guideline minimum baseline before considering a return. The first is that the very act of going into work for, say, four hours on three separate days will enable the client to re-establish important daily habits and routines around getting ready for work, commuting, getting to work on time, and fitting work back into their wider daily occupational pattern. It also allows the person sufficient time, once they are at work, to begin to re-establish their feelings of competence at their job. Importantly, they can take on pre-selected tasks, which co-workers may have been covering in their absence, allowing the client to perceive themselves to be a valued contributor to the team or department. It also allows them to start to identify, and put in place, their own coping strategies for dealing with issues such as pain and fatigue. Individuals often under-estimate the fatigue they will experience when they return to work, particularly when they have been absent for any length of time. Gaining this sense of mastery is important to re-building their confidence in themselves as a capable, valuable worker.

The second reason stems from the responsibility that we have to the others involved in, or affected by, this situation. A successful return to work is unlikely to be achieved without the co-operation and goodwill of the employer. The employer has a right to expect that the therapist will try to aim for a timely, efficient and safe return to full duties, within a reasonable period of time. An absent worker often places a significant financial burden on a company, as well as additional work on co-workers. Busy co-workers who have to shoulder the extra work are unlikely to be particularly receptive to someone who comes in for one or two hours a week to do simulated work tasks.

They are far more likely to respond in a positive manner if the person is able to resume some of their own work tasks and is seen to be pulling their weight. A hostile work environment is a barrier to a successful return to work, so inadvertently creating this type of situation should be avoided.

It may be that, at this point, you are working with a client who has a job to return to, is most likely ready to undertake a baseline number of hours at work, is motivated to return, and has a supportive manager who is willing and able to make any short-term adjustments to their job, as required. Mike, from earlier in the chapter, is a good example of someone who may be in this situation. He may well be able to return to work as part of his recovery, alongside continuing his medical treatment or rehabilitation. In this case, you would not need a pre-vocational programme and would move straight to stage four, the worksite meeting.

IDENTIFYING A WAY FORWARD WHEN THE PERSON IS NOT WORK-READY

In contrast to the scenario outlined above, the person may not yet be work-ready. There may be a whole host of reasons for this. For example, a person who has received incapacity benefits for a number of years may have lost their identity as a worker. This ability to retain a strong worker identity has been found to be a common theme amongst those unemployed disabled jobseekers who do manage to successfully enter or return to work (Mettävainio and Ahlgren, 2004). Without a worker identity, the person is unlikely to aspire to achieving a worker role. In this situation, they will not be work ready. Alternatively, the person may not, as yet, be sufficiently recovered from their illness/injury to safely return to the workplace. Or, they may clearly not be capable of returning to their former role.

Some individuals, particularly those who have sustained serious forms of illness or injury, may need a period of re-orientation, to take stock and re-evaluate their occupational priorities. As part of this process, they may need to find a new work identity and perhaps explore other career or work opportunities which are better suited to their current strengths and abilities. This may involve a period of re-training, or perhaps seeking work with an alternative employer.

Adapting to disability and making these life-changing adjustments and decisions can, for many individuals, take place over months and years, rather than in the shorter-term. The occupational therapist involved in supporting clients in this position, perhaps as a case manager, may be well placed to assist with these transitions and adjustments.

Alternatively, the person may decide, as a consequence of their illness experience, that there are other, more personally valued, roles which they wish to develop at this time. They may wish to pursue an unpaid work role, perhaps spending more time with their children, for example. Participation in VR is voluntary in the UK at present, and will hopefully remain so. It is important to respect the person's choice that returning to paid employment, at this particular stage of their life or recovery, is not the right option for them. You can validate this decision by ensuring that the door is left open for them in the future. In this way, you will be helping empower the person to resume work activities at a time which is right for them. Depending on the purpose and boundaries of your role, this may mean signposting or referring the person on to another service, if you are not in a position to maintain your involvement over this length of time.

In situations where the person wants to return to work, but is currently unable to undertake a minimum baseline number of hours, a time-limited pre-vocational programme may be indicated. We will continue by exploring this optional stage of the VR programme.

STAGE 3: THE PRE-VOCATIONAL PHASE

We begin this section by clarifying what is meant by 'pre-vocational', in modern times. In the past, pre-vocational programmes have not always been part of a planned and co-ordinated VR process. They have, rather, been an endpoint in themselves. They tended to take place in light and heavy workshops, often situated in hospital rehabilitation departments. While purporting to be developing and improving the work skills, behaviours, habits and routines of the attendees, there was often no clear progress route out of the pre-vocational programme and into some form of valued and meaningful work. Some have referred to these types of programmes as transitional (Inman *et al.*, 2007), yet nowadays most of these extended train-then-place programmes fall into the category of substitute work. You may remember that we learned about this form of work when we explored the meaning of work, earlier in the book. There is currently little political support for this approach, since it is costly and not compatible with the current social inclusion agenda. Current evidence suggests that this type of pre-vocational programme is not an effective way to secure entry to paid employment (Crowther *et al.*, 2001) and so supported employment, or the other service models of work which we have discussed previously, are nowadays seen as a preferred option for those who are moving towards work.

In the context of the VR process, a pre-vocational programme is an optional stage within a wider, planned course of action and is not the end point. There must be a clear route of progression to enable the person to move onto the following stage in the VR process. The pre-vocational programme is time-limited. It should preferably be as short as possible, especially where the person has an existing job to return to, since the employer is not going to hold the job open indefinitely. The purpose, then, of this third stage is fourfold:

1. to build work tolerance
2. to help a person retain their occupational identity, as a worker, during the early stages of their medical recovery/rehabilitation
3. to undertake further assessments
4. to undertake vocational exploration.

We will look at each of these indicators in turn.

BUILDING WORK TOLERANCE

A short-term programme, aimed at increasing work tolerance and preparation for work, may be an integral part of the VR process if the person is currently unable to complete a baseline number of hours of work. For the person who is returning to an existing job, this programme may comprise measures such as increased physical activity, perhaps through walking, swimming, or attending a local leisure centre. It may also include home-based work-related activities, such as periods of computer work. For some it may mean re-establishing normal routines and community participation. The following case study illustrates this point.

Gail is a 46-year-old social worker. She has been off work with depression for four months. She is on medication and has had counselling in the past, but does not wish to see a counsellor again at present. Although Gail has had episodes of depression before, this is the longest period that she has been absent from work. She has been referred to you, a member of an occupational health team, to help her return to work, as she is very worried about the possibility of losing her job. Gail comes to see you at the occupational health centre where you work. At the initial assessment Gail confesses that this is the first time she has left her home for over six weeks. She lives in a small community, and she is worried that if she is seen out and about people will think that she is not genuinely ill. Although Gail is still doing all her indoor household chores, relatives are doing all her shopping and paying her bills for her. She is very tearful and states that she feels like a prisoner in her home.

Gail's feelings of guilt are also preventing her from using the telephone. Her work manager, who is supportive, has left a couple of messages for her to find out how she is getting on, but Gail has not returned the calls. She states that her main goal is to return to work as soon as possible. Her job is very important to her and she has a strong worker identity. An additional concern is that she will no longer be entitled to receive her full salary when she has been off work for six months and, consequently, will not be able to pay her mortgage and other debts. This is adding to her anxieties. Before she is work ready, Gail needs to begin to re-establish her occupational routines and undertake some work preparation tasks. You explain this to Gail and agree a three-week pre-vocational programme with her. The programme includes:

- making a telephone call to her manager to tell her she is actively working towards returning to work
- making an appointment to see her GP for a review of her medication and to discuss her desire to return to work
- gradually taking back responsibility for doing her own shopping and other community activities.

Gail is able to identify friends and family members who will be able to provide encouragement and support her in undertaking these activities. If Gail is able to carry out these and other agreed activities with support, the plan is to then move onto the next phase of the VR process. This phase will involve undertaking a more detailed work assessment with her, as well as arranging a worksite visit, which will include a meeting with her manager.

The outcome of these actions is that Gail is able to commence a graduated return to work, with the support of her GP, her employer, her family and yourself, before the six-month deadline arrives.

The exact nature of the preparatory activities that make up a pre-vocational programme will depend largely on factors such as the nature of the client's condition, the length of time they have been absent from work, and identified barriers hindering their return.

For the client who is unemployed and is about to begin work, preparatory activities may include tasks such as purchasing suitable work wear and sorting out travel arrangements to get to the workplace on time. In both cases, undertaking these practical types of activities will help a person move forwards in their recovery, as well as mentally preparing them to engage, or re-engage, with the worker role. Frequently, this pre-vocational stage takes place alongside any medical rehabilitation, such as physiotherapy, or psychological interventions, such as counselling. In these situations, liaising and co-ordinating with others involved in the client's treatment will be a crucial component of the occupational therapist's role.

RETAINING A WORKER IDENTITY

The person who has sustained a severe injury or developed a serious long-term health condition needs help to retain a worker identity, since this can be an important part of their recovery. When a person, without warning, has had their worker role interrupted, they will undoubtedly have worries about work and their future. The person may wonder if they will ever be able to work again, or if this is to be a permanent role loss. Even if your client is likely to be away from work for several months, or longer, it is still essential to talk with them about their work. No-one can predict the future, so there will be few situations where you can advise a client, with absolute certainty, that they will never be able to work again. This is not to say you should give the person false reassurances, but you can encourage them to do practical things, such as keeping in touch with their workplace. It may be that the client would prefer you to act as an intermediary on their behalf, and you may then have regular brief telephone contact with their employer or with a contact in human resources, feeding this back to the client. The rationale for this approach is that, by keeping a two-way communication channel open, you can help ease the person's transition back to work, if appropriate, when the time becomes right to do so. It may become clear at a future date, that the person will not be able to return to their current role. In this situation, you can assist the person, through vocational exploration, to identify possible alternatives and help establish new opportunities for participation in valued and meaningful work.

UNDERTAKING FURTHER ASSESSMENTS

You may feel that it is necessary to carry out further assessments before the person enters, or returns to, work. Undertaking additional assessments will depend partially on the reason for referral, but more particularly on the complexity of the individual case and the potential level of risk involved in the person's return. In the light of this, further assessment may be directed towards the individual, their workplace or their actual work tasks. Quite possibly it may involve all three. Generally speaking, it is possible to achieve greater standardisation and generalisability when conducting a work-related assessment in a clinic situation than it is in the actual work environment. Workplace-based assessments tend to be more qualitative in nature (Innes and Straker, 2002). For this reason it is important to identify the purpose of the assessment. You will then be able to ensure that the method you select can provide the required information.

In some instances, the person may need to be referred to a specialist or perhaps for a standardised assessment. For example, a person who sustains a minor head injury in a weekend friendly football game and whose job it is to fly a rescue helicopter for a local charity, may well require a neuro-cognitive assessment from a specialist psychologist. Or perhaps a traveling sales representative who has suffered a mild stroke needs a driving assessment from a registered driving assessor before a return to work can be planned. The following examples of assessment tools are not condition-specific and may be used by occupational therapists to understand more about a particular client's situation. We will learn more about other tools and techniques, such as functional capacity assessments, when we examine condition-specific practice more closely in the following chapter.

The Worker Role Interview is based on the Model of Human Occupation, which we discussed in Chapter 4. This tool takes the form of a semi-structured interview. It is designed to be used during the initial assessment to help identify psychosocial or environmental factors which may enable or inhibit a successful return to work. Different formats of the tool are available, to be used with a worker who has suffered a recent injury or has a long-term disability (Braveman *et al.*, 2005). The worker role interview may assist the therapist to gain a more in-depth understanding of factors, such as the worker's views of their abilities and limitations, their sense of commitment to the worker role, how they feel the injury or disability has impacted on their other roles, their ability to modify their habits and routines, and their perceptions of their work environment (Fisher, 1999).

The Work Environment Impact Scale (Moore-Corner *et al.*, 1998) is also designed to be used as a semi-structured interview. It includes a rating scale which assists the therapist to understand how an individual with either a physical or psychosocial disability perceives their work environment. The therapist may use it with those people who are experiencing difficulties at work, as well as those who are currently away from work due to an injury or illness. In order to create the best 'fit' between the worker, their skills and the work environment, this assessment identifies the environmental characteristics which may facilitate a successful return to work, plus those factors which may be negatively affecting the performance and satisfaction of the worker.

Before your client is ready to resume work, you will also want to ensure that you have minimised the risk of harm to them or others. Risk management involves a problem-solving process based on the three steps of hazard identification, risk assessment and risk elimination or control (WorkCover NSW, 2001). In countries such as Australia, occupational therapists play a key role in occupational health and safety and in assisting employers to prevent workplace injuries. In the UK, preventative practice is not yet well established, so this is not a role commonly held by occupational therapists. Aspects of this function are more usually undertaken by health and safety advisors. However, as you are facilitating an entry into, or a return to, work you will still need to identify, and manage, any risk associated with this. In some instances, particularly where you need a clearer understanding of the actual work tasks, you may need to observe a fit colleague performing similar work duties or work collaboratively with a health and safety advisor, if one is present.

VOCATIONAL EXPLORATION

There may be a number of reasons why you might need to undertake some form of preliminary vocational exploration with a client. It may be the case, for example, that the person cannot return to their previous line of work. This client may therefore need assistance to explore a permanent alternative role within their company, which may involve redeployment, or a totally different career choice. In a different situation, you could perhaps be involved with a young school leaver with a disability who needs to explore the range of potential career options that may be right for him or her. To achieve this, you may be working collaboratively with a personal adviser in the Connexions service. Alternatively, you may be dealing with an adult who has long-term mental health problems and would like to work, but has so far been unable to do so. In a similar vein, many people who have been longstanding recipients of disability benefits may need some form of additional support and guidance to help them identify the steps they may need to take to begin to move towards work.

As a first step you may, in a very general way, want to ascertain the existing work abilities and residual skills of the client. Your assessments may investigate the person's interests, their education and training, any transferable skills they may have gained through previous work or life experience (O'Halloran and Innes, 2005), as well as their wider occupational roles, choices and patterns. All of these factors are indicators of the person's current employability. It will also be helpful for you to know about the demands of any work an individual has done previously, or, if the person is currently expressing an interest in moving into a particular field of work, the complexity, skill, level of responsibility, or other requirements of potential jobs within that field. Ask yourself how well these pre-requisites match your understanding of the individual's current skills, abilities and limitations. Thinking about the complexity of the different tasks involved in particular forms of work may help with this matching process. Figure 6.4 may help you with this process.

Nowadays, as expectations of workers and job demands continue to increase, work opportunities for people who are seeking less complex, more routinised forms of work within the open labour market are becoming scarcer. Many people wanting to move into work will first need to participate in some formal training, if they do not already have recognised skills or qualifications.

A career matching computer software programme which may prove helpful for occupational therapists involved in vocational exploration with clients is Adult

A limited range of very simple, repetitive tasks carried out according to set routines.

A number of simple tasks performed according to a formal routine. Several operations are required to complete each task. Some job-specific skill is required.

A number of the job tasks require skill or knowledge within the particular field. The worker has specific job-related responsibilities which require limited personal decision-making. An error may result in minor productivity losses.

Many varied tasks requiring specific skills and knowledge within the field. There is an increased range and complexity in decision-making situations. Education, training, and/or experience are required. Needs to work collaboratively with others. Errors may result in significant losses or potential harm to others.

Numerous different tasks and increased levels of specialised skills required. The actual job content is unstructured. Advanced problem-solving skills needed across a range of different activities. Supervisory responsibilities involved. Will often need formal training.

Figure 6.4. Levels of task complexity

Directions. The software is published by a company called CASCAiD in conjunction with Loughborough University. The programme provides up-to-date information on more than 1,800 current UK jobs, as well as over 3,000 photographs of people at work. The programme requires the individual to work through a series of on-screen questions and, in doing so, a list of jobs is produced which is consistent with their expressed likes and interests. It is also possible for specific health or disability factors to be taken into consideration during this matching exercise. Job details are given for the list and include such information as a basic description of what the job entails, the level of training required, the salary range and labour market information. More information about this product can be obtained at: http://www.cascaid.co.uk (accessed 15/10/06). An illustration of how occupational therapists might use this software is provided in the following example.

Samuel is a 26-year-old Nigerian man who has schizophrenia. In his teenage years he used to take street drugs which aggravated his psychosis. His illness seems to have stabilised somewhat in recent years and he has not required hospitalisation for his condition for over two years. Samuel is not well-engaged with statutory mental health services, but he regularly attends a local voluntary sector organisation for people from minority ethnic backgrounds. He has good support systems there and is well-liked. He is a long-standing member of a band which plays at the centre and occasionally gets to perform at local gigs. He also helps out in the kitchen by assisting with lunch preparation at the centre one day a week.

For the past six months, the occupational therapist has been running a monthly outreach session at the centre, called Job Shop. This is run in collaboration with a disability employment advisor (DEA) from the local Jobcentre Plus. The purpose of the session is to provide support to any of the centre attendees who decide that they would like to work. Samuel attends one of the sessions stating that he wants to get a job, but doesn't know where to start. He wonders if the occupational therapist is able to help him. After undertaking an initial assessment, the occupational therapist begins to assist Samuel to identify potential fields of interest. He works through the Adult Directions programme, which identifies a range of possible job matches; many of which reflect his interests in music and in catering. The DEA advises Samuel that there is a wide range of opportunities in catering within the local hospitality sector.

Since Samuel has no work history or relevant qualifications, he recognises that he may need to undertake some training. The DEA is able to fund a four-week part-time training place with a local training provider. This will enable Samuel to gain a Basic Food Hygiene and Safety Certificate. The particular course the DEA has in mind is delivered at a slow pace with plenty of opportunities for revision. If Samuel successfully completes the course, there will be several opportunities for him to enter part-time work, either via a supported employment route or in a local social enterprise scheme. He will still be able to continue to attend the centre. Samuel is concerned about how he will get to the course on the right days and at the right time. The occupational therapist agrees to help him work out and practice the route to the training venue, and provide telephone prompts to Samuel on the days the training is taking place. If Samuel has any problems while attending the training, he will contact either the occupational therapist or the DEA. Three months later, Samuel has successfully finished his course. He is now working ten hours a week in a social firm at a local tourist attraction. The business sells hot beverages and home-made produce to visitors. The DEA has done financial calculations with him and he is paid at the national minimum wage for his work. He continues to receive some benefits, so as to ensure he is not worse off through working. He is still able to continue with his music and attends the centre regularly.

In some situations you will work with a person who has multiple barriers preventing them from engaging in work. In these situations, there is a benefit to working collaboratively with other specialists wherever possible. For example, you may have a client with impaired social functioning, such as Asperger's Syndrome (also called high-functioning autism). In-depth specialist assessments may be required as part of their vocational exploration. An occupational psychologist in the Jobcentre Plus service may be able to carry out this type of assessment to help identify an individual's particular strengths and abilities. More information about the occupational psychologist can be found in Chapter 8.

STAGE 4: THE WORKSITE VISIT

By now, you will have some understanding of the person, both as a worker and an occupational being beyond the workplace. You will know about the value they place on their worker role and particular occupational identity. You will also have formed some views as to the functional performance limitations which their condition is placing on their day-to-day functioning. You will be familiar with their aspirations and goals, and, in your own mind, may have begun to formulate some strategies and approaches to assist and support them with achieving these. You may also have identified some barriers which may be preventing them from accessing or returning to work. Next, you will want to gain a further understanding of their work and their work environment. The person's work may be paid or unpaid, and your workplace assessment may therefore be conducted within any of the different service models we identified in Chapter 5. Undertaking a workplace assessment is an important part of facilitating the return to work process. Workplace assessments tend to be qualitative in nature (Innes and Straker, 2003), which reflects the wide variability of settings and job tasks that may need to be assessed. Regardless of the setting – the person may be returning to an existing job, entering supported employment or even a voluntary position – the workplace assessment will still focus on very similar elements.

During the initial worksite visit you should be gathering information about three main subjects:

1. the job itself
2. the wider work environment
3. the employer's views about the individual and their role, or potential role, within the organisation.

In all cases, you will first need to obtain permission from the employer to undertake a workplace assessment. As an external visitor you will often be restricted to the specific work environment of the particular client you are supporting into work. Unfortunately, this often constrains the VR practitioner in their ability to identify, and provide advice about, wider health and well-being issues within the organisation.

At this stage, the occupational therapist will usually undertake an initial worksite screening assessment, often combined with a meeting or telephone discussion with the employer or line manager. This preliminary assessment may raise the need for further assessments to be carried out. With this in mind, we will examine the type of information which you may be seeking from your initial visit to the worksite. It will be important for you to decide, based on your role and your current levels of expertise, which aspects of these assessments are of relevance and also which are within the scope of your competence.

Before we move on to the actual details of the workplace assessment, we will digress slightly in order to gain some insight into how jobs can be classified by their various characteristics. A broader understanding at this more general level may assist the therapist with the process of analysing a particular type of work or job. We will also touch briefly on the resources which may be available to occupational therapists wishing to understand more about the specific characteristics and job tasks of an identified type of work.

TYPES OF JOBS

The Standard Occupational Classification (SOC) was first published in the UK in 1990 and replaced earlier classification systems. It was revised and updated to produce SOC2000 and a new edition is due to be published later in 2007. The classification is based on two main concepts: the job and the kind of work which it entails, and the skills which are required to perform the tasks and duties of it competently.

The major groups of the SOC are:

- Managers and senior officials
- Professional occupations
- Associate professional and technical occupations
- Administrative and secretarial occupations
- Skilled trades occupations
- Personal service occupations
- Sales and customer service occupations
- Process, plant and machine operatives
- Elementary occupations.

More information about the SOC can be viewed at: http://www.statistics.gov.uk/methods_quality/soc/structure.asp (accessed 10/08/06).

Unfortunately, this job classification system is far less comprehensive than those used in other countries, such as America and Canada. Consequently it offers occupational therapists little guidance as to the actual work tasks of a particular job or form of work. In contrast to the SOC, the Dictionary of Occupational Titles (DOT), developed by the Employment Service in the United States of America, contains nearly 13,000 occupational definitions. These were used to match job seekers to jobs from 1939 to the late 1990s. The DOT also defines nine different categories of occupations, which you will see overlap somewhat with those of the SOC:

1. Professional, technical and managerial occupations
2. Clerical and sales occupations
3. Service occupations
4. Agricultural, fishery, forestry and related occupations
5. Processing occupations

6. Machine trades occupations
7. Benchwork occupations
8. Structural work occupations
9. Miscellaneous occupations.

Each of these nine categories is then systematically subdivided. To give an example, under 'Professional, technical and managerial occupations', there are a further 19 divisions, including 'Occupations in medicine and health'. This group contains a further ten divisions; one of which is 'Therapists'. Under this title 20 occupations are identified, including occupational therapist. You will find a general description of the tasks and duties of a person who practices OT, or whatever occupation you have selected. An on-line version of the DOT can be found at: http://www.occupationalinfo.org/ (accessed 10/08/06).

Recent attempts have been made to create a web-based alternative to the DOT. Known as O*Net, this interactive system allows the user to explore and search occupations. It identifies descriptors of the distinguishing characteristics of an occupation, such as occupational requirements, workforce characteristics and occupation-specific information. It also defines person-specific variables such as worker characteristics, worker requirements and experience requirements. The database can be accessed at http://online.onetcenter.org/ (accessed 10/08/02). Canada also has an on-line occupational classification system which details the main duties and employment requirements of different occupations. This can be accessed at: http://www23.hrdc-drhc.gc.ca/2001/e/generic/welcome.shtml (accessed 11/08/06).

Therapists need to recognise that there will be international, as well as national, differences between the job specifications of any given job. These systems may, however, provide a useful starting point for the therapist who wants to gain some basic, preliminary information about a job that is unfamiliar to them. It is also important to bear in mind that a job analysis may take many different forms and be carried out for a variety of different purposes. Occupational psychologists, for example, may be interested in the roles, functions, and skills required to perform a job (Blackmore, 1999), but often use these terms in quite a different way to the meaning which is inferred by occupational therapists.

Another source of information which may provide occupational therapists with some baseline information about a job is the job description. Job descriptions usually have three sections – the first will contain information about the company, the job title and the main objective of the job, as well as perhaps a simple organisational chart. The second section outlines the main responsibilities and job tasks of the post, and the third part often includes a person specification detailing the required expertise of the person that the company is looking for. Job descriptions are not always available, particularly in smaller companies or where the person is a long-standing employee. Frequently, the person's actual job has evolved over time, so that it no longer resembles the post they were employed to fill some years previously.

From the therapist's perspective, a recent, well-written job description may provide useful background information. It will not, however, tell you about the actual functional performance skills needed to carry out the job tasks, or the frequency or relative importance, of each part of the job. It is not unusual to find that a manager and client disagree about the fundamental elements of a given job. To overcome the barriers which this situation may create, occupational therapists may become involved in developing functional job descriptions for certain jobs. We will return to look at functional job descriptions in more detail later in the chapter.

The therapist who practises in a workplace environment may also come across the term job evaluation. This is not the same as job analysis, but is in fact a management technique used to compare the demands of different jobs within an organisation. This evaluation is then drawn on as the basis for developing a fair and equitable grading and pay structure. The aim of job evaluation, therefore, is to evaluate the position, rather than the person who holds the post (Armstrong and Baron, 1995). It is concerned with the demands of the job; for example, the experience and the responsibility which are necessary to carry it out. It is not concerned with factors such as the total volume of work, the number of people required to do the job, or the particular abilities of the post holder. Several job evaluation tools and techniques are commercially available, but they may be based on different criteria such as skill, level of responsibility or perhaps on working conditions (Chartered Institute of Personnel Development, 2007).

Having now increased our general awareness of how we may begin to understand jobs let us return to the VR process and to our workplace assessment.

THE WORKPLACE ASSESSMENT

While undertaking a workplace assessment the occupational therapist will primarily be aiming to:

* assess and identify those duties and tasks which may be suitable for a worker in terms of their physical, psychological, cognitive, social and environmental demands
* identify and negotiate ways in which work tasks may be modified to meet the needs and limitations of the worker
* in the case of injury or illness, identify and negotiate suitable work-place based strategies directed towards promoting the worker's recovery.
(WorkCover NSW, 2000)

In order to meet these objectives, the occupational therapist will draw on an understanding of occupational performance, functional skills and abilities, and task analysis. The therapist will also need to be able to identify the demands of the work within that particular workplace environment. Let us look more closely at some of these features.

Understanding the job and work environment

You will gather specific information about the person's job during the workplace assessment. This is called a job (or work) analysis. The job analysis is 'a study of the worker's activities and the skills required to perform them.' (Holmes, 1985, p.311).

It is a similar process to the task or activity analysis undertaken by occupational therapists in many health or social care settings. You will want to identify and describe the:

- activities and functions performed by the worker
- methods, techniques and/or processes entailed in the work
- discretion, responsibility or accountability involved in performing these tasks
- results of the work, such as the goods produced or services provided
- characteristics of the worker, including their knowledge, skills and ability to achieve the expected work tasks
- context of the work, including the environmental and organisational factors as we discussed above.

(Holmes, 1985)

Specifically, you will be asking yourself the following questions.

What are the physical demands of this work?

This may include identifying the functional positions in which the work tasks are performed, such as standing, sitting, walking, lifting, carrying, pushing, pulling, climbing, balancing, bending, squatting, twisting, crawling, kneeling, rotating, handling, fingering and reaching. It may also include any tools which are used, equipment which needs to be operated and any particular visual, auditory or tactile requirements of the work (Aja, 1996; Jacobs, 1999). We will look at occupational therapists' use of functional capacity assessments in the following chapter.

What are the cognitive demands of this work?

Functional capacity assessments frequently afford less attention to the cognitive demands of a job than to its physical demands. Cognitive aspects of the job that you may need to consider include perceptual requirements, stressors inherent in the work, work intensity, decision-making requirements, memory, concentration and the ability to shift attention amongst multiple tasks.

What are the social demands of this work?

This category may include the level of responsibility of the job, any supervisory duties, leadership requirements and whether the job is carried out autonomously or whether collaboration with others is needed.

What are the environmental conditions under which this work is performed?

This includes the design and layout of the work area, as well as temperature, noise, lighting, ventilation and any risks inherent in the working environment.

During your worksite visit, you will want to learn more about the wider work environment in which the individual works or may be planning to work. Consider the following questions.

What is this company's business?

Knowing the purpose for which a business exists will give you useful clues to the types of work performed and the work environment.

What is the size of this company?

According to the Department of Trade and Industry definition, a large company has more than 250 employees, a medium-sized firm has between 50 and 249 employees, and a small business has 0 to 49 employees (http://www.dti.gov.uk, accessed 17/04/07). Larger companies may well have more resources to be able to support a person with a health condition or disability in the workplace.

How diverse are the job types within this company?

Greater diversity may provide more options for a temporary alternative role, or change to existing duties, during a return to work programme.

How is absence managed within this organisation?

Employers may use different interventions for short- and long-term absences. Not all absence will be attributable to a health condition or disability and the vast majority of cases of absence will be dealt with by the employer or the line manager. It is, however, helpful for occupational therapists to gain an understanding of how organisations may manage attendance issues. Common interventions to manage short-term absence include:

- return to work interviews
- training line managers in absence management
- providing sickness absence information to line managers
- restricting sick pay
- attendance review and monitoring
- disciplinary procedures for unacceptable absence levels
- involving occupational health professionals.

(Chartered Institute of Personnel and Development, 2006b)

Occupational therapists are most likely to play a role in assisting with long-term absence management or in helping to prevent short-term absence becoming long-term absence. Organisations are beginning to acknowledge the need for a formal strategy to assist employees back to work after an absence caused by a prolonged period of ill-health or injury. Therefore, in addition to the management interventions outlined above, some organisations will recognise that changes may be required to the work pattern or the environment, or in some instances a rehabilitation programme may need to be implemented.

Is there an existing return to work or rehabilitation policy?

Some employers will have a policy in place to deal with the phased return to work. You may then be expected to design your graduated programme to fit in with the terms of this policy. If the policy is excessively prescriptive, or is not suitable for your client, you may wish to raise your concerns with the human resources department to try and negotiate a different approach.

Are regular annual staff appraisals undertaken?

Annual staff appraisals are not, strictly speaking, part of your concern as a rehabilitation professional. However, if an individual is off work with work-related stress, for example, and you have been asked to facilitate their return to work, you may find that role conflict or a lack of role clarity are contributing to the person's difficulties at work. An annual appraisal is an important way of focusing on the priorities for a job, and this helps the person to understand what is expected of them within that role, as well as identifying any training needs they may have. This meeting should also alert a trained line manager to any pressures or difficulties occurring within a particular team or department.

What is the employer's perspective?

As well as analysing the job, examining the required functional abilities and the wider environmental concerns, the occupational therapist will also want to gain the employer's views, expectations and opinions. He or she will have their own ideas about the person, their role and the planned return to work. The following questions may help you understand the employer's perspective:

- What are the main work tasks of the client?
- How well did the client previously perform their role?
- Would it be possible for you to observe a fit colleague performing the job tasks, if necessary?
- What is the availability of modified duties?
- Would it be possible to do some work tasks at home?
- Has there been regular contact with the absent employee?
- What is the employer's (or manager's) understanding of the reasons for the client's absence?
- Are they anticipating that the person will return to work? When do they think this is going to occur?
- Are they familiar with their responsibilities under the Disability Discrimination Act, if applicable?

After your visit is completed, you may want to reflect on the following questions, since each will have an impact on the success of any return to work plan which you develop:

- What were your initial impressions of the ethos within the organisation or department?
- Does the employer seem supportive of the person returning? Perhaps on a graduated programme?
- What was the perceived value of the person to this company, both in financial terms and in terms of their skills, abilities and role within the organisation?
- Do any co-workers you met seem supportive or hostile towards the client?
- What was the person's previous attendance pattern like and are there any outstanding capability or disciplinary matters?
- Based on your current knowledge of the client, what is the likely fit between the worker and their work?
- Could the person return to their job with modified duties and restrictions?
- Is there an alternative role they could perform on a temporary basis?
- Do you need additional information?

Following the workplace visit, you may decide that you have gathered sufficient information to enable the development of a return to work plan, which is the next stage in the VR process. Alternatively, you may have identified that you require additional information. You may need further, more specialised assessments to be carried out, perhaps by others, to provide you with this information. For example, you may have identified that a workstation assessment is needed. Some occupational therapists may have the skills or training to undertake this type of assessment, others will not and will therefore refer their client on to an appropriate source. We will return to the workstation assessment in the next chapter.

STAGE 5: THE RETURN TO WORK PLAN

This stage is the most important of the VR process. A return to work plan is a planned graduated programme which is developed by an occupational therapist, in collaboration with the client and the employer, to enable the worker to return to work on suitable duties with the necessary restrictions (WorkCover NSW, 2003). Within the return to work plan, the therapist will outline any modifications to the workplace environment, suitable duties, the hours to be worked, tasks to be avoided and any arrangements for supervision, additional training and support. The importance of gaining the agreement of all parties for a return to work plan is paramount and cannot be over-stated. Without this contract it will not be possible for the client's return to work to go ahead. It is important that, once agreed, the plan is monitored and regularly reviewed by the occupational therapist.

A written return to work plan should include:

- the job title and place of work
- an agreed goal

- the name of the supervisor
- the hours and days to be worked
- duties to be performed together with any restrictions or duties to avoid
- any medical appointments or treatments to be attended
- the commencement date of the programme
- the length of the programme
- review dates
- the documented agreement of all parties.

(adapted from WorkCover NSW, 2003, p.15)

A return to work plan should contain the precise details of the timings and tasks to be carried out by each party involved in the return to work programme. A sample return to work plan is outlined in Figure 6.5.

STAGE 6: INTERVENTION

In this section we will examine a selection of potential interventions that may be used by occupational therapists at this stage of the VR process. We do, however, need to recognise that the scope and range of these interventions will differ across different organisations. The case management approach, which is currently a popular mode of service delivery in VR across a number of sectors, presents the occupational therapist with limited opportunities to undertake clinical or therapeutic interventions themselves. This is not the primary purpose of the case manager role. We will return to discuss case management in more detail in Chapter 8. We will also discuss in the next chapter interventions, approaches and resources which are of specific relevance to clients with a particular disability or health condition.

SUPPORTING THE RETURN TO WORK

We are now at the stage of the person actually entering, or returning to, work. A comprehensive plan has been developed and agreed by all parties concerned. A return to work date has been agreed. It is common for individuals to feel increasingly fearful of returning to work once a date is set, especially if they have been away from the workplace for some time. It is important for the occupational therapist to recognise this, prepare the person for this experience and provide support through any concerns, as necessary. It is not unusual for people to experience disturbed sleep patterns and reduced appetite in the days prior to their return to work. Individuals may often question their ability to perform their work tasks competently and wonder how others in the workplace will respond to them. In most instances, reassurance and encouragement will be sufficient to help the person through these fears. Occasionally, the person may need to be assisted to develop better coping mechanisms; for example, basic anxiety management strategies and techniques.

SAMPLE RETURN TO WORK PLAN

Name: Job title:

Place of work:
Line manager:

Vocational rehabilitation goal: To return to full duties as a call centre supervisor, working from 3.30–11.30pm with a one-hour break, five days in seven.

Date of commencement of return to work programme:

Week	Objective	Person(s) responsible	Review action
1 and 2 (date)	To work from 7–11 pm on Tuesday, Thursday and Saturday (12 hours).	Client and OT	Telephone call (Monday and Friday).
	Perform the modified tasks and actions outlined in the attached guidelines, taking breaks as required (Appendix 1).	Client and line manager	Weekly meeting on Tuesday.
3 and 4 (date)	To work as for weeks 1 and 2 and also on Wednesday and Friday from 7.30–9.30 pm (16 hours).	Client and OT	Telephone call (weekly on Friday) and additional midweek calls if required.
	To commence limited supervisory duties, in collaboration with co-worker, as outlined in Appendix 1.	Client and named co-worker	
	To continue to take short breaks when needed.	Client and line manager	Weekly meeting on Tuesday.
	Review meeting	Client, OT and line manager	Discuss progress and review plan as necessary.
5 and 6	Daily attendance from 6.30–11.30pm (with a 30-minute break) (22.5 hours).	Client and OT	Telephone call (weekly on Friday).
	To continue with work tasks from weeks 3 and 4 (Appendix 1).	Client and line manager	Weekly meeting on Tuesday.
7	Daily attendance from 5.30–11.30 pm (with a one-hour break) (25 hours).	Client and OT	Telephone call (weekly on Friday).
	Resume independent supervisory duties for part of the shift, as negotiated with employer.	Client and line manager	Weekly meeting on Tuesday.
8	Full-time hours resumed.	Client and OT	Telephone call (weekly on Friday)
	To continue to negotiate resumption of additional duties.	Client and line manager	Fortnightly meeting on Tuesday.
9	Full-time hours and normal duties resumed.	Client and OT	Telephone call (weekly on Friday).
		Client and line manager	Meetings as required.
10–12	Full-time hours and normal duties.	Client and OT	E-mail contact or client to phone if necessary.
		Client and line manager	Meetings as required.

Agreement

This return to work plan will be monitored and reviewed at regular intervals. I confirm that I have been involved in its development and/or that I support the actions contained therein.

Employee: **Date:**

Employer/manager: **Date:**

Occupational therapist: **Date:**

GP/medical consultant: **Date:**

Other treating health professional(s):   **Date:**

Appendix 1

Included within this section of the return to work plan will be details about the modified work duties, together with any physical restrictions or specific tasks to be avoided. It may include details about any breaks which should be taken, or actions which the employee should take, such as varying their work tasks, doing particular exercises or ensuring that they arrange their workstation ergonomically at the start of a shift. It may also include training activities to be undertaken in the workplace, arrangements for shadowing others in a supernumerary capacity or pre-scheduled meetings with an identified 'buddy' who is able to provide day-to-day support in the early stages of the programme. If the job includes regular overtime or extended periods of travel, then these may also be included in the restrictions, as appropriate. These sorts of concessions may be of particular importance in a workplace with high levels of job intensity or workload pressures, particularly where they may have contributed to an employee suffering from work-related stress, for example.

Each return to work plan will be specific to the individual and their needs, taking into account their limitations, the type of work and the nature of their workplace. It is important to remember that you will need to secure the employer's agreement for any suggestions that you are making, particularly where a cost may be incurred.

Figure 6.5. Sample return to work plan

DEVELOPING IN-WORK SUPPORTS

One of the criticisms leveled at the Government's New Deal programmes and other employment initiatives, is that they have placed a far greater emphasis on assisting people to secure a job, than they have on helping those people to retain that job in the longer term. Ways to support job retention should be an important consideration for occupational therapists, since repeated loss of the worker role may have a detrimental effect on a person's well-being and disabled people frequently experience difficulties keeping a new job. A small study recently identified a range of non-financial supports aimed at helping people, particularly those who have moved from state benefits into paid employment, to retain their jobs (Kellard *et al.*, 2002). The strategies suggested include:

- Job coaching is on-the-job practical assistance provided to individuals for the tasks that they need to carry out to actually do their job
- Mentoring involves matching a new employee with a co-worker, or possibly an external volunteer, who then helps the new employee to adjust to the workplace and the routine of being back in work
- Peer support groups provide new workers with support by creating opportunities to share their experiences with others in similar positions
- Case management, where case management services are targeted towards specific client groups; such as, women returning to work, disaffected young people and disabled people (the authors of the study suggest that some small-scale studies have demonstrated the success of this approach)
- Post-employment education and training, career ladders and career guidance have been found to improve retention in some instances, but all can be potentially expensive to deliver
- Although there is no evidence for their effectiveness, telephone help lines may provide practical assistance to employers and employees, and possible strategies to help retention.

EMPLOYER EDUCATION

In the UK, few employers currently have a good grasp or understanding of the purpose or application of rehabilitation for work. They may have unrealistic expectations or even misperceptions of what it is about. Employers are not bound by the strong legislative framework which exists in a number of other countries, particularly in terms of their responsibility to accommodate injured workers, for example. This lack of understanding may be a barrier to a successful entry into, or return to, work. The VR practitioner therefore has a key role in the education of employers across a number of different situations:

- working collaboratively with a disability employment advisor to meet with local employers, in order to help create supported employment opportunities for people with a health problem or disability
- act as a mentor or a job coach to a person who has entered a job through a supported employment route
- advise an employer on their responsibilities under the DDA (2005)
- assist an employer to identify situations where rehabilitation may be of value
- provide an employer with information about a particular clinical condition – this must be undertaken in a way that maintains client confidentiality
- offer to run workshops for employees on issues such as back care or mental health awareness – again, this must be done in a way that maintains client confidentiality.

BORROWED KNOWLEDGE: ERGONOMICS AND COGNITIVE BEHAVIOURAL THERAPY

A number of parallels have been drawn between the development of the ergonomics profession and that of OT (Berg Rice, 1999). Therapists who specialise in working with people with musculoskeletal conditions recognise that a knowledge of ergonomics can be of value. Some occupational therapists gain additional qualifications to further their knowledge in this field, so achieving a dual qualification that enables them to also practice as a registered ergonomist. Many more occupational therapists in VR make use of an ergonomics approach within their practice, since there are numerous shared interests between the ergonomist and the occupational therapist (Jacobs, 1999; Hignett, 2000). On their website, the Ergonomics Society describes ergonomics, which is also sometimes called human factors, as:

> *The application of scientific information concerning humans to the design of objects, systems and environment for human use. Ergonomics comes into everything which involves people. Ergonomic design is a way of considering design options to ensure that people's capabilities and limitations are taken into account. This helps to ensure that the product is fit for use by the target users.*

Work situations where ergonomic principles may be applied include the design of:

- equipment and systems, such as computers, to make them easier to use and reduce the likelihood of the operator making errors when using them
- tasks and jobs so that they are effective and take human needs into account, while ensuring that the job fits the person
- equipment to improve working posture and ease the load on the body, thus reducing work-related musculoskeletal disorders
- work environments, including factors such as lighting and heating, to suit the needs of the users and the tasks performed.

More information about ergonomics and the Ergonomics Society can be found at www.ergonomics.org.uk (accessed 24/09/07).

We will return to look further at the application of an ergonomic approach in Chapter 7.

Another common approach which is currently used by occupational therapists is the cognitive behavioural approach. Again, we need to distinguish between cognitive behavioural therapy (CBT) and a cognitive behavioural approach. CBT is a form of psychotherapy which requires a postgraduate qualification and supervision. Some occupational therapists undertake this training to become a recognised cognitive behavioural therapist. More information about additional training may be obtained from the British Association for Behavioural and Cognitive Psychotherapies website: http://www.babcp.com (accessed 17/07/07).

Occupational therapists more commonly draw on a cognitive behavioural approach, which is highly compatible with the problem-solving strategies that are a core skill of many occupational therapists (Creek, 2003). Interventions are designed to help the person become more aware of their reasoning and how automatic thoughts may affect the way they respond or behave in certain situations, particularly when they are distressed. Occupational therapists may use this approach to assist the person to develop their skills to overcome their avoidance, or fear, of participating in certain activities or situations. Learning how, and why, they respond in a particular way may help some people to regain their sense of control, thus enabling them to move forwards. In the next chapter, we will return to explore some of the ways in which cognitive behavioural strategies may be used by occupational therapists with people with mental health problems.

DEVELOPING FUNCTIONAL JOB DESCRIPTIONS

If you work closely with a particular employer, perhaps in an in-house occupational health setting, your role as a return to work facilitator may be enhanced by developing functional job descriptions. As we discussed earlier, a standard job description will outline the main job tasks, but will seldom consider the functional abilities to perform the job. The functional job description is created by an occupational therapist, in discussion with employees who perform the role, and their line manager(s). It is based on the occupational therapist's observations while shadowing skilled workers who are performing their normal work tasks. Where a functional job description has been developed, it can be a useful basis for discussion during the planning and implementation of a return to work plan.

WORKING COLLABORATIVELY WITH OTHERS

A number of occupational therapists, particularly those working in the NHS, would like to be able to do more to address the work needs of their clients. This may not, however, be a service priority of the particular organisation which employs them. Resource constraints may prevent the occupational therapist from extending their role into this field. The following scenario, however, illustrates how this can, in part, be overcome by developing collaborative working relationships with other organisations, such as the Jobcentre Plus or voluntary sector providers.

Tony is a 48-year-old former barman. Five years ago he was diagnosed with ulcerative colitis, a disease which causes chronic inflammation of the bowel. He lost his job as a barman, shortly after the diagnosis was confirmed, because of his lengthy absences from work due to his ill-health. He has been out of work and claiming incapacity benefits ever since. For the last two years, Tony has also been treated for depression by his GP. Tony knows that he has relapses and periods of remission from his ulcerative colitis, and he does his best to manage his condition sensibly. He knows that his fluctuating health means that no employer is likely to want to employ him. He would not want to return to his occupation as a barman anyway, because he has found alcohol to be a relapse trigger for his colitis.

Tony has no formal qualifications. He keeps himself fit by going to the gym regularly, but the fact that he is unable to work gets him down and his GP recognises that his mood is quite low at present. He refers Tony to the local community mental health intake team for further advice. An occupational therapist sees Tony for an initial screening assessment, and it is plain that he has troubling symptoms of depression. The occupational therapist recognises that his lack of meaningful work is contributing to his current depressed state, and arranges a follow-up appointment to explore this further with him. At this second meeting it is very clear that Tony feels a need to work and has retained a strong worker identity, despite being away from the workplace for some time. The occupational therapist suggests that it would be worthwhile meeting with the disability employment adviser at the local Jobcentre Plus, with whom the occupational therapist has developed a good working relationship.

Tony is unsure about this, since he has significant financial pressures. He is worried that if he shows an interest in work he may be moved on to Job Seekers Allowance and this would reduce his income and increase his debts. The occupational therapist is able to re-assure him that this will not be the outcome and offers to attend with him, to allay his fears. He is agreeable to this arrangement. At the meeting, the DEA discusses the option of undergoing further training, with a view to becoming self-employed. She undertakes some Better Off calculations to check that entering paid work would not reduce his income. For Tony, being self-employed is an attractive option because it means that he would be able to take up work offers when he is in remission. Most importantly to him, this arrangement would mean that he wouldn't feel he was letting anyone down when he suffered a relapse. Removing this source of anxiety is an important consideration, because Tony knows that his condition is aggravated by stress.

Tony is interested in one of the suggestions put forward, which is to become a self-employed security guard. He enjoys working at night, is physically fit, and would meet the requirements for this line of work. There are plenty of opportunities in the local area, but he would need a recognised qualification. The DEA is able to fund a place for Tony on a training course to gain the qualification he needs. He is, however, very anxious about undertaking this six-week training programme because he has very poor memories of school, and has avoided any form of formal learning since then. The occupational therapist offers to provide regular telephone support to help Tony manage his anxieties about attending the course and if this proves to be insufficient, Tony could participate in the next anxiety management course being run by the occupational therapist in two months time. The occupational therapist keeps the GP informed of the interventions to date, and has also sent through a short report. The occupational therapist asks Tony to discuss his plans to return to work with his GP, so as to ensure that there is medical approval. The GP supports Tony's plan.

Following further discussions, and with some trepidation, Tony enrols on the course for security guards. He passes successfully, with regular telephone support from the occupational therapist and a couple of visits to see the DEA. He did not need to attend the anxiety management course. He is then put in touch with Business Link, which, as mentioned previously, is a public sector funded organisation which assists small businesses (www.businesslink.gov.uk). The advisor there helps him develop a business plan, obtain funding for a van and develop some publicity fliers, which he distributes around the local area.

Three months later, Tony has secured two medium-term contracts. One is with a local construction company, which is about to begin a new property development, and the other with a garden centre, which has recently become a target for vandals. He feels much better in himself, has less financial worries and has begun to reduce his anti-depressants, under his GP's supervision. The occupational therapist discharges him from their caseload.

This case study illustrates how collaborative working with others in different organisations, in this case the DEA and the GP, can effectively help your clients to move towards, or into, work.

The final part of this section outlines potential opportunities for entrepreneurial occupational therapists within the growing VR sector. This has been based largely on initiatives and interventions which continue to be successful for occupational therapists in other countries. Understanding the rationale behind these types of interventions, and what these terms mean, will also assist those readers who wish to consult the international literature in this field.

WORK HARDENING AND OCCUPATIONAL REHABILITATION

Although work hardening and occupational rehabilitation are not currently widely practiced in the UK, they are worthy of inclusion in this section, since they may present therapists with opportunities for service development in the future. Occupational therapists in countries such as America, successfully deliver a wide variety of work hardening programmes. These are rehabilitation programmes which are designed specifically to assist workers who have sustained a work-related injury. Their purpose is to regain sufficient functional performance skills to enable them to return to competitive employment. The majority of these programmes are funded through insurance coverage from workers' compensation schemes. They are generally based in clinic-type settings and make use of structured, graded, work-oriented activities (King, 1993).

In Australia and New Zealand, occupational rehabilitation is similarly concerned with workers who have suffered a work-related injury, and is also funded by workers' compensation insurance. It is defined as:

> the restoration of ... injured worker(s) to the fullest physical, psychological, social, vocational and economic usefulness of which they are capable, consistent with pre-injury status. It is a managed process aimed at maintaining injured or ill workers in or returning them to suitable employment. It involves early intervention with appropriate, adequate and timely services based on assessment of the injured worker's needs.
> (WorkCover NSW, 1993a, p.8 cited in Innes, 1995, p.148).

In contrast to the American form of provision, however, occupational rehabilitation is more likely to take place in the actual workplace, rather than a clinic setting. Instead of adopting a reactive approach to injury management, the occupational therapist involved in occupational rehabilitation routinely takes a more preventative role, which emphasises safe working practices and early re-integration into the workforce (Innes, 1995; Innes and Straker, 2002).

Injury management services are still in their infancy in the UK, probably because there is an absence of the legislative backdrop which can be found in other countries. Also, only a very small percentage of workers will require these types of intervention. The changing nature of workplace-related conditions, such as the rise in mental health problems and the agenda to keep older workers in work, means that occupational therapists would be well advised to retain a wider perspective on their potential contribution to workplace health and well-being, beyond injury management.

HELPING TO CREATE HEALTHY WORKPLACES

Canadian occupational therapists play a strong role in health promotion and workplace mental health. Cockburn *et al.* (2004) outline how occupational therapists may provide employees within an organisation with education about depression and stress. They may also undertake job matching and create job profiles, to ensure that workers are well matched with their jobs. They are able to provide ongoing support to managers and employees through developing suitable return to work plans for people with mental ill-health, while also helping to create a positive culture in the workplace. In the UK, the quality of work and the creation and development of healthy workplaces is attracting growing attention. In a recent publication, The Faculty of Public Health and The Faculty of Occupational Medicine (2006, p.6) identified the following benefits of a healthy workplace:

- *improved productivity and performance*
- *reduced absenteeism and other costs associated with ill-health*
- *fewer injuries and accidents, and insurance and compensation claims*
- *improved employee morale and staff retention*
- *employees who are more receptive to and better able to cope with change*
- *An enhanced business reputation and corporate responsibility.*

They identify how key performance areas, such as retention and rehabilitation, the reduction of stress, musculoskeletal disorders and substance misuse, combined with improved physical activity and eating habits, can help create a safe and healthy work environment.

GROUP INTERVENTIONS

The majority of VR interventions that are currently undertaken by occupational therapists within employment settings in the UK take place on an individual, one-to-one basis. Group work is a core skill of many occupational therapists, and this is an area where there is likely to be scope for further development in the employment sector in the future. The literature reflects the different purposes for which group work has been used in VR. For example, supporting older workers who are searching for employment (Kemp and Kleinplatz, 1985) or certain supported employment initiatives, such as a small mobile crew of two to three individuals working together to undertake service jobs, like cleaning and gardening, in a community setting (University of North Carolina, 2006). Some occupational therapists employed within the Government-funded Condition Management Programmes introduce groups based on a cognitive behavioural approach to build confidence, manage anxiety and encourage supported self-help, for example. We will examine these interventions in the next chapter, when we look more specifically at mental health problems.

STAGE 7: EVALUATION/OUTCOME

The success of the VR process may often, rather crudely, be measured by what are called hard outcomes; such as whether or not the person enters or returns to work, or how many people the occupational therapist successfully enabled to return to work across the course of a year. These measures are understandable, because the service objectives will usually be directed towards achieving this goal, and, sometimes, the funding for the service will be dependent on it. The Government's planned payment by results strategy may increase the number of occupational therapists, and other providers, whose success is determined by these types of markers. Hard outcomes such as reduced number of days of absence, increased chances of returning to work and improved benefit-to-cost ratios have been reported amongst different groups (Arnetz *et al.*, 2003; Dean & Dolan 1999). Measuring and analysing outcomes is, in fact, a complex task, particularly in view of the wide ranging variables which may influence the success of the rehabilitation programme (King, 1993).

There is however, also a need for the recognition of soft outcomes, such as taking a step towards work, perhaps by doing a training course, engaging in voluntary work, maybe achieving a better quality of life or greater job satisfaction. These measures are particularly important for those who are furthest away from the labour market, and may need a greater number of stepping stones to eventually reach this destination. These less tangible improvements are, of course, far harder to measure or demonstrate. Gaining the views and opinions of programme participants is perhaps an under-utilised form of outcome measurement. Satisfaction surveys, for example, can be a valuable source of feedback about the strengths and weaknesses of the service. However, further research to measure and effectively demonstrate the value of different types of outcomes is still needed.

STAGE 8: DISCHARGE

We have reached the final stage in the VR process: discharge. Expert practice suggests that, in the case of a return to work, this should ideally take place about three weeks after an employee has resumed their full hours and duties. Sometimes, the employer makes a false assumption that once the person is back to full capacity, they are now fully recovered. They may therefore believe that there is no longer any need to be concerned, and that things can now be forgotten. The occupational therapist should ensure that an employer is aware that this is not necessarily the case, and that care should to be taken to reduce the likelihood of a relapse occurring.

Making a decision about when is the right time to discharge a client often requires sound judgement. Ideally this should be when the client's goals have been met or the therapist is no longer able to add any value to the client's situation (Chapman *et al.*, 2006). Occupational therapists practising within a commercial environment may find there is sometimes a sense of pressure to discharge the client at the earliest possible opportunity. Alternatively, if an individual is not making sufficient progress there is a similar obligation. This does, of course, make sound business sense and within the current health economy there is a need for rehabilitation to be cost effective. Sometimes, however, the occupational therapist may be left with the feeling that they could possibly have done more or given more time.

For the person with a health condition or disability who has entered work for the first time, or after a long absence, ideally provision should be made for ongoing, long-term support. Earlier in this chapter, we discussed the forms that this support may take. Discharge, in this situation, should be gradual and over an extended period of time, ensuring that alternative supports are in place, as necessary. This will be of particular importance where an individual has a fluctuating medical condition, or perhaps significant psycho-social stressors outside of the work environment.

We have now worked our way steadily through the VR process from the point of referral to discharge. In the next chapter we will be examining common approaches and interventions for people who have a particular type of health condition or disability.

7 Vocational Rehabilitation for Specific Health Conditions and Disabilities

So far, we have learned about a range of service models, approaches and interventions that may be of value to our clients, as workers. We have thought about how we might understand work from an occupation-focused perspective. We have explored the work needs, and the barriers to work, for clients who may have any number, or combination, of disabilities, health problems or other disadvantages. In doing so, we have discovered that vocational rehabilitation (VR), in itself, is not illness or disability specific. That said, it is important to recognise that many occupational therapists are employed in services which are targeted towards clients who have a particular medical condition or disability. This section, therefore, focuses specifically on what is currently known, and understood, about particular conditions, work, and VR. It may serve as a useful starting point for the reader who wishes to find out more specific information about VR with their client group.

The literature relating to specific conditions remains strongly focused on medical treatment and interventions. For people of working age, vocational recovery should be taking place alongside, and as an integral component of, this medical recovery. In many situations, this is currently not the case (British Society of Rehabilitation Medicine, 2000). Disappointingly little research has been directed towards successful vocational strategies and return to work outcomes for different patient populations. Seldom are these variables seen as indicators of successful rehabilitation. The field of mental health has, perhaps, seen the most advances in this area. This is partly as a result of the social inclusion agenda and the focus on community management of mental ill-health. Many other conditions remain locked into a medical model of care.

The conditions discussed in this section have been very loosely grouped under the headings of mental health disorders, musculoskeletal disorders, cardiac and respiratory disorders and neurological disorders. There has been a need to be selective, since each of these conditions could easily fill a book of its own. This chapter attempts to combine current trends and policy drivers, with existing occupational therapy (OT) research evidence. It also highlights practical strategies, interventions and further resources for each of these four broad condition-related groupings.

An assumption has been made that you will already have a degree of familiarity with many of the functional difficulties faced by your particular client group. However, it is worth noting that clients with different conditions often share a number of common troublesome symptoms which can impact on their work abilities. Pain, fatigue, fear, stigma, discrimination, and a lack of understanding, will frequently have to be faced. Similarly, early intervention, education, problem-solving and condition self-management are common intervention themes. In the light of this, you may find potentially useful information of relevance to your particular clients beyond the margins of the particular condition in which you are interested.

VOCATIONAL REHABILITATION WITH CLIENTS WITH MENTAL HEALTH PROBLEMS

There is a very high prevalence of mental health problems within the population, yet only a minority of this group are in any form of employment. We read earlier about how people with mental health conditions now form the largest group of incapacity benefit (IB) claimants. Mental illness comes in a variety of forms, and there are particular barriers and obstacles to work for each person with this condition. So, there is an array of issues which need to be explored within this section on VR in mental health. This section has, therefore, been divided as follows:

- severe and enduring mental health problems
- common mental health problems
- substance abuse problems.

Of course clients may have multiple barriers to employment, such a dual diagnosis or mental health problems combined with a forensic history, so we will touch very briefly on some of the issues for these client groups as well.

WORK AND THE CLIENT WITH SEVERE AND ENDURING MENTAL HEALTH PROBLEMS

Satisfying work, as we know, can provide a central role in life and contribute to a sense of social and community inclusion. We are also keenly aware that there is a strong political drive to increase the number of people who are entering employment. People with serious mental illnesses, such as schizophrenia, bipolar affective disorder and the more severe forms of depression, however, often have difficulties choosing, getting and keeping a job. Only a minority of people from this client group is, at present, able to secure and sustain competitive employment within the open labour market (Reker et al., 2000). Figures cited in the literature suggest that just 15 per cent of people with chronic, serious mental health problems are employed (Evans and Repper, 2000; Tsang et al., 2000). This is despite the fact that surveys, case studies and personal narratives have consistently suggested that many people with these types of conditions want to work (Evans and Repper, 2000). Vocational rehabilitation and work participation have become a growing focus of concern for mental health professionals. This is particularly so for occcupational therapists, since this group often forms a significant percentage of their caseload in an NHS community mental health setting.

Improving mental health has been given a high priority, and The National Service Framework (NSF) for Mental Health (Department of Health, 1999a) provides a clear directive to promote social inclusion, combat discrimination, and take action to address employment, training and needs for other occupation. This message has been reinforced by The National Institute for Clinical Excellence (NICE) (2002), which has developed clinical guidelines recommending that, as part of good practice, a comprehensive assessment of the occupational status and vocational aspirations of people with schizophrenia should be undertaken as part of their treatment under the Care Programme Approach. Also, that a range of local employment schemes should be developed, through partnership arrangements, which suit the different employment needs of people with severe mental health problems. Combined with a wider social inclusion agenda, this seems to have provided occupational therapists in mental health with an additional platform from which to pursue VR within the NHS. It reinforces the need for a range of different pathways to accessing work opportunities across the continuum of VR, as we discussed in an earlier chapter. These access routes are not necessarily based on the traditional ways of entering employment. Therefore, occupational therapists need to be familiar with the different designs of service models that may best meet the work needs of their clients who want to move into work.

Despite some notable successes, however, a number of obstacles to implementation remain. There are service barriers, such as a lack of communication and co-ordination, benefits barriers, such as the complexity of the system and a fear of loss of benefits, and stigma, including the negative attitudes of some health professionals and family members (Henry and Lucca, 2002). Consequently, progress towards supporting clients' vocational aspirations from within community mental health teams, has reportedly been slow to develop (Seebohm and Secker, 2003).

Depending on the availability of services in your local area, it may be necessary to engage in collaborative ventures with other organisations to help establish a wider range of meaningful work and employment options. These will provide important alternatives for occupational choice, and for engaging in satisfying work for those who are not yet ready for the demands of obtaining a job through a competitive interview process. Additionally, when developing new services, or evaluating the relevance and effectiveness of old ones, it is important to bear in mind that the current evidence base points quite strongly away from pre-vocational training, such as developing basic work skills and work habits. Better outcomes have reportedly been achieved through initiatives such as supported employment (Crowther et al., 2001).

South West London and St George's Mental Health NHS Trust is offered as an example of good practice by the Department of Health (2005) because it has successfully increased its employment rate for people with severe and enduring mental health problems. A vocational services strategy was developed, based on the individual placement and support approach – a type of supported employment which we discussed earlier. Occupational therapists, together with mental health and employment co-ordinators working within clinical teams, enabled people with severe mental health problems to access open employment and mainstream education. Care plans were focused towards individual choice and included ongoing support. The success of the strategy was such that, after one year, the employment rate rose from ten to 40 per cent. The percentage of those not engaged in some form of education, training or employment dropped from 55 to five per cent. Over the course of a year, 271 people were successfully supported into open paid employment. This demonstrates the effectiveness of a co-ordinated approach to assisting this group into employment.

There is a host of approaches and interventions which you may use when exploring and creating work opportunities with your clients, and next we will overview a selection of them.

Occupational choice

When setting out to assist a client to obtain work it is important to gain a clear idea of what the person is aiming for, so that you are able to begin the VR process with a shared understanding of their rehabilitation goal. Put another way, understanding a client's volitional narrative can help the therapist to identify and seek out meaningful work opportunities and experiences for that person (Barrett *et al.*, 1999; Strong, 1998). As well as helping to discover the person's motivations and beliefs, creating a vocational profile in this way may also assist in pinpointing those factors which may be acting as a barrier to work (Davis and Rinaldi, 2004). These are crucial elements in the recovery process.

However, since there may be both benefits and drawbacks to entering employment for people who have mental health problems (Honey, 2004), the person's views of what they perceive to be valued and meaningful work need to be explored at the outset. If the person is thinking about employment, talk with them about their reasons for deciding now is the right time to pursue this option. Do they feel that they have an understanding of their condition and how it affects them? Do they feel ready to take on new challenges? Have they thought about how they might manage any setbacks and the strategies they might use to maintain their health? What do they think about disclosing their mental health condition to a prospective employer? What support networks might they use (Commonwealth Rehabilitation Service Australia, 2004)? These are all issues which you will want to address with the person as you move through the VR process outlined in the previous chapter.

Combating stigma

It has long been known that stigma is one of the greatest barriers to work which is faced by people with mental health problems (Combs and Omvig, 1986; Henry and Lucca, 2002). The actual diagnosis or severity of the psychiatric symptoms experienced by an individual is a poor indicator of whether, or not, the person has the ability to engage in work (Anthony, 1994). However, despite this fact, just four out of ten employers would consider employing people with mental health problems, compared to six out of ten who would contemplate taking on someone with a physical disability. People who have mental health problems do not only face discrimination in trying to get a job, more than a third of people who have been in work and developed mental health problems report that they have been dismissed or forced to resign from their job (Office of the Deputy Prime Minister, 2004).

In order to create work opportunities for clients with mental health problems, the occupational therapist who undertakes VR needs to recognise and pro-actively make efforts to tackle these issues of stigma and discrimination. A good starting point may be to identify people or groups who may be interested in change. Education through both informal and formal channels needs to address the common myths which are frequently held by people about mental illness and those who have it. These myths may include:

- *recovery from mental illness is impossible*
- *people who have a mental health problem tend to be second-rate workers*
- *people with a psychiatric disability aren't able to tolerate stress on the job (this is also a common concern of health professionals – this stress most often occurs where there is a poor match between the individual worker and the work or the workplace and where the person has inadequate support)*
- *people with mental health problems are unpredictable, potentially violent and dangerous.*

(Mental Health Association in Pennsylvania, undated, p.1)

Early intervention and prevention

Conditions such as schizophrenia, schizophreniform psychosis, schizo-affective disorder and drug-induced psychosis often present during adolescence or young adulthood. This is a crucial life stage when the young person is moving towards independence and is about to enter work or further education. The OT literature describes how early intervention and prevention programmes can help prevent relapse, as well as assisting young people to enter paid employment, voluntary work or further education (Parlato *et al.*, 1999). Strategies and interventions which may be used by the occupational therapist include:

- psycho-education
- the development of a positive therapeutic relationship to help maintain communication with families and peers
- enabling the young person to develop mastery over the illness (see self-management and recovery in the next section)
- provision of services away from the mainstream psychiatric unit to prevent stigma
- collaborative group work to help engage young people
- active participation in activities designed to assist optimal functioning.

Self-management and recovery

Enabling a person to take control of, and manage, their own condition in the context of their life as a whole, is a central theme in the process of recovery (Gould *et al.*, 2005). A key turning point is when a person takes an active decision to recover. This is not, of course, a cure, since the condition may be of a long-term nature, but rather it is the very personal process of facing and overcoming the adverse effects of experiencing mental health problems. Recovery, in this sense, centres around personal development and growth. Feelings of hope and optimism for the future need to be nurtured and strategies need to be developed in collaboration with others to enable change to allow the person to move forwards.

Recovery involves the person taking steps to live their life as fully as possible, rather than feeling that they are ruled by their condition. As part of this process, the person needs to be able to see themself as being capable of taking charge of their condition and of recovery. This state of mind contrasts strongly with a viewpoint of being merely a passive recipient of health and social care interventions.

Although much of this recognition takes place at a personal level, it may undoubtedly be facilitated and supported by a commitment amongst organisations, as well as individual frontline staff, such as occupational therapists, doctors, and community psychiatric nurses, to adopting a recovery-oriented approach. Concepts such as the lived experience, the recovery journey and recovery narratives, the need for a supportive environment, and taking small steps towards recovery (Rethink, 2005), will be familiar concepts to many occupational therapists who work within the mental health field. Helping the person adjust to the sense of loss which is often caused by the onset of a mental illness, as well as helping them develop their confidence and self-esteem, are important objectives (Bassett *et al.*, 2001; Gould *et al.*, 2005). Taking these steps towards, and into, work may be seen as an integral part of the recovery process. For young people who have a psychiatric condition, it has been suggested that the recovery framework should include:

- evidence-based employment
- educational assistance
- mental health care
- brief vocational counselling
- illness management skills
- training in stigma countering and disclosure strategies
- context specific social skills and skills in social network development.

(Lloyd and Waghorn, 2007)

Many of the ideas and beliefs that underpin the notions of recovery and self-management are also of relevance to others who have a long-term condition, not only those with a mental health disability.

WORK AND THE CLIENT WITH A COMMON MENTAL HEALTH PROBLEM

A second, large group of people who may need VR are those suffering from what is frequently termed a common mental health problem. This may include conditions such as anxiety, depression and stress-induced mental ill-health. These conditions may, or may not, be work related. The fact that they are widespread does not mean that common mental health problems are trivial; they can lead to significant disability and hardship for large sectors of the population. In contrast to people with severe and enduring mental health problems, many people in this group may have a job but be absent from work, or may have worked previously and now be receiving disability benefits.

The majority of the treatments and interventions received by this group will fall under the remit of primary care services. However, therapists are seldom deployed in a VR capacity in this setting (Joss, 2002). People with these conditions are therefore, at present, unlikely to be seen by an occupational therapist, or receive any other form of VR service from within the NHS (Office for National Statistics, 2003). A few exceptions may, of course, be found. Robdale (2004) describes a successful employment retention scheme that brings together at an early stage the various parties who will be involved in the return to work process. Other examples include clients who may be seen by an occupational therapist in an occupational health setting, or in a facilitated return to work scheme as part of an income protection insurance policy (in the insurance sector), or where the occupational therapist delivers a Condition Management Programme for IB claimants. While there is considerable literature about common mental health problems and work, there is reportedly little evidence on vocational outcomes following some form of rehabilitation for this group (Waddell and Burton, 2004). It is unsurprising, therefore, that research suggests neither primary nor secondary care healthcare practitioners, including GPs, practice nurses, psychiatrists, psychologists and community mental health nurses, have a clear strategy on the management of common mental health problems (Nolan *et al.*, 2003).

Stress at work

It may be helpful to begin by clarifying the particular sources of stress, symptoms and coping mechanisms of an individual who has work-related or occupational stress. Stein *et al.* (2006, p.210) identify a series of questions which may usefully be raised during the VR process. Gaining these additional insights will help the therapist design an individualised stress management programme. The suggested questions include:

- *What are the job stressors, how severe are they, and how frequently do they occur?*
- *What are the personal stressors, if any, outside of the work environment?*
- *What are the symptoms of job stress and/or personal stress carried into the job and how do they interact?*
- *What are the coping skills and personal resources used by the worker in dealing with stress?*

- *What is the lifestyle balance of the person experiencing stress?*
- *What is the plan to reduce the job stress, decrease the symptoms of stress and increase the coping mechanisms in the person's life?*
- *What is the commitment of the employers/management to reducing occupational stress?*

As well as individual characteristics, there may also be organisational factors within the workplace itself, which may be contributing to an individual's feelings of distress. The Mental Health Foundation (1999, p.5) identifies the following work-related features, which can negatively affect well-being. With prolonged exposure, they may play a contributory part in stress-related, or other health conditions, such as heart disease. These include:

- *lack of control over work*
- *under-utilisation of skills*
- *too high a workload with the imposition of impossible deadlines*
- *too low a workload with no or few challenges*
- *low task variety*
- *high uncertainly due to poorly defined roles and responsibilities, a lack of clear priorities and targets or job insecurity*
- *low pay*
- *poor working conditions, for example, noise, overcrowding, excessive heat or inadequate breaks*
- *low interpersonal support, for example, through inadequate or insensitive management, or hostility from colleagues*
- *undervalued social position.*

You will note that many of these factors cannot be adequately addressed by intervening solely at the level of the individual struggling to cope with stress. The nature, quality and characteristics of the work being undertaken, and the workplace itself, are important considerations too. A health survey undertaken by the Department of Health found that 19 per cent of men and over 30 per cent of women worked in jobs where they had low levels of control over their work. Furthermore, a third of men and half of the women who took part in this national survey were in monotonous jobs with little variety. A third of both men and women also reported working in jobs where the pace and rate of work were high (Department of Health, 1996). All of these factors, as noted by the Mental Health Foundation earlier, may negatively affect the well-being of workers.

It is becoming increasingly important for organisations to build clear policies on stress management and well-being into the workplace. These should be combined with well-designed and evaluated interventions at an organisational level. In this way, the organisation will be better placed to address stress-related ill-health. Particular difficulties within an organisation may be identified through a system of comprehensive recording of absence and an analysis of the type, and size, of the problems that their workforce are experiencing (Rick *et al.*, 1997). Stress audits, often carried out through confidential on-line surveys, are progressively becoming a feature of corporate stress-awareness initiatives. They are able to profile stress levels across the different parts of an organisation, thus giving indicators of where preventative action may be needed. There are a wide range of resources available for work-related stress, both at an individual and an organisational level. The Health and Safety Executive (2005) has developed standards for managing stress in the workplace, together with practical guidance on ways in which employees may work with their employers to begin to tackle the problem (International Stress Management Association, 2004). The NICE is also currently developing guidance for the workplace on the promotion of good mental health in employees, which is due for publication in 2008.

Supported self-help using a cognitive behavioural approach

Self-help materials, which are readily available in bookshops or through mental health charities, often make use of a psycho-educational strategy to help people better understand their condition and how it affects them. Publications of this nature, chiefly those based on a cognitive behavioural approach, may be useful resources to occupational therapists. This is particularly the case where they are working with clients who need additional assistance to be able to access, and make effective use of, materials of this kind. Being able to feel in control of, and manage, a long-term condition is an important precursor to work, and may be included within a pre-vocational programme, as we discussed in an earlier chapter.

Some occupational therapists working in Condition Management Programmes, for example, use the Five Areas Approach (Williams, 2001), either with individuals or with groups who are unemployed and moving towards work. The approach is targeted specifically at people with depression (Williams, 2001) or anxiety (Williams, 2003), and comprises a series of worksheets aimed at helping people understand their condition and the strategies through which to manage it. These strategies include: problem-solving and assertion; recognising and making changes to unhelpful thought patterns, such as negative thinking; changing behaviours, like avoidance; increasing activity levels and overcoming sleep problems. As with any approach, the Five Areas Approach will not be suitable for everyone; particularly those who are not interested in self-help approaches, have literacy problems, very poor concentration or other cognitive impairments which make reading and writing difficult. However, it may provide a useful starting point for a condition self-management programme, particularly in a group setting.

A further element of this approach used by occupational therapists is an individual or group stress management programme, including relaxation techniques, to help participants learn to recognise their own stress reactions, both in the workplace and in their wider lives outside of work. In this way, the individual may be assisted to develop better coping strategies, improved occupational role balance and more effective occupational performance within their various roles and day-to-day activities, including work. There is moderate evidence that stress-management programmes can play a role in preventing common mental health conditions (British Occupational Health Research Foundation, 2005).

WORK AND THE CLIENT WITH A SUBSTANCE ABUSE PROBLEM

The third group included in this section about mental health and work, is made up of those who have a substance abuse problem involving either alcohol or illicit drug use. This is a significant and growing problem within our society. The UK has the highest rate of drug use in Europe. Around seven per cent of the population is alcohol dependent and two per cent is drug dependent. Alcohol abuse in the workplace is of particular concern, with 20 per cent of fatal accidents at work involving victims who were above the legal drink-driving limit (Royal College of Psychiatrists, 2003).

While little has been written from an OT perspective about substance abuse and work, occupational therapists in various VR settings have told me of the particular difficulties they face in working with this client group. This may be when they are trying to assist people with these problems into work through, for example, a Condition Management Programme, or facilitating a return back to work when the person's absence is covered by an insurance policy. Substance abuse has also been found to be a major barrier to engaging young people with psychosis in vocationally-focused, early intervention OT programmes (Parlato et al., 1999).

Research commissioned by the HSE found that illicit drugs were used by 13 per cent of the workers in their study, but that this figure was highest in those under 30 years of age, where nearly a third had used some form of illegal substance in the previous year. The demographic characteristics of these study participants were well-educated, single, young men with neurotic personality traits, who also often smoked and drank heavily (Smith et al., 2004). Problematic alcohol abuse was similarly most likely to be found in young single or divorced men, with low self-esteem and depression, and with higher than usual levels of stress. In contrast to the profile of the drug users, however, they more commonly had a lower educational and skill level than those reported in the HSE study.

Evidence further suggests that the rate of consumption of alcohol and drugs varies according to the type of work which is undertaken. Alcohol use, in particular, is high amongst those who have easy access to it, such as publicans and those within the alcohol industry. In other occupations there may be either a social pressure to drink or high levels of occupational stress, as found in groups such as medical practitioners (Alcohol Concern, 2006). Workplace characteristics found to be associated with alcohol misuse included long work hours, work with a high risk of injury, high levels of physical demands, monotonous work, tight deadlines, job insecurity and poor supervision (Midford et al., 2005).

Consumption of alcohol and drugs is highest amongst those who are unemployed but, in contrast to other mental health conditions we have considered thus far, the majority of users are in employment, but this gap appears to be narrowing (Smith et al., 2004). The severity of the problem is determined by distinguishing between substance abuse and substance dependence. Substance abuse is diagnosed where the person is having significant problems, yet still continues to use the substance. For example, they may be having legal or financial problems, frequent absenteeism from work or use the substance in dangerous situations, such as when working with heavy machinery. Alcohol abuse has been linked to work-related problems such as poor job performance, inconsistent patterns of functioning, lower work output, mistakes being made, disciplinary issues and even theft from the employer. It can also result in difficulties in interpersonal relations and managing conflict, and in unpredictable behaviour, such as leaving the workplace unexpectedly (Strada and Donohue, 2004). Drug misuse can lower alertness, create a less positive mood, cause slower concentration and attention reaction times, as well as poorer memory and reasoning performance (Smith et al., 2004). If the person has substance dependence, then they have developed a physical and/or psychological addiction to it.

From a commercial perspective, between eight and 14 million working days are lost through alcohol-related absenteeism each year and it is estimated that between three and five per cent of all absences from work are as a result of substance use. In addition to lateness and absenteeism, it also results in reduced work performance and productivity, potential damage to customer relations, increased risks to health and safety, and damage to workforce morale (Health and Safety Executive, 2006c). Alcohol abuse in the workplace may also result in unemployment, accidents, lower occupational attainment and premature death (Alcohol Concern, 2006).

A key management tool in the management of drug and alcohol misuse in the workplace is the adoption of a written policy (Faculty of Occupational Medicine, 2006). This should be developed through consultation and communication with staff, as part of an overall health and safety policy. The policy should include: how the problem will be recognised, the help which may be offered and at what point, and in what circumstances an employee's drinking or drug use will be treated as a matter for discipline rather than as a health problem (Health and Safety Executive, 2006c; 2004b). Some employers introduce routine or random alcohol or drug screening as part of this policy and recent guidance has been introduced in this area (Faculty of Occupational Medicine, 2006). While this action may help identify the extent of the problem, it will not, in itself, solve or treat it.

Substance abuse and work

Clearly, from an occupational therapist's perspective, substance misuse can have adverse effects in terms of health, well-being and continued occupational participation. In terms of functional performance skills, drugs and alcohol can cause impairments in cognition, perception and motor skills. Different types of substance have different effects on the body, with a particular impact where these substances are used in combination (Smith et al., 2004). The effects may be grouped into three main categories:

1. depressants
2. stimulants
3. hallucinogens.

Depressants, for example, alcohol, tranquillisers, barbiturates, heroin, methadone and solvents, slow down the central nervous system and therefore can negatively affect abilities such as co-ordination, attention and reaction times. Alcohol can induce feelings of relaxation and disinhibition, which may lead to inappropriate behaviour in the workplace. Due to slow reactions, depressant use is particularly dangerous while driving or operating machinery.

Stimulants include amphetamines, also known as speed, ecstasy, cocaine and caffeine. These substances increase the heart rate and provide a sense of increased confidence, alertness and energy. Some stimulants may cause people to become aggressive. Stimulants may be used by workers to enable them to work long shifts, however repeated regular use can lead to dependence.

Hallucinogens, such as, cannabis, LSD and magic mushrooms, alter the way people think, feel and perceive their environment. They can also cause feelings of anxiety or paranoia. They may distort a person's sense of time and their perceptions and are therefore potentially dangerous in jobs where safety is a critical factor. Hallucinogens may cause a psychological dependence on the effects, rather than a physical dependence as found with depressants and stimulants. The most commonly used illegal drug in the UK is cannabis (DrugScope, 2005).

INTERVENTIONS

Finding, or providing, effective interventions and treatments for the worker with an alcohol or drug problem may present the occupational therapist, and other healthcare professionals, with significant obstacles. The nature of the condition means that the person is often evasive about the extent of the problem. Substance abuse is frequently progressive, and the high level of stigma attached to the condition can compound a person's denial. Local drug and alcohol services are often targeted towards those with a high degree of motivation, but are seldom focused towards job retention (Royal College of Psychiatrists, 2003). Employers, and others such as family members, may see resolution as simply a matter of willpower, and may therefore fail to have an understanding of the difficulties faced by the individual in abstaining. Some individuals in need of an in-patient detoxification programme will face a lengthy wait for admission.

It is important to recognise that work-related factors, as discussed earlier in the section, may play a contributory part in the development of the illness. Therefore, wherever possible, these factors should be confronted and raised with the employer by the occupational therapist. Helping to create healthy workplaces, as we discussed in an earlier chapter, may, in the future, prove to be an important preventative element in the reduction of both mental distress and substance abuse.

Interventions which we have already covered in this section so far may also be of relevance in substance misuse. These include: combating stigma, particularly through education; self-management and recovery; stress management; and self-help initiatives. Strategies and approaches for working with the individual who has a substance abuse or dependence problem as taken from the American literature include:

- motivational interviewing, which is a type of brief psychological therapy
- social skills training, which improves communication, support networks and coping skills to help with drink or drug refusal, conflict resolution and assertiveness
- a community reinforcement approach, where the individual, with the therapist, learns to identify the triggers for using the substance and the situation in which they occur, such as the social, recreational, family or work environment and then develops the skills that they need to face, and respond to, the situation in a different way
- behavioural interventions, such as behaviour therapy
- family therapy, where relationship conflicts play a role in the substance abuse
- self-help groups may provide a vital source of support, as evidenced by the 12-step programme of the international Alcoholics Anonymous organisation (for further information on Alcoholics Anonymous see: http://www.alcoholics-anonymous.org.uk, accessed 16/01/07)
- relapse prevention uses established support networks and a cognitive behavioural approach to identify and manage high-risk relapse situations
- ongoing support from within or outside of the workplace, including employer education
- for some, entering employment may help abstinence
- work is viewed as an important part of the recovery process, therefore programmes based on a therapeutic community model, for those who are unemployed, will often require community members to take on some responsibility for helping to run or manage elements of the facility.

(Strada and Donohue, 2004)

Further resources

There are a number of prominent organisations which produce publications and fact sheets about mental health, work and employment. These include, but are not limited to:

- the Sainsbury Centre for Mental Health (http://www.scmh.org.uk)
- the Mental Health Foundation (http://www.mhf.org.uk)
- Rethink (http://www.rethink.org)
- the HSE (http://www.hse.gov.uk)
(all websites accessed 19/07/07).

VOCATIONAL REHABILITATION WITH CLIENTS WITH MUSCULOSKELETAL DISORDERS

In this next section we will examine some of the central elements and the core principles behind VR for people who have musculoskeletal problems – a common source of OT referrals. A number of conditions can be included under this broad category. A musculoskeletal condition may be the result of an injury, such as when multiple fractures are sustained in a road-traffic or work-related accident, or as part of a chronic disease process, such as arthritis. Pain in the lower back, neck, hips, knees, or upper limbs, due to various causes, may also affect the person's work ability. It is not possible to cover all conditions in any depth, therefore some common categories that result in work difficulties and absence from work have been selected to form the basis of our discussion. We will begin with some information about these conditions.

UPPER LIMB DISORDERS AND WORK

This group of conditions is often more widely known in the UK by the somewhat misleading term 'repetitive strain injury' (RSI). It refers to those disorders which affect the muscles, nerves and tendons, particularly of the neck, shoulders and upper limbs. It includes specific conditions such as tenosynovitis, carpal tunnel syndrome, bursitis and injuries with a more diffuse presentation where pain and symptoms exist without a definitive medical diagnosis. Symptoms of upper limb disorders can include aching, pain, swelling, numbness, tingling, weakness and cramps. These symptoms may be precipitated, or aggravated by, excessive repetitive movements, static or poor posture and stress.

There have been increases in the prevalence of upper limb disorders in recent years, with health and social care staff having the highest incidence of the condition. It is a common disorder which affects nearly half a million workers. In 2003/2004 it resulted in a loss of nearly five million working days (Health and Safety Executive 2007a). The HSE have produced guidance for managers who have a responsibility for workers who may be at risk of developing limb disorders. It identifies the hazards and risks and suggests ways to control them (Health and Safety Executive, 2002b). It has also produced a useful leaflet for small businesses explaining how to identify, manage and prevent the condition in the workplace (Health and Safety Executive, 2003b). Upper limb disorders may be associated with working at a poorly designed workstation or computer, and we will be looking at workstation design and usage later in the section.

Interventions

The most effective strategy in dealing with upper limb disorders is prevention. This may be achieved through the use of suitably varied work tasks, regular risk assessment audits and early identification of potential problems. The occupational therapist may use a variety of interventions, including education; biofeedback; relaxation and micropausing (the affected limb is placed in a resting position for a very short time, then the length of time between breaks is gradually upgraded); posture; lifestyle review; health promotion including positive mental health; and developing coping strategies (McNaughton, 1997). It may also include work station redesign and suitable exercises to reduce muscle tension build-up from static postures.

ARTHRITIS AND WORK

More than seven million adults in the UK (15 per cent of the population) have long-term health problems due to arthritis and related conditions. Almost nine million people in the UK, nearly a fifth of the population, visit their GP each year for arthritis and related conditions. Within the workplace itself, arthritic conditions resulted in 206 million working days being lost in the UK in 1999–2000, which equates to a loss of production of £18 billion (Arthritis Research Council, 2002). There are over 200 different kinds of rheumatic disease but here we consider the main features of the most common forms.

Osteoarthritis is caused by the deterioration of the cartilage in between the joints which causes the bones to rub, resulting in pain, inflammation, swelling and stiffness of the affected joint(s). The main joints which are affected in osteoarthritis include the hips, knees and spine. It is found mainly in older workers, particularly women and people who are obese, since the additional body weight increases the wear and tear on the joints. As well as causing pain, it can also cause restricted movement and mobility problems.

Rheumatoid arthritis often develops earlier than osteoarthritis and usually presents between 30 to 50 years of age. It also affects mainly women. It is an auto-immune condition which causes inflammation and damage to the affected joints and tendons. It is usually found in the small joints of the hands and feet, most commonly on both sides of the body. The disease causes pain, stiffness, loss of strength and movement in the inflamed joints, and causes the person to feel unwell and fatigued. It often has a progressive deteriorating course, therefore it may gradually impact on the person's ability to perform their work tasks.

Ankylosing spondylitis is a condition which causes inflammation of the joints of the spine. It often starts at the base of the spine, in the sacroiliac joint. Over time, if not treated, the disease can result in the fusion of the vertebral joints causing limitations in the movement of the spine. This condition is usually found in young men, so it is important to support the affected person to maintain a worker role, wherever possible.

Other arthritic conditions include fibromyalgia – where pain and stiffness are experienced in the muscles, tendons and ligaments rather than in the joints – gout, polymyalgia rheumatica and systemic lupus erythematosus, also known as SLE or lupus (Arthritis Care, 2006).

Juvenile idiopathic arthritis is a form of arthritis which begins in childhood and affects around 12,000 children in the UK. While OT has been recognised as being well-placed to address the vocational needs of adolescents with this condition, this is hampered by an identified lack of confidence and knowledge amongst practitioners (Shaw *et al.*, 2006).

Interventions

A significant majority of those who suffer from arthritic conditions are covered by the Disability Discrimination Act (DDA) (2005). This means that employers are required to make reasonable adjustments to employment practice, or to their premises, if these features of the workplace put the person at a substantial disadvantage. Reasonable adjustments for the person with arthritis may include:

• reasonable time off for assessment, rehabilitation or treatment
• flexibility in working arrangements, such as avoiding the rush hour, part-time working, or perhaps doing some work at home
• modification of job tasks
• provision of aids and adaptations
• ensuring the best posture is achieved, appropriate to the work tasks.
(http://www.arc.org.uk, accessed 30/08/06)

Clinical guidelines for occupational therapists working in rheumatology (College of Occupational Therapists, 2003), highlight the fact that people with inflammatory arthritis have high levels of job loss, together with an associated reduction in income. While the review group found limited research and evidence for effective interventions used by occupational therapists in reducing work disability, some of the guidelines put forward included:

• using a range of assessments and assessment tools
• early intervention and specialist work rehabilitation
• the use of a cognitive behavioural approach to keep people in work
• joint protection based on an educational behavioural programme
• the use of assistive devices, such as wrist supports and working splints
• consulting with the disability employment adviser (DEA) at the Jobcentre Plus, where appropriate
• graded return to work following an extended absence
• workplace accommodations, such as ergonomic adjustment and job modification where necessary.
(College of Occupational Therapists, 2003).

Like other people with musculoskeletal conditions, people with arthritis may also benefit from learning pain management strategies, as well as understanding ways in which to plan and pace work tasks. A randomised controlled trial examined VR with employed people with rheumatic diseases who were at risk of job loss, and found intervention to be successful in delaying job loss (Allaire *et al.*, 2003).

Further resources

Charities such as Arthritis Care (http://www.arthritiscare.org.uk, accessed 30/08/06) and the Arthritis Research Campaign (http://www.arc.org.uk, accessed 30/8/06) produce useful fact sheets about arthritis and about arthritis and work.

WORK AND BACK PAIN

Back pain, particularly in the lower back, is a very common condition amongst working-age people, and may affect up to as many as 40 per cent of adults in any one year (Department of Health, 1999b). The condition may be acute (six weeks or less), sub-acute (six–12 weeks) or chronic (more than 12 weeks) in duration. A systematic review of non-surgical treatments for acute and chronic low back pain was carried out by the NHS Centre for Reviews and Dissemination (2000). The review identified that sufferers should continue ordinary activity with short-term use of medications, such as non-steroidal anti-inflammatory drugs. Evidence shows that bed rest is ineffective. During an acute phase, returning to normal, everyday activity can result in less time off work, as well as reducing the likelihood of a chronic disability developing. A search using OTSeeker, an OT evidence database, supported these findings, and suggested that multidisciplinary rehabilitation, including workplace visits, back schools, workplace exercise and advice to stay active and/or return to normal activities, are considered the most effective options (McCluskey *et al.*, 2005). When a person has chronic pain, they may benefit from activity pacing. Interventions used by therapists in activity pacing include: breaking activities into manageable parts, limiting the duration of activities, prioritising activities, gradually increasing the amount of activity, alternating tasks, taking short frequent rests, alternating positions during activities and delegating tasks (Birkholtz *et al.*, 2004).

Within the workplace, specific tasks that require repetitive or heavy lifting, excessive bending and twisting, exerting too much force, poor working conditions, and high job demands with a lack of control, are known to be specific risk factors for back pain. Back pain is most commonly found in occupations which involve:

- heavy manual labour and handling
- manual handling in awkward places, such as delivery work
- repetitive tasks, for example manual packing of goods
- sitting in front of a computer for a long period of time, particularly when the workstation is not correctly arranged or adjusted to suit an individual's needs
- driving long distances or driving over rough ground, particularly if the seat is not, or cannot be, properly adjusted.

(Health and Safety Executive, 2007b)

Let us examine some specific issues which these points raise.

Heavy manual labour and handling

Assuming, in this instance, that all parties concerned have agreed that it is desirable for the person to resume an existing job, and that they are work ready to do so, it will be important to take environmental design factors into account when planning the return to work. In doing so you need to consider:

- the task to be performed
- the person or human operator who will be expected to perform the task
- the equipment that needs to be used
- the environmental factors that may influence the performance of the task, including vibration, noise, light and temperature.

(Picone, 1999)

You will be paying particular attention to the functional abilities required while undertaking the manual handling tasks, and noting any ways in which the tasks can be modified to prevent future injury. Manual handling is defined as 'any transporting or supporting of a load (including the lifting, putting down, pushing, pulling, carrying or moving thereof) by hand or bodily force' (Manual Handling Operations Regulations (amended), (Department of Employment, 1992, paragraph 2)). While no specific requirements are set by the regulations regarding a safe weight to lift, the HSE has produced several useful fact sheets and information about manual handling. Recommended actions include:

- making the load smaller or easier to lift
- modifying the work area so as to reduce carrying distances, twisting movements, or lifting things from floor level or above shoulder height
- making manual handling easier and safer by creating optimum environmental conditions with regard to lighting, flooring and air temperature
- ensuring the person doing the lifting has been trained to lift as safely as possible
- making use of appropriate lifting and handling aids, such as rotary and tilt tables, and mechanical hoists.

(Health and Safety Executive, 2004)

Interested readers can find more information at: http://www.hse.gov.uk/contact/faqs/manualhandling.htm (accessed 22/11/06).

The person who is suffering from more chronic lower back pain, may sometimes be re-assigned to 'light duties' at work, on the advice of a GP or other health professional, until they are fit to resume their normal duties. While this may be an important consideration during the early stages of a return to work, over an extended period of time it is likely to result in greater physical de-conditioning. This may, in turn, further reduce the likelihood of the person returning to their former role. Consider the following case study.

Jesir is a 38-year-old storeman for a large catering firm. Eleven months ago he injured his back when he stepped awkwardly off a wheeled platform step while holding a light, but bulky container. Following a period of absence from work, his GP suggested he could go back on light duties. His employer had a temporary vacancy in the office, as one of his staff was off on maternity leave, so arranged for Jesir to cover this position, anticipating that he would recover and be fit to return to his normal duties. That was six months ago. Jesir has not returned to his employed role as his back seems to be worse than ever. The sedentary nature of the office work has caused him to put on weight. He gets high levels of discomfort from sitting for long periods of time. He misses his work colleagues and doesn't enjoy the predominantly female office environment. The temporary vacancy will soon cease to exist as the postholder is due to return from maternity leave.

You will see from this example that Jesir's return to work was not actively managed. There was no graduated return to his normal duties. The use of light duties did not result in an improvement in his condition. He became physically more de-conditioned and his well-being at work decreased. It is a common misconception that physical activity should be avoided until the person is pain free.

In order to prevent this scenario from occurring, the occupational therapist may undertake a functional job analysis, together with Jesir and his line manager, in order to identify suitable work tasks, and then gradually upgrade them, as we discussed earlier. In doing so, the therapist may also make use of their knowledge of biomechanics, in order to help them understand the actions of the human body, and the forces acting on its parts during normal work activities (Vincello, 1999). This knowledge base can also tell us about the limits that the body can safely endure, for example in lifting and manual handling activities. The biomechanical approach will be familiar to many therapists, since it is often a core component of medical rehabilitation programmes. In certain circumstances, the occupational therapist may also decide to undertake a functional capacity assessment, and we will briefly turn our attention to this form of assessment.

The functional capacity assessment (evaluation)

The majority of functional capacity assessment tools and techniques originate from the United States of America, so they are more commonly known as functional capacity evaluations (FCEs). The FCE is a 'comprehensive, objective test of a person's ability to perform work-related tasks' (Saunders and Piela, 1998, p.1). Therefore, this type of assessment is most commonly used in situations where an objective measurement of the client's residual physical functional capacity is required, especially within a legal context, or as an outcome measure to demonstrate clinical effectiveness (McFadyen and Pratt, 1997). The baseline components included in an FCE include lifting, pushing, kneeling, fingering, standing, pulling, crouching, feeling, walking, climbing, crawling, talking, sitting, balancing, reaching, hearing, carrying, stooping, handling and seeing (U.S. Department of Labor, Employment and Training Administration, 1991).

Some form of additional specialist training or equipment is generally required to undertake FCEs. They are, therefore, perhaps less likely to be of relevance to the novice practitioner who has a more general interest in learning about VR. Consequently this discussion has been limited. At the present time, FCEs are used far less routinely in British practice than in some other western countries. In America, they are most commonly used in workers' compensation cases, often when there is a question hanging over the person's work capabilities. An FCE may, potentially, be requested by a physician, employer, insurer, solicitor, case manager or injured worker. Each will have their own motives for making the request (Saunders and Piela, 1998).

FCEs can be divided into physical capacity evaluations – such as strength testing and range of movement measurement – and work capacity evaluations – for example lifting, pulling, standing, sitting, climbing, and so on (Velozo, 1993). The OT literature suggests that the physical capacity evaluations may have little bearing on actual functional performance or levels of disability of an individual (Gibson and Strong, 2003). Equipment used by occupational therapists to carry out these assessments include, for example, Baltimore Therapeutic Equipment (BTE), and the ERGOS work simulator. The ERGOS work simulator uses computer-based technology to measure physical performance components, such as strength and range of motion, as well as more functional performance abilities, including standing and sitting tolerance, while simulated work tasks are performed (Pratt, 1997; Velozo, 1993). More information can be found at: http://www.simwork.com (accessed 22/11/06).

Occupational therapists may also use work samples, such as Valpar component work samples, to assess functional work performance. For a number of years, the Valpar International Corporation has produced a range of tools which can be used to measure aspects of an individual's ability to perform particular work tasks. The work sample which is most commonly used by occupational therapists in the UK, is the whole body range of motion (work sample no. 9). This tool requires the person to move three shaped forms, attached by screws, between four different levels: above their head, at shoulder height, waist height and in a crouching position. This allows the evaluator to assess various physical and cognitive functional performance skills, including identifying any pain or limitations associated with assuming these positions. A method–time–measurement analysis allows comparison of the client's performance on the test with competitive industry standards. The practitioner who uses this assessment method also makes use of resources such as the Dictionary of Occupational Titles (U.S. Department of Labor, Employment and Training Administration, 1991), which you may remember from an earlier chapter, contains the job descriptions of nearly 13,000 different occupations. The Valpar International Corporation has more recently introduced a range of computer-based vocational assessment and exploration software, designed to test an individual's aptitudes for the purposes of career matching. Occupational therapists have described in the literature how this type of standardised assessment helps them make clear recommendations about an individual's work abilities (Jackson et al., 2004). Further information on Valpar in the UK can be obtained from http://www.khavalpar.co.uk (accessed 19/07/07).

While FCEs have particular popularity with some insurers, there are a number of recognised limitations to their usage. They are time-consuming and therefore expensive to undertake (Saunders and Piela, 1998). They also only assess physical tolerances and abilities. Another criticism which can be leveled at them is their disregard of environmental factors, which may present a significant barrier to returning to work (Velozo, 1993). Their objective nature means that subjective elements and viewpoints, such as the person's occupational identity and their illness experiences, which we touched on earlier in the book, are not taken into account. Additionally, not all components of an FCE will be relevant to the particular functional abilities required of an individual in performing their particular job. This may result in unnecessary assessment being undertaken. For these reasons, it is important that an FCE is undertaken as part of a more comprehensive occupational assessment.

Work and computers

Computers have increasingly become a central element of people's day-to-day working lives. It has been recognised that the health and safety risks associated with this activity need to be assessed and managed. Under the Health and Safety (Display Screen Equipment) Regulations (1992) employers are required to undertake an analysis of all the workstations used by their staff to assess and identify any health and safety risks to the computer user. They are also required to plan, or provide for, short frequent breaks or changes in activity within the work routine. These should preferably involve performing other tasks away from the keyboard.

The poorly designed computer workstation increases the risk of the worker developing back, neck, shoulder, elbow, forearm, wrist, hand and leg injuries. Occupational therapists may be involved in undertaking workstation assessments where an ongoing problem has been identified, which the employer has been unable to resolve. Some will carry out assessments and produce reports with recommendations for the Access to Work Scheme, which you may recall is accessed through the DEA, as part of the Jobcentre Plus provision. The cost of any equipment and/or adaptations is shared between the jobcentre and the employer.

The workstation assessment

When undertaking a workstation assessment, the occupational therapist will want to assess the fit between the individual worker and their workstation. To do so, they will draw on their understanding of ergonomic principles. Ergonomics, as we learned in the previous chapter, involves taking into account the design of work spaces, tools and equipment, to ensure that the product or area is fit for its intended use. They may also use a basic understanding of anthropometric principles. Anthropometry is a key element of ergonomic study which involves the measurement of the human body (Pheasant, 1996). It is important for the understanding of why a particular workspace is failing a particular individual. The types of situations where anthropometric data may be helpful include determining:

- vertical and horizontal reach
- 'visual' reach: being able to see what you are doing when carrying out a work task; e.g. the distance of the computer monitor away from the operator
- clearance: the amount of room needed to allow the person(s), or a part of their body, to enter a designated space freely; for example, the door width required for the entrance to a busy supermarket, or the space required for a mechanic to be able to reach into a car engine to remove a certain part
- posture: the best orientation of the various body parts while in the sitting or standing position – this is generally considered to be what is called a neutral posture and we will be discussing this shortly
- precision and strength.

(Baker, 1999)

In considering the above points when undertaking the workstation assessment, the therapist will want to examine the following types of issues:

- Is there adequate space under and around the desk?
- Is there excessive clutter?
- What shape and height is the desk? For example, does the person have a desk that is specifically intended for use as a computer workstation, or is the computer perched on a narrow counter? If they have to write at the desk as well, or make frequent telephone calls, is there adequate space to do so?
- Does the person have their own workstation or do they 'hotdesk' (use whatever desk is available, or allocated to them, when they arrive for their shift)?
- Is there adequate lighting?
- Is there excessive glare?

In the case of a client with a musculoskeletal complaint, you will want to ensure that their workstation is set up correctly.

- What is the height of the computer monitor? The top of the screen should be level with the person's eyes, so they are looking straight at it. Monitors placed directly on to a desk are invariably too low, so a screen raiser will be needed.
- Where is the monitor situated? When working at the computer, it should be situated directly in front of them, not off to one side.
- Does the person wear glasses to do computer work? Varifocal and bifocal glasses are often not suitable for computer use because of the neck position required in order to focus on the screen.
- Does the person use a document holder? This is relevant if the person is required to do copy typing, since a holder can help reduce repetitive inclinations of the head. Correct positioning of the document holder will depend on whether, or not, the person is able to touch type.
- How is the person's posture? This is a particularly important consideration. The neutral sitting posture should be a relaxed, symmetrical position with the feet flat

on the floor (or a footrest), and the elbows and knees flexed at 90 degrees. Further information about adapting and adjusting the computer workstation to achieve a comfortable posture is available from several equipment suppliers (see 'Further resources' at the end of this section). Rather than sitting with a straight, fully erect spine, it is suggested that leaning slightly back (to 105 degrees), allows the worker to gain greater support from the back of the chair (Baker, 1999). Unfortunately, however, the typical office chair is not easily adjustable, and may provide inadequate support if there is a poor fit between the user and the design of the chair (Hermennau, 1999). Additionally, it may have been designed, using anthropometric data, to accommodate an average sized person. Since there is, of course, an enormously wide range of average, both in terms of height and build, it follows that the standard chair will not meet the seating needs of a significant number of people, particularly those who are at the extremes of being particularly tall or short.

- Does the person use a footrest? A shorter person is more likely to need to use a footrest to maintain a neutral posture and to be working at the correct height in relation to the desk.
- Does the chair have arm rests? Arm rests are often a matter of personal choice, but to be most useful they should be height and position adjustable. Fixed arm rests often prevent a person from getting near enough to the desk and contribute to a poor posture. Adjustable arm rests can be helpful in supporting the upper limbs where a person has neck or shoulder pain.
- Does the desk have the optimum layout? The therapist should also advise on the optimum desk layout, for example, the position of the keyboard, mouse and telephone, paying attention to horizontal reach, to avoid awkward postures.
- Does the person have work task variety and perform exercises? Wherever possible, work tasks should be organised to achieve a mix of sitting and moving about. The Chartered Society of Physiotherapy (2005) recommends that a computer user should undertake a few gentle exercises every hour to reduce the chances of developing the discomfort and pain which may be caused by a static posture. Exercises which they suggest are outlined in the box.

While standing:

- Put the heel of the hands into the lower back and draw the elbows back and down. Slowly arch the back and look up towards the ceiling, keeping the head and neck steady with the chin tucked in.

While sitting:

- Shoulder shrugs: keep the shoulders back, then lift them towards the ears while breathing slowly in. Tighten the shoulder muscles for five seconds and then drop the shoulders slowly while breathing out. Repeat three times.
- Neck turning: rotate the head left then right, aiming the chin at the shoulders while keeping the eyes on the horizon. Focus on something in the distance (to help prevent eye strain). Repeat three times.

- Elbow flare: loosely grasp the hands behind the neck, keeping the head and neck erect. Squeeze below the shoulder blades while taking the elbows back. Care should be taken not to press on the neck. Hold for five seconds.
- Back of forearm and wrist stretch: with the elbow straight, tuck in the thumb to make a gentle fist. Bend the wrist forward gently stretching the forearm muscles, wrist and fingers. Hold for five seconds.
- Side to side turning: sitting slightly forward in the seat, rotate the mid- and upper-back to the right, while holding on to the backrest of the chair with the left hand. Hold for five seconds. Do the same in the opposite direction.
- Shoulder retractions: stand or sit up straight. Pull the shoulders back behind you, squeezing the shoulder blades towards each other. The stretch should be felt across the chest. Hold for five seconds.
- Forward press: with gently interlocked fingers, press the palms away from the body. Gently stretch the forearm muscles, fingers and the muscles between the shoulder blades. Hold for five seconds.
- Chin tuck: sit tall and visualise being suspended from the crown of the head by a piece of string. Keep the eyes level with the horizon and tuck in the chin to make a double chin. Hold for five seconds.

Visual demonstrations of additional exercises, can be viewed on-line at http://www .habitatwork.co.nz/ (accessed 24/04/07).

Specialist seating

Higher specification seating is frequently required where a person has an identified musculoskeletal problem. Adjustable lumbar support can often be helpful for the person who has low back pain, for example. In some instances chairs may also need to be custom built to meet the specifications or functional limitations of the user.

Kris is a 54-year-old adviser in a citizen's advice bureau. Eight months ago she had a total hip replacement due to osteoarthritis. The operation has significantly reduced her pain, but despite rehabilitation, she has failed to regain a full range of movement in her hip and she now walks with the aid of a stick. Kris is an obese woman, who has gained significantly more weight because of the inactivity caused by her condition. She wants to return to work, but is unable to sit in her standard office chair, because she cannot flex her hip sufficiently. She has tried raising her chair to its full height and perching on the edge of it, but her desk is then too low to be able to move her legs under it properly. She cannot reach her keyboard or see her monitor properly. Her posture is awkward and uncomfortable. Additionally, her chair base is too narrow to provide adequate support for her build. The therapist suggested a custom-built chair with a split seat which could be adjusted to accommodate her restricted range of movement. Additional reinforcement was also recommended to ensure the chair was safe for her to use. A height adjustable desk is also likely to be required.

Breda is a 34-year-old call centre worker who slipped on an icy pavement and fractured her coccyx. Now seven months post-injury, she is still suffering considerable discomfort and is unable to sit at her desk for longer than ten minutes at a time. She has tried using cushions and different chairs in the office, but is unable to relieve the pressure she feels at the base of the spine. The therapist recommended a custom-build chair, with a cut-out in the seat base to relieve the pressure in the region of the coccyx.

When undertaking an assessment for seating, the therapist will need, as a minimum, to take the following key measurements shown in Figure 7.1.

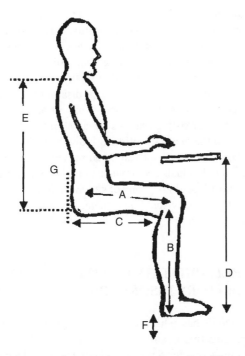

Figure 7.1. Key measurements for a seating assessment. A = Hip to knee measurement; B = Knee joint to floor; C = Rear of pelvis to back of knee (place a book behind the person's buttocks and measure from the cover); D = Desk height (top of surface to the floor); E = Top of shoulder to the top of the chair seat (sitting up straight); F = Usual shoe height; G = Lower back curvature – flat, medium or deep.

This has given a brief introduction to a selection of factors which the therapist may look out for when undertaking a workstation assessment. Possible solutions have also been offered for illustrative purposes. These are by no means exhaustive and the reader interested in workstation assessments is advised to follow up cited references for more comprehensive information.

Further resources

The websites of a number of equipment suppliers provide a wealth of information about
aids and equipment which are available on the market, as well as suggestions and advice
for addressing and overcoming particular difficulties. See:

http://www.posturite.co.uk
http://www.advanceseatingdesigns.co.uk
http://www.ergonomics.co.uk
(all websites accessed 24/03/07).

Occupational therapists working with computer users may find AbilityNet
(http://www.abilitynet.org, accessed 15/4/06) useful. This national charity specialises
in computer accessibility for people with a wide range of disabilities. They have expertise in adapting computers and suggesting alternative ways of using them, for a
person who finds it difficult to use standard computer equipment in a regular fash-
ion, because of difficulties caused by pain or a disability. Their website includes
downloadable fact sheets, details of equipment suppliers and advice on how to adapt
your computer, often using existing features already built in, to help make the computer more accessible to the needs of different individuals. They can also advise on
equipment such as voice-activated software, and provide a range of assessment and
consultancy services to individuals and organisations. They can make suggestions for
suitable technology and adaptations (many of which are free) which may be of help to
people with varying degrees of visual impairment, upper limb disorders, pain and/or
loss of function, and dyslexia.

VOCATIONAL REHABILITATION WITH CLIENTS WITH
CARDIO-RESPIRATORY DISORDERS

In recent years, the NHS has put considerable resources into reducing mortality
and providing more effective treatments for people who have heart disease. The
National Service Framework for Coronary Heart Disease (Department of Health,
2000a) outlines the standards for service provision for people who have this condition.
The central focus is on surgical and medical interventions, most of which are delivered
from within the acute hospital sector.

One exception, perhaps, is a standard which has been set regarding the provision
of multidisciplinary cardiac rehabilitation programmes. The aim of such programmes
is to reduce the risk of subsequent cardiac problems and promote a return to a full
and normal life. There are now some 400 cardiac rehabilitation programmes across
the country. Despite the broader intended aim of these programmes, much of their
focus is currently directed towards medical rehabilitation, often based around exercise, education and relaxation (Waddell and Burton, 2004). This is not surprising,
since the evidence base shows that regular exercise, or exercise with education and

psychological support, can reduce the likelihood of dying from heart disease (Jolliffe et al., 2007).

Regrettably, however, VR is largely omitted from most of the discussions about rehabilitation. There is mention in the NSF, in each of the identified phases of the rehabilitation programme, that the person should receive advice, including vocational advice, about employment. For example, before the person is discharged they should receive lifestyle advice including smoking cessation, physical and sexual activity, diet, alcohol consumption and employment (Department of Health, 2000a). Unfortunately, advice is unlikely, of its own, to provide sufficient support to facilitate a successful return to work for many who could benefit from it. Furthermore, this strategy fails to recognise, and address, the central role of the employer in any successful return to work programme.

There is currently limited evidence available about vocational outcomes from this, or any other, type of intervention which actively facilitates a return to work for this client group (Waddell and Burton, 2004). Little is known about who might most benefit, when, and in what circumstances. However, it is hoped that in the future there may be greater scope for those occupational therapists within cardiac rehabilitation teams to argue for a stronger, more timely, and pro-active role in addressing the individual work needs of participating clients.

CARDIAC CONDITIONS

Since many people are affected by cardiac diseases, we will briefly touch on some of the main conditions, as identified by the British Heart Foundation (2007), which occupational therapists may come across in VR with a person who has a heart condition.

Coronary heart disease is the narrowing of the coronary arteries due to atherosclerosis. It can cause pain (angina) or a myocardial infarction (heart attack) if one of the arteries becomes blocked. Coronary heart disease kills more than 110,000 people in England every year. Furthermore, over 1.4 million people suffer from angina and 275,000 people have a heart attack annually. Despite the fact that it affects so many people, it is also, largely a preventable disease. Government targets aim to reduce the death rate from coronary heart disease, stroke and related diseases in people under 75 by at least 40 per cent by 2010 (Department of Health, 2007).

Arrhythmias (irregular heart beat) include tachycardia, where the heart beats too fast, and bradycardia, where it beats too slowly.

Cardiomyopathy is where there the heart muscle is diseased without there being an obvious cause.

Valvular heart disease is a disease or damage to the mitral, tricuspid, aortic or pulmonary valve that reduces the efficacy of the heart. Valve stenosis occurs when a valve doesn't open fully, and valve incompetence is when the value doesn't close properly.

Heart failure is when the heart is unable to pump blood efficiently around the body, particularly as a result of permanent damage caused by a heart attack, or perhaps by poorly controlled blood pressure, valvular heart disease, or cardiomyopathy.

Congenital heart disease is a condition where a heart abnormality has been present since birth. The limitations will vary depending on the nature and severity of the abnormality. Further information can be obtained at: http://www.bhf.org.uk (accessed 19/07/07).

RESPIRATORY CONDITIONS

Chronic obstructive pulmonary disease is an umbrella term covering a range of conditions, including chronic bronchitis and emphysema. This is a long-term condition that results in damaged and narrowed airways, causing breathing difficulties because it is harder for air to get in and out of the lungs. It is estimated that up to 100,000 miners and ex-miners in the UK may have developed this condition as a result of their work (Department of Health, 2000b), and thousands have recently received compensation. While smoking is the main cause of this disease, it can also be developed as a result of occupational risks such as dusts, smoke and fumes. There are approximately 30,000 deaths each year from the disease in the UK (National Institute for Clinical Excellence, 2004), however many more people will have a mild or moderate form. Since about 40 per cent of people with this condition are below retirement age (Health and Safety Executive, 2007) there is a clearly identifiable need to actively facilitate, and maintain, an individual's ability to remain in work, if this is their objective. The National Service Framework for Chronic Obstructive Pulmonary Disease is currently under development and is due to be published in 2008.

There are many other respiratory conditions which have adverse effects on people's functional abilities, including their ability to perform their work activities, such as asthma. However, the evidence base in these conditions, similarly, remains focused on medical interventions. Further research and development is needed to gain an understanding of the role of VR with people who have chronic respiratory conditions.

WORK INTERVENTIONS WITH CARDIO-RESPIRATORY DISORDERS

The diagnosis of a cardiac or respiratory condition does not, of itself, give any indications of the severity of the condition, nor of current and future functional performance limitations. In common with many other potentially life-changing events, people who receive this diagnosis may begin to review the present priorities in their life. For some, this will mean that they wish to change the existing balance of their present daily occupations. They may choose to spend more time with their family, for example, or perhaps take steps towards fulfilling a lifetime ambition, such as travelling. Others may wish to return to their normal daily routine, including their usual work, as soon as possible. Returning to work can be an important part of the recovery process. Some people will be able to return to their existing job, others may need to retrain, or look at alternative work options.

In each situation, there is a need for a considered and well-thought-out plan. Early vocational intervention will provide the greatest likelihood of success, although this is likely to be very dependent on the person's pace of recovery. The optimal time, although this is not specific to cardiac or respiratory conditions, is currently thought to be between one and six months after the work absence, since after this time there are more obstacles to the return and VR will be more difficult (Waddell and Burton, 2004).

The British Heart Foundation (2005) has identified a number of factors which should be taken into account by the person with a heart condition when they are considering returning to work. As part of your further assessment during the VR process, you will want to explore some of the following factors.

- What type of condition does the person have? Is it stable and controlled by the medical treatment? Many people have angina that occurs with a particular amount of exercise, but otherwise is well controlled with medication.
- What type of treatment has the person received, and what is still needed? How long is it likely to take to recover after that treatment? For example, major surgery may require restricted physical activity for two to three months, whereas less invasive treatments will need a shorter recuperative period.
- What type of work does the person do? How much physical exertion is required? Some forms of work, particularly where the job regularly requires high levels of stamina and physical effort, will be unsuitable.
- Does the person need a driving licence to do their job? If so, what sort of licence do they need? There are restrictions on driving with certain types of heart conditions. There are also higher medical standards in place for those who drive lorries and buses because of the size and weight of the vehicles involved and also the length of time drivers may spend at the wheel in the course of their occupation. The Driver and Vehicle Licensing Agency (DVLA) publishes, and regularly updates, specific information about driving with particular types of medical conditions (Driver Vehicle Licensing Agency, 2007).
- How stressful does the person find their job? While there is no evidence to suggest that stress causes heart disease, prolonged exposure is recognised as a risk factor. Earlier in this chapter, we identified a number of workplace factors which may contribute to the development of stress-related conditions. The quality of the person's work is therefore an important consideration. Perceptions and experiences of stress are, however, often uniquely individual. It is important to explore the person's feelings in relation to their own job. It is also important to remember, and share with the client, that it is about finding the right balance for them. Boredom, and a lack of meaningful and fulfilling activities, can also be stressful and therefore may, potentially, be just as damaging to their recovery.
- How far do they have to travel to get to work? Again, there is no indication that travelling long distances causes heart disease, but commuting can be a particularly stressful activity for many people. As part of a graduated return to work programme, it may be possible to negotiate off-peak travel with the employer during the early phase of the return to work plan.

- What is their level of confidence? A person's confidence about their ability to do their job competently is quickly eroded following the onset of many health problems, including a heart condition. These doubts may set in relatively soon, and therefore positive encouragement during the early stages of the cardiac rehabilitation programme can help maintain the person's worker identity.
- Do they feel particularly anxious about their condition? A planned and supported return to work, as part of a gradual increase in activity levels, can help re-build confidence and self-esteem and thereby reduce feelings of anxiety or depression associated with the heart condition.
- Does their workplace, or any organisation which regulates the type of work they do, have specific regulations about whether and when they may return to this sort of work with their specific heart condition? Some occupations, particularly where critical safety factors apply, such as pilots and armed forces personnel, require particular standards of medical fitness. This will be an important consideration in any decisions which are made about prospects for returning to their current work.
- Does this person come under the DDA? This will depend on the impact and severity of their condition. If the person does not fall under the terms of the DDA, then the employer does not legally have to make changes to accommodate them. The employer's willingness to allow the person to return on modified duties, or a graduated return to work programme, will therefore have to be ascertained by either the employee or the therapist, with the person's consent. We will discuss the DDA further in a later chapter.
- Are they getting community support? A local heart support group can provide valuable support and encouragement and may be able to give the person practical suggestions or ideas about returning to work.
- Do they need to change work? Your further assessment may reveal that the person is not able to return to their existing job. If, for example, they have a pacemaker fitted to correct an arrhythmia, they will not be able to handle certain types of electrical equipment. In this situation, you will want to undertake a vocational exploration with the client. You will be exploring the following factors.
- Would redeployment with their existing employer be an option? Do they need retraining? Are they looking more towards voluntary work? For some clients who have done the same type of job all their working lives, facing change may be a daunting prospect. Your vocational exploration needs to focus, in particular, on their strengths and on the transferable skills they have learned. It may be helpful to do this collaboratively with the DEA.
- Based on these discussions and other considerations, the person may undertake a re-evaluate of their occupational priorities. They may decide that they wish to take early retirement. In this situation they should be encouraged to seek guidance from their employer and the Jobcentre Plus regarding the financial implications of this decision. The DEA should also be able to help the person identify, and apply for, any other benefits they may be entitled to. Early retirement should be a planned and considered choice, not a forced decision taken because the person does not see that they have any other option.

VOCATIONAL REHABILITATION WITH CLIENTS WITH NEUROLOGICAL CONDITIONS

CONDITIONS AND INTERVENTIONS

There is a wide range of conditions which may negatively affect the functioning of the brain, and, consequently, may impact on a person's ability to achieve their vocational potential. The occupational therapist may be involved with either a specific client group who has one particular type of brain injury or cognitive impairment, or with clients who have a wider spectrum of conditions. The National Service Framework for Long Term Conditions (Department of Health, 2005a) sets 11 quality requirements aimed at supporting people with long-term neurological conditions to live as independently as possible. It recognises that people with a neurological condition often experience major barriers when trying to find suitable, flexible employment. Therefore, one of the quality standards is directed towards VR. The aim is to enable people with a long-term neurological condition to work, or engage in alternative occupation. VR should include vocational assessment, rehabilitation and ongoing support to enable the person to find, remain in, or engage in work, or alternatively to access other occupational and educational opportunities.

The NSF presents evidence-based markers for VR and highlights the fact that current provision in the UK is probably only about ten per cent of the estimated requirement. A range of local, specialist residential, and intensive day rehabilitation programmes are needed. In order to increase supply, better co-ordination is needed between health, social services, Jobcentre Plus, and the independent and voluntary sectors. It has been suggested that the NSF is applicable to other conditions which are long term in nature, thereby potentially broadening the recognition of the need for VR to a wider range of people. Anecdotally, the NSF does not appear, as yet, to have provided the impetus for expanding the current range of VR services available to people with long-term conditions, whether neurological or otherwise.

Cognitive difficulties are present in many neurological conditions and Japp (2005) has brought together a wide range of these conditions under the umbrella term of 'brain injury'. Instead of adopting a traditional classification, based on the medical origins, the presentation, or nature of the condition itself, they have been grouped according to the ways in which certain characteristics may have a particular effect on work performance, and how they are likely impact on an individual's ability to undertake day-to-day work tasks. These characteristics include, whether the condition was acquired or congenital, stable or likely to deteriorate, continuous or intermittent, and whether the brain injury is permanent or transient in nature.

On the one hand, this method of grouping them is helpful, because it transcends the traditional split between those conditions which are viewed as health-related, and those which traditionally have been seen as more disability-related. It also serves to heighten our awareness of how many people may, potentially, face difficulties in the workplace because of the cognitive or behavioural consequences of their condition. Many will have problems entering work because of the functional performance difficulties associated with their brain injury. On the other hand, however, making generalisations in this way does produce some anomalies. Epilepsy for example, is not necessarily a congenital or a developmental condition. Nevertheless, with this proviso in mind, let us now examine VR within each of the five broad categories which Japp has identified.

Acquired brain injury

An acquired brain injury may have been caused by a traumatic insult to the brain, either through an external force, as seen in a work-related accident, a road-traffic accident or sporting injury, or through weakness or disease within the brain itself; that is, an internal cause, such as that which is caused by a stroke or a brain tumour. Following medical recovery from the acute event, the individual is usually left with residual cognitive impairments. These may be mild, moderate or severe, but further deterioration is unlikely.

A significant number of people will experience an acquired brain injury. For example, over 130,000 people in the UK have a stroke each year. While most people affected by this condition are beyond retirement age, strokes can happen at any time, and around 1,000 of these people will be under the age of 30 (The Stroke Association, 2007). Young people have difficulties coping with the loss of their worker role and with the resulting financial hardship (Stroke Association 1996). A number of small studies have commented on the difficulty of returning to the worker role after a brain injury (Chappell *et al.*, 2003) and the great variability of the rates of return following a stroke. A common finding, however, is that the majority of people express a desire to return to work. Even so, in the absence of a return to work facilitator, the actual pathway back to work is often unclear (Corr and Wilmer, 2003). A guide about getting back to work after a stroke has been produced by the Stroke Foundation and can be found at: http://www.stroke.org.uk/campaigns/current_campaigns/getting_back_to.html (accessed 21/02/07).

Each year over one million people attend hospital as a result of an acquired brain injury, of which around 100,000 are left with a significant disability. It is the leading cause of death and disability in young people and children and the largest cause of acquired disability in the working-age population in the UK today. Road-traffic and sporting accidents account for a significant percentage of injuries. It is estimated that between a quarter and a third of road-traffic accidents involve somebody who is using the road for work purposes. This means that about 1,000 people are killed, and a further 8,000–10,000 are seriously injured in work-related road accidents in Great Britain each year. Over 80 per cent of those sustaining a severe brain injury will be unemployed after five years, and without intervention, few will have a chance to work again (Rehab UK, 2007). Rehab UK is a charity that provides a range of rehabilitation, including VR and training, throughout the UK and Ireland. They have recently produced an on-line handbook, which includes a section on returning to work following a brain injury. Further information about the types of services they provide can be found on http://www.rehabuk.org/brain_injury.htm (accessed 19/07/07).

As with any other condition we have studied so far, the therapist working with a client with an acquired brain injury will follow the VR process outlined in an earlier chapter. However, recognition is needed of the potentially greater complexity and multiple consequences of a brain injury, since the major long-term difficulties, particularly in relation to employment, will often centre around cognitive, intellectual, behavioural and emotional problems (Barnes, 1999). Cognitive problems may include loss of memory and concentration, as well as difficulties with higher cognitive functions, or executive skills as they are also known, such as planning, organising, decision-making and problem-solving. Some individuals may experience varying degrees of co-ordination and movement difficulties; loss of sight, taste and smell; communication problems; and emotional and behavioural problems, including disinhibition, aggression or unpredictability. Each of these impairments will have an impact on the occupational performance of the individual, and on their ability to return to their work or studies. Potential litigation may also hamper rehabilitation and return to work interventions. We will return to this when we discuss case management in a later chapter.

Inter-agency guidelines for vocational assessment and rehabilitation after acquired brain injury (British Society of Rehabilitation Medicine *et al.*, 2004) recommend that:

- health rehabilitation assessments should routinely include questions about occupational status, aspirations and needs
- those seeking a return to their previous employment, or educational activities, should receive a neuropsychological or OT assessment to determine work readiness and other rehabilitation needs
- assessment should include the person's personal and family situation, sensory, motor and cognitive skills and behavioural and emotional control.

Occupational therapy assessment may include cognitive functioning abilities such as attention; following directions; immediate memory and recall; temporal awareness; visual and auditory memory/sequencing; money and mathematical skills; foresight; planning; concrete and abstract problem solving; judgement; abstract thinking; divided attention; multi-tasking and so on. Physical functional capacity and manual handling assessments may also be carried out (Chappell *et al.*, 2003). The exact content of these assessments should be targeted so as to be of specific relevance to the nature and requirements of the individual's work, particularly if they have a job to return to.

Vocational rehabilitation interventions, amongst others, may include:

- education, such as brain injury awareness
- the development of necessary skills and behaviours
- re-establishing work-related routines
- increasing attention and work tolerance

- developing coping strategies
- the introduction of activities which are of relevance to the skills and abilities required in their particular job
- cognitive rehabilitation.

When a client is assessed to be work ready, the workplace visit, return to work plan, and actual return to work will follow the pathway outlined earlier in the chapter about the VR process. With this client group, however, there may also be a particular need for longer-term follow-up (Corr and Wilmer, 2003), since clients may not fully appreciate the extent or the implications of their difficulties at the time (British Society of Rehabilitation Medicine *et al.*, 2004), and they may also experience difficulties such as fatigue. There is a need for opportunities to address problems as they arise in order to develop job stability and prevent avoidable job loss. As discussed previously, however, there are currently few services which offer, or are able to provide, this type of longer-term support. A study which examined job stability, and undertook a four-year follow-up, found that groups who are most likely to be unemployed include those who are from minority groups, people who did not complete their secondary education and those who were single.

The ability to sustain work was significantly influenced by being able to resume independent driving. Job stability could be predicted by taking into account the person's age, the length of their unconsciousness, and the severity of their disability one year after the injury. Early identification of those who are most at risk of poor employment outcomes should mean that the necessary rehabilitation planning, and interventions, may be put in place (Kreutzer *et al.*, 2003). Another longitudinal study which examined outcomes and work adjustment, found that as well as neuro-cognitive and physical factors, more subjective variables such as self-esteem, the individual's own appraisal of his or her situation, perceived social support and levels of emotional distress, all impacted on the success of the individual's vocational adjustment (Kendall, 2003). A small, phenomenological study which examined the meaning of work for people with a brain injury, found that work may take on a new, less central role. While it may be experienced as less central, the meaning attached to the social dimensions of work is increased. The person's own view of their competence may become less certain and their work identity may be altered, so there is a need for the person to discover a new identity as part of their recovery (Johansson and Tham, 2006).

Assessment by a work psychologist in the Jobcentre Plus and collaboration with the DEA may be the best route to follow when seeking alternative work options for clients who are unable to return to their previous work role. Some individuals with complex needs may require specialist residential brain injury VR services, as provided by the Papworth Trust, the Queen Elizabeth Foundation and the Brain Injury Rehabilitation Trust. While extensive research on the vocational outcomes after a traumatic brain injury shows that results can vary quite dramatically, positive outcomes have been reported from specialist brain injury vocational programmes, such as these (British Society of Rehabilitation Medicine *et al.*, 2004).

Progressive neurological conditions

Progressive neurological conditions include illnesses such as Parkinson's, Huntington's disease, ataxia and multiple sclerosis. Where an individual has a progressive, deteriorating condition of this type, interventions and adaptations to the work, and the work environment, will need regular review. Fatigue commonly occurs and, for some, symptoms may worsen with certain environmental conditions.

Gordon is a cost estimator with a local building supplies firm. He works in a prefabricated building which is accessed by several wooden steps. Gordon has had multiple sclerosis for seven years now, and his condition has gradually deteriorated over that time. His employer is supportive of Gordon, who has worked for the company for over 20 years. He is perfectly satisfied with the quality of Gordon's work, but he currently has concerns about the health and safety implications of Gordon's decreased mobility. Three main difficulties have been identified:

1. he is struggling to manage the stairs to get in and out of the building
2. he has difficulties with the temperature extremes of the building, particularly in summer when it gets very hot
3. he has twice fallen off his chair, particularly when he is fatigued from the heat.

The following plan is agreed to minimise the risk of injury and to enable Gordon to continue at work:

- The steps to the building will be replaced with a ramp. Gordon's employer is happy to organise this, particularly as the steps can get icy in winter and, although no-one has been injured, others have reported slipping on them.
- A portable air-conditioner will be installed alongside Gordon's desk.
- If the temperature exceeds a certain agreed limit, Gordon will take his work home with him – he is already doing this on an informal basis at the moment.
- Although Gordon refuses to consider a wheelchair, he is agreeable to a more supportive office chair with a central locking mechanism, to prevent it rolling away from him, as well as a head rest and adjustable arm supports, to provide additional postural support.

These accommodations will be jointly funded by the Jobcentre Plus and Gordon's employer. Ideally, since Gordon is likely to experience further difficulties in the future because of the deteriorating nature of his condition, there should be long-term, ongoing support available to Gordon and his employer. This should be from a named person, such as an occupational therapist, perhaps in the local primary care team. However, this type of support is unfortunately currently seldom available.

Developmental or congenital brain injury

According to Japp (2005), developmental or congenital brain injuries may include conditions such as dyslexia, attention deficit hyperactivity disorder, cerebral palsy, Down's syndrome, autism, epilepsy and general learning difficulties. With the exception of epilepsy, as mentioned earlier, these are lifelong conditions that will have a particular impact on an individual's work participation. For example, a survey of adults with learning disabilities found that about 17 per cent had a paid job and six per cent had an unpaid job (Emerson *et al.*, 2005). However, UK estimates suggest figures nearer one in ten (Department of Health, 2001). For many young people there is little in the way of support once they leave formal education. Depending on the nature of the disability, they may struggle to gain employment or access further education. Those with significant limitations will be offered a day centre place instead of individualised support into suitable employment. These types of services have long since been criticised by disabled activists because of their emphasis on care rather than on promoting participation in ordinary adult society (Barnes, 1990). While some day centres are focused on employment and are supported by dedicated employment placement teams, many others continue to offer little, or no, employment-related activity. Identified barriers include links to mainstream services, such as Connexions and Jobcentre Plus, and sometimes carers, and day centres themselves, may not be supportive of the idea of paid work (Beyer *et al.*, 2004). For effective VR, the barriers presented by each of these conditions, as experienced by the particular individual, will first need to be understood by the therapist.

The Government White Paper *Valuing People* (Department of Health, 2001) sets out the way to help people with learning disabilities live full and independent lives as part of their local community. More recently, a lifespan perspective was adopted in the report *Improving the Life Chances of Disabled People* (Department for Work and Pensions *et al.*, 2005). The report lays out a vision of a more co-ordinated approach that emphasises improvements to the support and incentives for assisting people with different disabilities to get, and stay in, employment. It highlights the need to improve opportunities for young people who are leaving school. These improvements include:

- effective early support and guidance, including rehabilitation, to overcome barriers to work
- enhanced employability through improving skills and access to in-work support
- making the transition to employment less risky and complicated
- engaging employers to improve attitudes to disabled people and increase their understanding of what it means to employ a disabled person
- building information networks to bring together and disseminate important information to disabled people, employers, family and friends, and carers
- A strong focus on delivering personalised, tailored support
- Specialist case managers able to provide guidance and assistance through all the stages.

(Department for Work and Pensions *et al.*, 2005)

Occupational therapists who work with children and young people with these types of conditions may be well placed to take some of the pro-active steps identified in collaboration with others, such as Connexions, to facilitate and ease this transition into work or training. Other potential entry routes include schemes such as Entry to Employment (E2E), which is provided by the Learning and Skills Council for

16–18 year olds. This programme funds local colleges and other providers to improve basic and key skills, vocational skills and personal development. Much of the work is workplace- and community-based, rather than classroom-based. Confidence building, improved literacy and numeracy, team building and supported work experience placements may be included. Some charitable organisations, such as Mencap (http://www.mencap.org.uk, accessed 19/07/07), provide information and services to assist people with learning disabilities who want to move towards work. The Disability Rights Commission has produced a booklet about the rights of people with learning disabilities at work (Disability Rights Commission, 2006).

People with autism have limited social and communication skills, as well as difficulty handling change and low levels of frustration tolerance. These features will often limit their employment options. However, some may also have high levels of abilities in areas such as maths, computer knowledge and memory skills. Research shows that few people with Asperger's syndrome, which is also sometimes called high-functioning autism, will find suitable employment without receiving specialist support (Powell, 2002). This is despite the fact that a significant percentage of people with this condition are of average, or above average, intelligence. They may also have positive personal traits such as reliability and persistence. This combination of strengths and barriers points to the need for a careful match between the demands of the work and the workplace, and the strengths and capabilities of the individual. Capo (2001) suggests that the occupational therapist, working within an interdisciplinary team, may help to bridge the school to work transition, enabling the young person with autism to enter work through a supported employment route. The National Autistic Society (http://www.nas.org.uk, accessed 19/07/07) holds an extensive range of publications for purchase, including books, videos and leaflets, about employment for people with autism.

Viral and bacterial infections

Viral and bacterial infections include conditions such as meningitis, Creutzfeldt-Jakob disease (CJD) and acquired immune deficiency syndrome (AIDS) (Japp 2005). It would also include chronic fatigue syndrome (CFS), sometimes called post-viral fatigue syndrome or myalgic encephalomyelitis (ME), since this condition is classified by the World Health Organization as a neurological disorder, although not all would agree with this aetiology. It is a common disorder which is characterised by persistent fatigue, cognitive impairment, malaise, pain, sleep and digestive disturbance (Action for M.E., 2006). People with this condition may also have heightened sensitivity to environmental conditions such as bright lights, loud noise and extremes of temperature. The literature reflects that there has been little research in the area of work-focused rehabilitation or employment outcomes for people with CFS. This is despite the condition causing significant work-related disability. Reported rates of unemployment range from 35–69 per cent, and job loss from 26–89 per cent (Taylor and Kielhofner, 2005). Further research suggests that an out-patient lifestyle management programme, run by occupational therapists and aimed at improving coping strategies and condition self-management, may produce positive return to work outcomes with clients who have this chronic condition (McDermott *et al.*, 2004).

Neuropsychiatric conditions

Neuropsychiatric conditions, for example schizophrenia, severe depression and early onset dementia, may cause impaired cognitive functions, such as reduced concentration, memory problems and poor decision-making ability. We have already examined these under mental health conditions earlier in the section, but it is important to recognise and bear in mind that certain individuals may be cognitively affected by their illness.

DISABILITY MANAGEMENT STRATEGIES IN THE WORKPLACE: WORKERS' VIEWS

We have, very briefly, touched on key considerations for occupational therapists in VR working with clients with different mental health, musculoskeletal, cardio-respiratory and neurological conditions. There are many other conditions which, potentially, could have usefully been included here as well. Before moving on to the next chapter, it is appropriate that this one end with some research findings about effective management strategies, which disabled people themselves have identified, as being helpful in the workplace.

Research published by the Joseph Rowntree Foundation, which sets out to identify how disabled workers got by and managed to be successful in the workplace (Roulstone *et al.*, 2003), found that the strategies used are diverse and wide ranging. Furthermore, what works for one worker may not be suitable for another in a different situation. However, some common strategies which were identified from the study included:

- being assertive in asking for support and being open about the nature of the impairment and barriers faced
- empathy, a 'give and take' attitude and formal and informal mutual support from both inside and outside of work, was central to the enjoyment of work (sources of this support were identified as colleagues; Jobcentre Plus Access to Work provision; family and friends; employers and managers; organisations of and for disabled people; and trade unions)
- getting to know an organisation first and then gradually developing suitable strategies was helpful
- gradual strategies were necessary in order to understand employment environments, management styles, personnel changes and corporate priorities.

8 Team Structures in Vocational Rehabilitation

Occupational therapists traditionally work as members of a multi-disciplinary team and are skilled in team working. Within the employment sector and industry, however, occupational therapists may work alongside practitioners from different professional backgrounds to those in traditional health and social care settings. In addition to these different roles, the structure of the team may also differ. This chapter will introduce you to some of the different professions, roles and perspectives of the potential members of a multi-disciplinary team in vocational rehabilitation (VR), as well as the ways in which a team may be organised or structured.

THE ADMINISTRATIVE TEAM

Occupational therapists working in non-traditional settings, such as a private rehabilitation company, an insurance company, or even a Condition Management Programme, tend to have their own allocated caseload of clients. This happens in much the same way as a key-worker or care co-ordinator role is assumed within, perhaps, a community mental health team. The amount of direct contact that the occupational therapist has with the client in these different settings will vary. A model of intervention called case management is a common service delivery structure, and we will learn more about this type of approach later in this chapter.

The caseload size varies across these different organisations, but each occupational therapist assumes responsibility for, and has a duty of care to, the individual clients on his or her caseload. It differs somewhat from a more traditional setting in that it tends to be a more autonomous role. That is, it is unusual for more than one therapist, or other heath professional employed by the respective organisation, to be directly involved with the service provided to any given client. Since the VR role is a generic one, the job tasks are similar across different professional groups within a particular employing organisation. Practitioners in VR may have different job titles, such as VR consultant, rehabilitation co-ordinator, rehabilitation case manager, condition management practitioner, and so on. Professionals who fill these roles may come from an occupational therapy (OT), physiotherapy or other allied health professional background. They may alternatively have a psychology or a nursing qualification. Occasionally, you may come across a practitioner performing this role who has a recognised qualification and role in VR from a country outside of the UK, such as a rehabilitation counsellor.

In larger organisations, a group of therapists is generally organised into a team under a team manager. The purpose of these teams is administrative rather than therapeutic, since practitioners within them will work as individuals, often with individual targets to meet, rather than as part of a group or a team who are supporting a client to meet their work goals. The manager will be responsible for tasks such as actively managing caseloads and working towards achieving service targets. This team structure also provides varying degrees of formal and informal peer support to individual practitioners. This is a particularly important function since the role may potentially be quite isolating, particularly for those practitioners who work from home. Team members can seek out advice on aspects of intervention with a particular client, and may draw on the experience of a colleague with expertise in a particular field or clinical condition. It is good practice for mentoring arrangements to be put in place to support new employees within these teams. This usually involves pairing an experienced team member with a new recruit.

In some settings the skills and expertise of the occupational therapist will be used to benefit others in different parts of the organisation. For example, within the insurance sector, the occupational therapist may also be a member of a small claims management team. In this capacity, the occupational therapist serves as a resource to the claims managers, advising on the suitability of an individual for rehabilitation, for example. More information about the claims manager and their role is presented later in this chapter.

THE VOCATIONAL REHABILITATION TEAM

When a person needs assistance to enable them to participate in work, this support is likely to come from a customised VR team. The VR team is a working group of people who will engage in a planned, shared effort to overcome the barriers and enable the particular individual concerned to successfully achieve their goal to enter, return to, or remain in work. Each client becomes an integral part of a co-ordinated, supportive, frequently multi-agency team. You may, at this point, be wondering where you might find such a team. It does not just materialise, rather it needs to be created, developed and nurtured.

The purpose of a VR team is to give the individual the optimum chance of successfully achieving their work goal. This means involving those people – professional or otherwise – who are most likely to help facilitate this objective. According to Raper (1995) it needs to be recognised that rehabilitation for work is not a simple process. For the person who is returning to work after a long absence, things will have changed and moved on during their time away from the workplace. The person needs to be prepared for this and allow time to adjust and adapt to these changes. They will need a period of work re-conditioning, preferably through a planned, supported, graduated work entry, to help them regain their confidence in their abilities as a competent worker. Colleagues and co-workers will also need time to become comfortable with having the absent person back at work.

As we begin to think about who may be part of this VR team, we need to be mindful of three important facts. Firstly, we need to take a client-centred perspective, so the person themselves will be the central, core member of the VR team. The VR team will be built around them and their particular needs and we will be working collaboratively with them on shared work objectives. Secondly, we know that successful and effective work outcomes are often hampered by a lack of co-ordination and collaboration between key agencies and service providers. Therefore, our VR team needs to act as a conduit, or a bridge that cuts through these organisational barriers to overcome this significant obstacle. We need to look carefully at what is currently available: at the facilities; resources; knowledge and skills of existing services; and whether these services are statutory or from voluntary or private providers. We need to ask ourselves who may have a valuable contribution to make towards the specific work needs and objectives of our client. This will then allow the occupational therapist, or any other VR practitioner acting in this role, to set about building a VR team around the individual, which will help them overcome the identified barriers and will work towards meeting the client's particular goals.

This brings us to the third important point: each VR team needs a leader. This is the person who brings the necessary people together, ensures that the agreed actions materialise, that the plans are enacted, and that the team continues to work effectively with, and on, the client's behalf. For the purpose of this chapter, an assumption has been made that the occupational therapist is this person. In this capacity, the occupational therapist acts as the return to work facilitator, and so takes on the responsibility for developing and leading the team. In reality, this is a generic facilitation role that any person, from any of the settings we have discussed, may potentially take on. Some of the skills that may be needed to perform this role include leadership, administrative skills and enhanced communication competencies. These proficiencies are often beyond those which are acquired during traditional graduate education courses (Ahrens and Mulholland, 2000), therefore some occupational therapists may need to expand and develop their repertoire of skills in these areas.

MEMBERS OF THE CORE VOCATIONAL REHABILITATION TEAM

For the person who is returning to work, the most simple of VR teams will consist of the client, the employer, or employer representative, and the return to work facilitator. For our purposes, we will make the assumption that the return to work facilitator is an occupational therapist.

Within a more complex team, there may also be other health or rehabilitation professionals involved, perhaps an insurer or a solicitor, as well. The client's medical practitioner or medical specialist may also need to play a contributory role. In certain instances, a co-worker may become a team member, providing valuable formal or informal support in the workplace. If you wish to be reminded of the parties who may potentially be involved in the return to work process, return to the discussion about the disability management model in Chapter 4.

If your client is out of work, then your team may well have a different configuration. You will need to involve a member of the Jobcentre Plus staff, most commonly the disability employment adviser (DEA). More details about the DEA and their role can be found later in this chapter. In this case, the core VR team may consist of you (the occupational therapist), your client (the work seeker) and the DEA. It may be extended to include input from other health professionals, training providers or voluntary sector workers, as required. Ideally, the potential employer will also become a member of the team as the planning for entry into a particular workplace takes place and the job is commenced. There is currently a need for far better support and mentoring during the work entry process and beyond. This is necessary to avoid early work loss and encourage job retention for people with disabilities.

MEMBERS OF THE EXTENDED VOCATIONAL REHABILITATION TEAM

We have identified some core members of a possible VR team for a person seeking entry to work or a return to work. Other potential team members within an extended team, who may, perhaps, be more familiar to the occupational therapist, include a treating physiotherapist, an osteopath and/or a psychological therapies provider, such as a clinical psychologist, a counsellor, or a cognitive behavioural therapist. Occasionally, in cases of complex brain injury, additional assistance or advice may be sought from a sub-specialist, such as a clinical neuro-psychologist. These are clinical psychologists who have specialised in working with people with a neurological illness or injury. This person would undertake assessments of cognitive function, such as general intellect, attention, information processing, perception, memory/learning and executive function as well as behaviour, emotion and social skills. They would devise a rehabilitation programme to address the related difficulties and provide advice about return to work, education and training (British Society of Rehabilitation Medicine *et al.*, 2004). The team may also extend to include an alternative or complementary therapist, depending on the actual nature of the client's health problem or disability. If the barriers which prevent the person from working are of a more social nature, the team may include a housing officer, financial adviser, or an adviser from the citizen's advice bureau, for example.

However, at this point we need to temper our discussion with a little reality. The larger the team, the more unwieldy it becomes and consequently, potentially less effective. It also needs to be acknowledged that the team membership will be dependent on the funding source of the client's VR programme. Resources are, of course, always finite in any setting. What the funding organisation will provide on behalf of a particular individual, as well as the availability of services and providers within the client's local area, will all impact on what is feasible and achievable. It is also highly unlikely that all these team members will be able to regularly meet together, if at all, to discuss their particular role within the VR team. Therefore, the return to work facilitator will need to co-ordinate the respective contributions. This person frequently acts in a case management capacity. We will return to discuss the role of the case manager later in the chapter.

There are numerous possible VR team configurations and numerous people, who may not necessarily be service providers or professionals, who may play a potentially vital role in facilitating a return to work. The client remains the lynchpin within this team and should be afforded as much control as possible over the proceedings. Let us use a case study to illustrate this point further.

Mr Rawson is the 58-year-old owner of an out-of-town garden centre. He suffered a heart attack three months ago, and has been off work since the incident. Following the necessary medical treatment and rehabilitation, he is continuing to work on improving his physical health. He has lost weight and is participating in an exercise-based cardiac fitness programme at his local leisure centre. While he still becomes easily fatigued, he now feels ready to return to work. He is, however, becoming increasingly frustrated at being discouraged from doing so by the staff in his primary care team.

You are an occupational therapist working for an insurance company as a VR consultant. Mr Rawson has an income protection insurance policy which covers his medical condition and you are asked by the claims manager to see him to discuss if, and how, his return may be facilitated. At your initial assessment meeting, Mr Rawson indicates that he would like his wife to be present as well. You enquire about his current daily activities at home and he reports that although he has slowed down significantly, he is able to carry out most of his previous activities with few restrictions. You also find out during your discussions that Mr Rawson is not able to resume driving as yet, and there is no public transport to his place of work. His wife volunteers to drive him there and back in the meantime if this would help.

As far as his job is concerned, Mr Rawson has a high level of control over his work tasks. Much of his work involves supervision of staff and serving and advising customers, which he enjoys. Since he has a number of staff working for him, the client is confident that he will be able to avoid any heavy lifting or other physically strenuous activities. He agrees for you to carry out a worksite assessment and job analysis with him, and likes the idea of going back to work on a planned, graduated return. He learned about activity pacing and energy conservation in his cardiac rehabilitation programme and would like assistance to extend these techniques to his workplace. When you develop this plan you will make sure that it is built around the timings of his fitness programme. You arrange a time to meet the client next week at his place of work.

In the meantime, you ask him to discuss these proposed actions with his GP. You give Mr Rawson your contact details should the GP wish to contact you with any queries or concerns. You obtain Mr Rawson's written consent to talk to his GP, should this become necessary. Following your worksite assessment, when you have agreed a return to work plan with Mr Rawson, he will go on to discuss the specific details of the plan with his GP. You will need him to obtain signed consent to the plan from his medical practitioner before you proceed with the planned course of action. Obtaining medical agreement is particularly important when the person has a chronic medical condition which is currently preventing them from working.

You can see from this example, that Mr Rawson's wife becomes a member of his VR team in this situation, since her involvement helps to facilitate his return to work. Co-workers will also be an important source of assistance. In addition, it will be important to actively engage with, and gain the support of, the appropriate primary- or secondary-care health professionals as well. Ideally, responsibility for this should be retained by the client himself, but in some instances it may be necessary for you to communicate directly with members of the medical team. As indicated in the case illustration, you will first need to obtain the client's authorisation to do so.

THE ROLES OF THE CORE VOCATIONAL REHABILITATION TEAM MEMBERS

Let us now continue our discussion by looking more closely at the roles and responsibilities of the core team members of the VR team. It is likely that the occupational therapist acting as a return to work facilitator, will do so in a case manager capacity. We therefore need to undertake a more in-depth discussion of this role.

The case manager

While case management is not specific to VR, it has become a common mode of delivering these services in the UK. Case management has been defined as 'collaborative process which assesses, plans, implements, co-ordinates, monitors and evaluates the options and services required to meet an individual's health, care, educational and employment needs, using communication and available resources to promote quality cost effective outcomes' (Case Management Society UK, 2005, p.70). As the complexity of individuals' healthcare and support needs have increased, so too has the range and number of services which may potentially meet and address these needs. The case management approach has been steadily recognised as enabling people to access the right services for their needs, from the ever-expanding, often fragmented, range available. Occupational therapists may take on the role of case manager from within any of the different settings which offer these services. It is suggested that health professionals assuming a case management role may experience greater breadth of responsibility and autonomy than when working in more traditional roles, however it may also mean the potential loss of profession-specific expertise (Allen, 2005).

Case management is considered by many to be a generic professional skill. It has been used in a variety of diverse settings, such as health, older people services, rehabilitation, long-term care, the employment sector, prison services, and the insurance sector, but is often applied very differently. For example, in the long-term condition model, developed in the NHS and social care setting (Department of Health, 2005a), effective case management is seen as a key element in improving quality of life and outcomes for those who have a long-term condition. As a result, a competency framework for case managers has been produced (Modernisation Agency and Skills for Health, 2005).

The spectrum of case management activities that are provided will vary. At the one extreme it may be purely delivering a brokerage service, often done over the telephone. This is where the case manager determines the services that the client should receive and then sources, manages and co-ordinates the delivery of those services. At the other end of the spectrum, case management could be an extension of a clinical role. In this situation, the therapist provides a therapeutic service to the client, alongside assisting them to access and link into other suitable community resources (Allen, 2005). Most commonly, practitioners specialise in providing a particular type of case management. These are predominantly concerned with the care needs and medical case management of an individual within their home environment (Department of Health, 2006), but they may also be directed towards people who have a particular type of impairment, such as brain injury case management. Occupational therapists may work as medical or brain injury case managers in different settings, however, our particular interest in this area is more specifically directed towards the application and uses of vocational case management by occupational therapists.

Vocational case management activities may include counselling and encouragement, referral to services, co-ordination of service provision, and support and facilitation into work. The central steps in the case management process are:

- intake and assessment
- planning
- implementation
- monitoring
- case closure
- evaluation.
(Allen, 2005)

Ideally, caseloads should be kept to a minimum in order to provide the intensive assistance required by a given individual (Kellard *et al.*, 2002). The Case Management Society in the UK has published *Standards of Practice* (2005) for case managers. These are intended to enable practitioners to benchmark the quality of the service they provide, as well as emphasising their duty to develop their knowledge and skills for safe and effective practice. To this end, they have also produced best practice guidelines (Chapman *et al.*, 2006), which stress the importance of developing a therapeutic relationship with the client based on trust, respect and empathy. We discussed the client–therapist relationship earlier in the book, but will return to this subject again shortly.

As any experienced case manager will know, there are always potential conflicts inherent in this role. It is essential to recognise the duty of care which exists towards the client, which has to be balanced against the central goal of advancing the rehabilitation process and co-ordinating the rehabilitation plan. An effective case manager sometimes needs to be able to face and resolve situations where there may be conflicting influences, expectations and demands. Ethical issues are often brought to the fore in vocational case management. In other situations, the therapist may be required by a solicitor or insurer to justify the rationale for the rehabilitation package that they have put in place (Chapman *et al.*, 2006; Allen, 2005). The therapist who assumes a case management role needs to be aware that these situations will require enhanced communication, negotiating, and sometimes conflict-resolution skills. A central role of the case manager is to seek out a variety of possible resource and service options to meet the individual's needs. In most settings outside of the NHS, this will be done by identifying and accessing the services of other professionals, rather than acting in the capacity of a treating therapist. In cases where the required therapy cannot be sourced, or there is perhaps an extensive waiting list, this hands-off approach has been known to cause an element of frustration for some therapists.

Having identified that it is the role of the return to work facilitator to create the VR team, let us now examine how we might set about doing this. The first team member we need to engage with will, of course, be the client. We have already extensively covered the ways in which we may understand the person as a worker, and what work may mean to them, so here we will look specifically at how we might foster our relationship with them.

The client

Successfully connecting with the client will be the first step in developing a VR team. During the earliest stage of the VR process, usually during the initial interview and assessment, the occupational therapist needs to build a rapport and establish a collaborative working relationship with the client. Both therapist and client will need to gain a clear understanding of the goals that the client is aspiring to achieve regarding accessing, or returning to, work. During first encounters, it is important to question what you are trying to achieve. A marker of success in achieving this collaboration is shown when the therapist confidently begins to talk about what **we** are trying to achieve, rather than what I (as the therapist) will be doing. Reflect on whether you feel that you have reached this level of understanding of your client's objectives.

Some clients, particularly those who have been away from the workplace for some time because of ill-health, will lack confidence or be unsure of their abilities to enter, or return to, work. In these circumstances, occupational therapists have reported that using motivational interviewing techniques may be helpful to move forward. Some of the general principles underpinning motivational interviewing are:

- Express empathy – it is important to recognise that the person may feel very trapped by their current situation
- Many people will have mixed feelings about returning to work – you will want to highlight this by pointing out any ambivalence that the person is displaying, without trying to resolve it
- Avoid argument – you risk alienating the person, and you will be unable to work collaboratively with someone with whom you are in conflict
- Don't be put off by resistance – fear of returning to work is a natural response and can present as resistant behaviour or a lack of motivation
- Support self-efficacy – it is particularly important not to create a dependent relationship and therefore you will at all times want to work alongside the client, in partnership with them.

(Miller and Rollnick, 1991)

It is interesting to note, on these final two points, that very few occupational therapists who work in VR refer to the person as a client, patient, or service user. Instead, they talk about: the person, this guy, this lady, the employee and so on. Being able to see the individual in this light will help foster a more collaborative partnership, as well as reinforcing the value and importance of that individual's own knowledge, resources and skills.

When a collaborative working relationship has been established, and the goals identified, the next step involves putting a plan together. This is where the occupational therapist and the client decide on the actions that need to be taken to enable the client to successfully return to work. These actions may include commencing a pre-vocational programme if the client is not yet ready to return to the workplace (see the chapter on the VR process for more details about how this conclusion is reached). It may also involve onward referral for specific additional assessments or interventions to be carried out by others, as we discussed earlier in this chapter. Also as we mentioned earlier, the other core member of your team will depend on whether your client wants to access work, in which case it will be the DEA, or return to an existing job, which will mean that this person will be the employer. Let us begin with the former.

The disability employment adviser

Each individual who is out of work is assigned a personal adviser (PA) at their local Jobcentre Plus (we will return to the PA role later in this chapter). An individual's personal adviser may refer the person with a disability on to the DEA if they feel that extra assistance is needed because of an individual's health condition or their disability. The DEA provides specialist support to help jobseekers with more severe and enduring disabilities find and retain a job. DEAs help in the search for a suitable job, provide advice and support while the person is looking for a job, and offer advice and information on specialist training opportunities available. The DEA will draw up an action plan with a particular individual. As we have discussed previously, the DEA may also be able to provide assistance to people who are already in work, but may be at risk of losing their job because they have a health condition or disability.

A DEA's services may include an employment assessment to help identify abilities and strengths, and consideration of how the disability or health condition may affect the type of work the person wants to do. They are able to provide a job-matching service and inform the person about local jobs that match their experience and skills. In some instances, a DEA may approach an employer on the individual's behalf. DEAs are able to provide access to a range of local training or employability services, or to specialist training programmes and organisations for disabled people. These specialist programmes include, for example, the Job Introduction Scheme and WorkPath Programmes which we discussed earlier in the book. DEAs may receive support and supervision from a work psychologist. We will touch briefly on this person's role a little later.

Few occupational therapists will, as yet, have well-developed working relationships with DEAs, although this does vary around the country. For example, the job clinic model is an interagency model of VR used by occupational therapists in mental health within Northern Ireland (Devlin et al., 2006). It involves partnership working between occupational therapists from the healthcare trust, the DEA from the Jobcentre Plus and an employment officer from a voluntary sector organisation called Action Mental Health. The occupational therapist provides a link between the worlds of mental health and employment as a member of both the mental health team and the job clinic team.

Working across agency boundaries in this way will increase the opportunities for the client to successfully gain a work role. It is important to realise, however, that these working relationships will not just happen. Time should be spent getting to know, and understand, what the DEA can, and cannot, offer and recognising the constraints within which they are expected to work.

The line manager

We will now assume that your client has a job to which they are planning to return. In a larger company, your initial employer contact will probably be a staff member in human resources. This person's continued involvement in the return to work process is subject to considerable variation across organisations. In smaller organisations you will probably be dealing directly with the business owner. The person who is most likely to be involved in the planning and implementation of the return to work plan will either be the line manager of your client or the head of their department. We will assume that this person is their line manager.

The line manager has an important role to play in the return to work process. They are often tasked, either directly or indirectly, with managing absence amongst their staff. In order to do this effectively, they will need a sound understanding of the organisation's absence policies and procedures. They should also be aware of their role within the absence management programme. They need an understanding of the legal and disciplinary aspects of absence and the role of the organisation's occupational health services, if they have one. The line manager must be knowledgeable of how any trigger points operate. For example, they may be expected to make a telephone call to an employee if they have been absent for a certain number of days, or alternatively to make a referral to occupational health. However, it is reported that only around a half of organisations train their line managers in the skills they need to fulfill this role effectively (Chartered Institute of Personnel and Development, 2006b). Therefore, the occupational therapist needs to be aware that a line manager may not necessarily be experienced in, or have a good grasp of, either the role of a return to work facilitator, or how a return to work may actually take place. In these instances, education will be an important element of engaging the line manager with the VR team. It is important to involve the employer in this capacity as soon as possible, so as to set up a collaborative spirit between employer and employee (MacDonald-Wilson, 1995). A positive attitude of the manager or supervisor toward early return to work and the return to work process will need to be emphasised (Ekberg, 1995), since this may be a key element in the success, or failure, of your return to work programme. Having a positive and committed manager within your VR team can, in turn, provide a good starting point to developing natural supports within the workplace. The creation of these support systems may contribute to developing a healthy workplace and also to promoting mental health and well-being (Secker and Membrey, 2003). Too few rehabilitation programmes involve the workplace (Ekberg, 1995), yet from this discussion you can see that there are many benefits to successfully including the line manager within your VR team.

It is very important to include a timely reminder here about confidentiality. While the employer is a key member of the VR team, how much you can, or cannot, disclose to them about the client's health condition or disability will be determined by the client. You will need to have discussed this matter with the person beforehand, and certainly a spirit of openness is to be encouraged, but many employees will not wish to have private, personal information discussed with their employers. This is their right, so you will need to be very mindful of respecting their wishes in this regard. You will also need to ensure that you do not contravene the Data Protection Act, which we will come to in the next chapter.

We have now examined the roles of each of the core members of the VR team. Sitting down together, with the client and either the DEA or the employer, will be a significant step forwards. During this meeting, the issues will be looked at and various proposals and suggestions may be put forward and discussed. In the case of a work return, this is where the graduated return to work plan will be formulated and agreed (see the earlier chapter about the VR process for more information about the return to work plan). Ideally this meeting should be positive, enabling and supportive. As the return to work facilitator you will want to inspire the confidence of both the employee and the employer in the VR process. For the return to work plan to be successful, all the VR team members need to be actively engaged in, and committed to, the process of supporting that person to return to work. It is also desirable for the client to leave this meeting perceiving the employer to be supportive of their return to work, and signed up to the process which will enable them to do so.

OTHER TEAM MEMBERS IN DIFFERENT SETTINGS

There are numerous other practitioners who are involved, directly or indirectly, in VR services. A selection of perhaps the most common roles which the occupational therapist may encounter in different settings is included below.

The **claims manager** works for an insurance company. Any new claim under an insurance policy, such as an income protection policy for example, will come through to this person. He or she will then check the eligibility of the claim and assess the claim to see if a decision can be made on it. If appropriate, the claims manager may discuss the case with a rehabilitation professional, such as an occupational therapist, to assess the potential for VR. The claims manager will remain involved in the case while any VR programme is being delivered.

The **safety practitioner** may also be called a safety officer, or a health and safety officer. They are most commonly found in larger organisations, and some provide their services on a consultancy basis. The safety practitioner may come from a variety of different backgrounds, often from a science or engineering profession. They will have undertaken additional formal study and gained a recognised qualification in health and safety. The practitioner is trained to interpret health and safety legislation, identify hazards in the workplace and give general advice on matters of safety. A central element of their role will include accident reporting and prevention, carrying out risk assessments, and providing health and safety training (Chambers *et al.*, 2001). The safety officer will also have membership of a professional body such as the Institute of Occupational Safety and Health (IOSH). The purpose of the IOSH is to regulate and steer the profession, maintain standards, and provide guidance on health and safety issues. Further information about the IOSH can be found at: http://www.iosh.co.uk (accessed 22/04/07).

The **occupational physician** is medically qualified as a doctor. However, since there is no formal obligation to gain additional qualifications in occupational medicine, the person may, or may not, have undertaken specific training in occupational health matters. Many general practitioners negotiate part-time occupational physician work with companies on a sessional basis. However, companies which employ part-time non-specialist practitioners are increasingly being required to ensure that whoever is appointed has the necessary competence.

The Society of Occupational Medicine, a specialist society of The Royal College of Physicians, was involved in the foundation of the Faculty of Occupational Medicine (FOM). This body is responsible for standards, training and qualifications in the specialty. The FOM advises that employers who take on a physician to carry out this type of sessional work should ensure that they have undertaken some training. Particularly since much of the required knowledge in the field of occupational medicine is not covered in undergraduate or general professional training (Wynn *et al.*, 2003). Furthermore, the FOM recommends that formal training is needed in order to meet the requirements for competence currently demanded by many aspects of current health and safety legislation.

A doctor may gain different levels of qualifications in occupational health. A diploma in occupational medicine is considered to be a basic level qualification, particularly for general practitioners who work part-time in occupational medicine. It provides the doctor with an understanding of the main issues affecting health and work. An Associateship of the Faculty of Occupational Medicine is a training qualification specifically for doctors who are interested in pursuing a full-time career in occupational medicine. It includes a core knowledge in occupational medicine theory and practice. Finally, Membership of the Faculty of Occupational Medicine is a specialist qualification which is required for appointment as a hospital consultant in this field. More information about the Society of Occupational Medicine can be found at: http://www.som.org.uk (accessed 30/4/07).

The **occupational health nurse** is responsible for the health and wellbeing of employees in the work place. He or she is a registered general nurse, sometimes with an additional qualification in occupational health nursing. In common with occupational physicians, there is no legal requirement for nurses to undertake further training to work in the occupational health field. However, it is strongly recommended by the relevant professional bodies that further training is undertaken, and this is often required by potential employers (Garvey, 1995). The Society of Occupational Health

Nursing is a specialist section of the Royal College of Nursing which is specifically concerned with health in the workplace, the importance of improving the working environment, and the health of the working population. More information can be found at: http://www.rcn.org.uk (accessed 3/05/07).

While some nursing degree courses may incorporate training in occupational health, postgraduate study is more usual. At least two years post-qualifying nursing experience is usually expected before postgraduate occupational health training is undertaken. This training may be at certificate, diploma or degree level, on either a full- or part-time basis via face-to-face provision or distance learning. Courses in occupational health may include topics such as behavioural science; health promotion; epidemiology; research and management; the effects of health on work and work on health; the public health strategy; and risk and health assessment in the work setting. Good interpersonal and management skills are needed, so communication and teaching; managing people and resources; team-building skills; and management of change are also often key elements of any programme of training (Garvey, 1995).

The nature of the duties of the occupational health nurse will often be dependent on the setting in which he or she works, since there will be different hazards and risks within different types of work settings. Therefore, a sound understanding of the organisation is needed in this role. The occupational health nurse may work in large businesses and organisations, for private consultancies, as part of an occupational or environmental health and safety team or, in small enterprises, sometimes alone. The nurse will be expected to undertake some, or all, of the following typical work activities:

- pre-employment medicals or physicals, including hearing and vision screen, and health and fitness advice
- provide advice to people who are returning to work after an accident or serious illness, and assist injured employees returning to work from medical leave
- counselling
- identify potential health hazards in an employer's workplace and communicate any safety concerns to the appropriate managers
- take preventive action to avoid illness
- promote the good health, welfare and safety of the workforce
- provide health education, health support and guidance
- organise health education campaigns
- co-operate with other health and safety professionals
- advise staff and management on safety measures and on how to comply with health and safety legislation
- regular health screening checks for staff
- use expertise to ensure that organisations meet their legislative requirements, such as conducting assessments and inspections on display screen equipment (DSE), personal protective equipment (PPE) and the control of substances hazardous to health (COSHH)
- provide first aid and medical treatment, maintain first-aid kits, order new supplies and dispose of out-of-date items as necessary

- contact doctors and/or hospitals, as necessary, to arrange further treatment
- maintain employee health records and prepare accident reports
- monitor employee exposure to hazardous chemicals
- keep up to date with legal and professional changes associated with occupational health and safety.

(Prospects, 2007)

The **occupational hygienist** is most likely to be found in the manufacturing sector and, in common with the safety practitioner, often comes from a background in a profession such as chemistry or engineering. They will have gone on to undertake additional training to perform this role. He or she is responsible for assessing risks in the workplace such as the level of fumes, noise and dust. The British Occupational Hygiene Society reminds us that workplaces have many hazards, both seen and unseen. These may be chemical, for example dusts and vapours, physical, including heat, light and noise, or ergonomic, such as posture and motion. These hazards may also be biological, for example bacterial or viral, or psychosocial, such as stress, violence or bullying. The role of the occupational hygienist is, therefore, to understand how these hazards may affect the health of employees, measuring how significant the effects may be, and then finding practical and cost-effective ways of controlling the identified risks to health (The British Occupational Hygiene Society, 2007).

Occupational hygienists gain their knowledge in subjects such as toxicology, physiology, occupational diseases, epidemiology, ergonomics, and occupational health and safety law. They need an understanding of the principles of hazard control, such as the ways in which a process may be modified, ventilation, the use of personal protective equipment, and associated administrative measures which may be introduced. Many hygienists provide training to others with the objective of achieving a healthier workplace (Australian Institute of Occupational Hygienists Inc., 2005). In industries outside of the manufacturing sector, a similar role may be performed by an ergonomist.

Cullum (1997) describes the benefits of a team approach within the workplace and suggests that professionals who may be involved in the management of health and safety include: the safety practitioner, the occupational health physician, the occupational health nurse, the occupational therapist, the physiotherapist, the back care adviser and the occupational hygienist. Some organisations may also have a range of additional team members depending on the size of the organisation and the type of work performed. Increasingly, larger organisations are extending the range of services provided to employees and these may include a qualified counsellor or psychologist, sessional physiotherapy or complementary therapy practitioners.

The **personal adviser** works in the Jobcentre Plus. When a person of working age who is not in employment, makes a claim for benefits, he or she is put in touch with a personal adviser. The personal adviser's role is to assist that person to look for work. They have access to a range of training or support services to assist the person to develop the skills they need to be employable. These services were discussed earlier in the book. Personal advisers can also give the person advice on financial incentives, which they may be entitled to through participating in certain schemes. Personal advisers receive on-the-job training to enable them to fulfil this role. They are not, however, always equipped to deal with the difficulties of the people for whom they are providing a service. Some personal advisers receive additional training to enable them to become incapacity benefits personal advisers (IBPA) and specifically work with people who are claiming this benefit. This role will be changed when welfare reform changes come into effect, and the incapacity benefit is replaced in 2008.

Work psychologists also work for the Department for Work and Pensions and can be found in some jobcentres. Work psychologists undertake a consultancy role to the DEAs, as well as providing specialist professional assessments and recommendations for work seekers with complex needs, particularly those who have cognitive difficulties. Work psychologists can also be found within the private sector. Key knowledge areas of the work psychologist include:

- the person–job fit and occupational choice
- selection and assessment of employees
- work-related attitudes and perceptions
- work motivation and satisfaction
- learning and training at work
- stress at work
- group dynamics and leadership
- organisational structure and change.

(Furnham, 2005; Doyle, 2003)

9 Working Within the Law in Industry

There are all kinds of external agendas and pressures that determine the scope and boundaries of our practice – the most obvious being legislation. While occupational therapists are not expected to have an in-depth understanding of the law and the legal system, it is important that the practitioner is familiar with the most relevant legislation that governs their particular specialty, and practices within the law. The employment sector has additional legislation which will be of relevance to the occupational therapist working in vocational rehabilitation (VR). Policies that the practitioner will need to be familiar with may usefully be grouped under 'health and safety' and 'disability rights'. This chapter provides an overview of the pertinent legislation and regulations in these two areas, as well as the bodies responsible for producing and enforcing the various regulations and laws. This chapter will also touch briefly on some other relevant Acts.

Health and safety legislation, which is primarily designed to safeguard and protect workers in the UK, is a particularly wide field, therefore this discussion is limited to looking at the legislation which is applicable to all workplaces, irrespective of the type of work that is undertaken. It is important to be aware that this chapter is by no means exhaustive, and that within industries where there is a higher risk of health and safety problems, such as agriculture and construction, additional regulations will apply. Policy is regularly updated, so occupational therapists involved in VR are advised to take steps to stay abreast of these changes.

THE HEALTH AND SAFETY AT WORK ACT

The Health and Safety at Work etc. Act (1974) forms the basis for the system of regulating health and safety at work in the UK. For this reason, the occupational therapist who practises in the workplace needs a sound understanding of this piece of legislation, since it has implications for the return to work process. The Act itself sets out basic principles of occupational safety, designed to protect all workers, regardless of the industry in which they work. In doing so, it imposes statutory duties on companies, managers and their employees. Before its introduction, only certain groups of workers, in certain types of industry, had any sort of protection under the existing laws. The main purpose, therefore, was to produce a thorough system of law to raise the health and safety standards for workers across the board. This law also covers members of the public who are not at work, but may be affected in some way by the actions of the workers, such as customers and passers-by (Foot and Hook, 2005). Importantly, the Act also allows for older laws and outdated safety regulations to be overhauled and updated, producing new codes of practice which are applicable within the modern, ever-changing, working world.

THE HEALTH AND SAFETY COMMISSION AND THE HEALTH AND SAFETY EXECUTIVE

The Health and Safety Commission (HSC) is a government body which came into being as a result of the Health and Safety at Work Act (1974). It has statutory responsibilities for regulating health and safety in the UK, and its main function is to safeguard the health, safety and welfare of people at work and the public. This is done by proposing new laws and standards, carrying out research, and providing advice and information (Health and Safety Executive, 2002a). The HSC, together with an employer organisation called the Confederation of British Industry and the Trades Union Congress, is responsible for national health and safety policy (Howard, 2000).

The Health and Safety Executive (HSE) is a separate organisation which advises and assists the Commission, as well as having its own specific responsibilities. The HSE recommends standards and provides guidance to the HSC, particularly where new problems are encountered, or where potential hazards are inherent within a particular type of industry, for example, within the nuclear power industry. The HSE is responsible for enforcing the requirements of the Health and Safety at Work Act, as well as a number of other Acts and statutory instruments which are relevant to the working environment. The guidance, approved codes of practice, and regulations which are produced by the HSE can be accessed from the extensive publication library contained on their website: http://www.hse.gov.uk (accessed 06/05/07). Local authorities complement the work of the HSE by enforcing the Act in specific sectors. They appoint inspectors, usually known as environmental health officers, who are responsible for distribution, office and retail, and leisure and catering services (Health and Safety Executive, 2002a).

EMPLOYERS' RESPONSIBILITIES UNDER THE HEALTH AND SAFETY AT WORK ACT

Employers are bound by seemingly vast volumes of legislation and regulations which, as we have just learned, are enforced by the HSE. Essentially, this reflects the fact that they have a duty of care to ensure the health, safety and welfare of their employees. They also have to ensure the workplace is safe, and safely organised, and that any equipment has been correctly maintained. They must ensure that there are safe ways for people to get into and out of buildings. They must provide training and information about health and safety and make sure that accidents don't happen because of incorrect handling, storage or transportation within the workplace. They must also make adequate welfare provisions for their staff. They may appoint a health and safety officer to ensure that they are fulfilling their responsibilities.

However, employees must also take responsibility for their own health and safety and that of their colleagues. They must not act in a way that may cause health and safety problems for others, and this may include failing to act. They must not recklessly interfere with, or misuse, any machinery or equipment and must co-operate with employers about health and safety initiatives.

OTHER HEALTH AND SAFETY REGULATIONS

A directive from the European Union in 1992 resulted in the introduction of six further sets of regulations.

- The Management of Health and Safety at Work Regulations 1992
- The Health and Safety (Display Screen Equipment) Regulations 1992
- The Manual Handling Operations Regulations 1992
- The Workplace (Health, Safety and Welfare) Regulations 1992
- The Provision and Use of Work Equipment Regulations 1992
- The Personal Protective Equipment at Work Regulations 1992.
(Foot and Hook, 2005)

These regulations extended the existing health and safety law, and also placed additional requirements on employers. Since their introduction, several amendments to these regulations have become necessary. The following paragraphs do not, therefore, present a full synopsis of the regulations or amendments, but just highlight those aspects of the regulations which may have a particular relevance for occupational therapists in their work.

The management of Health and Safety at Work Regulations 1999

These regulations updated those introduced in 1992, to make more explicit what employers are required to do to manage health and safety. The employer's main requirement is to carry out a risk assessment (you may remember that we discussed the risk assessment process in an earlier chapter). Additionally, employers are required to make arrangements to implement the health and safety measures identified during the risk assessment and appoint a competent person(s) to help implement these arrangements. They must also provide information and training to employees on health and safety (Health and Safety Executive, 2003a). The competent person identified here may well be an occupational therapist with the necessary skills and expertise. This role is regularly fulfilled by occupational therapists in other countries.

The Health and Safety (Display Screen Equipment) Regulations 1992

This legislation was most recently amended by the Health and Safety (Miscellaneous Amendments) Regulations 2002. Under the Health and Safety (Display Screen Equipment) Regulations (1992) employers are required to undertake an analysis of all the workstations used by their staff to assess and identify any health and safety risks to the computer user. They must ensure that workstations meet at least the minimum requirements. They are also required to plan, or provide for, short frequent breaks or changes in activity within the work routine. These should preferably involve performing other tasks away from the keyboard. Where a routine audit carried out by an employer identifies problems, particularly musculoskeletal ones, an occupational therapist may be called upon to undertake a comprehensive workstation assessment to address these issues.

The Manual Handling Operations Regulations 1992

Also amended by the Health and Safety (Miscellaneous Amendments) Regulations 2002, the Manual Handling Operations Regulations 1992 aim to reduce the levels of injury and ill-health associated with manual handling of loads at work. You may recall that we examined some of the details of these regulations in an earlier chapter. The effects of the legislation will vary across workplaces, depending on the nature of the work being undertaken (Foot and Hook, 2005). When trying to determine the potential risk involved in each manual handling activity, the employer must take into account factors such as: the physical suitability of the employee, the clothing worn, the knowledge and training which has been received, findings from previous risk assessments and the level of risk involved in the activity. The HSE (2006a) has produced a short guide that contains helpful details about good practice in manual handling. This is available on-line at: http://www.hse.gov.uk/pubns/indg143.pdf (accessed 20/04/07).

The Workplace (Health, Safety and Welfare) Regulations 1992

These regulations were also updated in 2002. They provide clear information about what facilities the employer is expected to provide for employees, including a good, clean working environment with adequate space, temperature control, ventilation and lighting. Where a job requires the person to sit, the seating should be suitable for the work being done, and for the person using it. It should provide adequate back support and a foot rest should be supplied where needed. Under the amendments, employers are also required to ensure that the design of equipment, such as workstations, and facilities such as passageways, stairs, rest areas and washrooms, which are used by disabled people at work are organised to meet the specific needs of those workers. An on-line HSE guide (2006b) on this subject is available at: http://www.hse.gov.uk/pubns/indg244.pdf (accessed 21/04/07).

The Reporting of Injuries, Diseases and Dangerous Occurences Regulations 1995

These regulations require the employer to report work-related accidents, diseases and dangerous occurrences to the HSE or local authority. For example, if a person who is on the employer's premises, whether an employee or a member of the public, is killed or taken to hospital, it must be reported. This action must also be taken when an employee is absent for more than three days following a violent incident or injury at work, or an employee is diagnosed with a reportable work-related disease. The relevant authority must also be notified in the case of a 'near miss' (Chambers *et al.*, 2001).

Other relevant employment legislation

The Chartered Institute of Personnel and Development (2006a) suggests that the main legal tools for employers facilitating absence management are the Employment Act 2002 and the Employment Act 2002 (Dispute Resolution) Regulations 2004. The former relates mainly to statutory leave arrangements and the latter to grievance and disciplinary procedures. Further information on these, and other employment matters, can be obtained from the Department for Trade and Industry, which has responsibility for employment legislation of this nature (http://www.dti. gov.uk/employment/index.html, accessed 03/05/07). A useful on-line resource, which brings together a wide range of public service information and services, and provides straight-forward advice for employees about work employment rights and responsibilities can be found at: http://www.direct.gov.uk (accessed 03/05/07).

THE DISABILITY DISCRIMINATION ACT

The Disability Discrimination Act (DDA) was passed in 1995 to address the discrimination that is faced by many disabled people. In 2004 it was estimated that around 700,000 children and 10 million adults in Britain were considered to be disabled and were therefore covered by the terms of the Act. At the time, about one in five was a person of working age. More recently, the number of working age adults has risen by half a million, to 5.7 million people, reflecting a general trend in the population to report milder health conditions and disabilities (Department for Work and Pensions, 2006b). By far the greatest majority of this group will have acquired their disability at some point during their life, since just a small percentage (17 per cent) of those who are disabled will have been born with their particular condition (Disability Rights Commission, 2006).

Different parts of the DDA legislation have taken effect at different times, and, in common with other legislation, there have been a number of amendments to the original Act. For example, in 2004, four kinds of discrimination were identified: direct discrimination, failure to make reasonable adjustments, disability-related discrimination and victimisation. The following year, The Disability Discrimination Act 2005 introduced a disability equality duty into the Act. This duty came into effect in December 2006, and is aimed at overcoming systemic discrimination. It requires public authorities to promote equality of opportunity for disabled people in the way they conduct their business. The scope of the DDA was also extended to include people with HIV infection, cancer or multiple sclerosis, and the requirement that a mental illness must be 'clinically well-recognised' was removed.

As far as public understanding of the DDA goes, it has been suggested that employers, particularly those in smaller companies, tend to have a narrower perception of what constitutes a disability than that stated in the DDA. Disability is often understood in terms of visible, physical impairments. There remains a need for general education, to raise awareness about the nature and breadth of disability (Roberts *et al.*, 2004), and occupational therapists may be well-placed to provide this education.

A person is disabled under the terms of the DDA if:

- they have a mental or physical impairment
  AND
- the impairment has an adverse effect on the person's ability to carry out their normal day-to-day activities in at least one of the following areas: mobility; manual dexterity; physical co-ordination; continence; ability to lift, carry or move everyday objects; speech, hearing or eyesight; memory or ability to concentrate, learn or understand; understand the risk of physical danger
  AND
- the adverse effect is substantial and long term, in that it has lasted for 12 months, or is likely to last for more than 12 months.

When determining if someone is disabled under the terms of the Act, any treatment or correction (such as a prosthesis) should not be taken into account (except glasses and contact lenses). If the impairment is no longer substantially affecting the person's ability to carry out their normal day-to-day activities, but it has done so in the past and is likely to do so in the future, it still counts as a disability under the DDA. Furthermore, if the person has a progressive condition which will substantially affect their abilities in the future, it is covered by the DDA from the moment it has some effect on normal everyday activities. Some conditions, namely cancer, HIV infection and multiple sclerosis, are automatically covered, as are people who have been certified as blind or partially sighted by a consultant ophthalmologist.

Section 2 of the Act is concerned with employment. It requires employers to make reasonable adjustments for a disabled person put at a substantial disadvantage by a provision, criterion or practice, or physical feature of the premises. What counts as 'reasonable' depends on a number of factors, such as the size and resources of the organisation, how practical it is, how disruptive, the costs involved, and how effective the adjustment might be in overcoming the disadvantage (Disability Rights Commission, 2004).

Some suggested reasonable adjustments in the amended DDA (2004) include:

- alterations to premises
- re-allocating certain duties to others
- altering working hours
- allowing time off for rehabilitation, treatment and assessments

- providing additional training and modifying equipment (Howard and Cox, 2000)
- mentoring, providing supervision or a reader/interpreter
- modifying instructions or manuals.

However, as is witnessed from this list, the majority of accommodations that are described in the literature concern physical rather than psychiatric disabilities (MacDonald-Wilson et al., 2002). Barriers to providing accommodations for this group are identified as: resources, issues around disclosure, the attitudes of co-workers, and communication difficulties. Providing accommodations for people with a mental illness is often inexpensive, but they do require observation, flexibility and good management (Pollet, 1995). Further American studies have suggested the following accommodations at work for people who have a mental health problem:

- training of supervisors
- modifications of the non-physical work environment (Fabian et al., 1993)
- emotional support
- flexibility
- supervision
- wages and benefits
- addressing co-workers' attitudes.
(Parrish, 1991)

In addition, it is suggested that guidance and information about psychiatric disabilities needs to be provided to employers, especially in the area of interpersonal relationships (Marshall, 1995). Further up-to-date information about the DDA can be found on the Department for Work and Pensions website http://www.dwp.gov.uk (accessed 19/07/07).

THE DISABILITY RIGHTS COMMISSION ACT

The Disability Rights Commission Act (1999) led to the establishment of the Disability Rights Commission in 2000. The Commission's statutory duties include:

- working to eliminate discrimination against disabled people
- promoting equal opportunities for disabled people
- encouraging good practice in the treatment of disabled people
- advising the government on the working of disability legislation, such as the Disability Discrimination Act 2005
- enforcing the law in the public interest (it is therefore able to provide support for certain individual cases, as well as conducting formal investigations).

The Disability Rights Commission has produced a comprehensive Code of Practice on Employment and Occupation (2004). This code contributes to the Commission's mission to eliminate discrimination against disabled people. It gives practical guidance on how to prevent discrimination against disabled people in employment, or when they are seeking employment. It describes the duties of employers and others, and is intended to assist employers to prevent workplace disputes. It also helps to explain what the law means for disabled people and what they can do if they feel that they have been discriminated against. The Code can be accessed on-line at: http://www.drc.org.uk/library/publications/employment/code_of_practice_-_employment.aspx (accessed 28/04/07).

OTHER RELEVANT LEGISLATION

There is other relevant legislation which protects the rights of people as individuals, irrespective of whether they have a disability or not. Let us consider, very briefly, how these might apply to the occupational therapist in VR.

The Data Protection Act

The Data Protection Act (1998) governs the use of personal information by businesses and organisations. Some information, such as a physical or mental health condition, is classified as sensitive information and is subject to tighter controls under the terms of the Act. Such information may only be used when there is an essential need to use it or where the individual has given their explicit consent. Therefore, you must ensure that you, as a health professional, ensure the confidentiality of the personal details which your client shares with you. You may not divulge this information to another person, particularly the client's employer, without their consent. It is important to discuss with the client what they are prepared to let their employer know about their health condition or disability.

Employees may be fearful of revealing this type of information if they feel that it may jeopardise their job. Since the unscrupulous employer may indeed use this information for other purposes, their concerns may well have validity. On the other hand, however, the employer cannot be expected to make reasonable adjustments, under the terms of the DDA, if the employee refuses to make known that they have a disability. On this point, it is worth noting that it is not impossible to encounter a situation where the employer has been informed, by an occupational health physician, that they need to make adjustments for an employee who is protected by the DDA, but they have not been told what accommodations are needed. This seems, to me, to be a rather untenable situation for both parties. There is far less risk of potential conflict between the two positions where a basic level of trust underpins the relationship between the client and their employer. This is what you should be aiming to achieve, wherever possible. For further information, the Data Protection Act can be found on-line at: http://www.opsi.gov.uk/ACTS/acts1998/19980029.htm (accessed 01/05/07).

Additional laws which are of relevance are **The Human Rights Act (1998)**, which includes working rights, and **The Employment Equality (Age) Regulations (2006)** which makes it unlawful to discriminate on the grounds of age, unless there is a justifiable reason for doing so. The regulations cover recruitment, terms and conditions, promotions, transfers, dismissals and training.

IMPLICATIONS OF LEGISLATION FOR THE OCCUPATIONAL THERAPIST IN VOCATIONAL REHABILITATION

As stated at the outset, this is not a comprehensive outline or list of the laws affecting VR, nor could it possibly be so. Laws must be interpreted, and so as each new case is brought before the courts it adds a further dimension to how that law is intended to be applied and understood.

Having read through the laws and regulations which have been outlined above you will no doubt have recognised the need to strike a delicate balance. This balance must be, on the one hand, between the rights of any individual not to be discriminated against and to have every opportunity to participate in meaningful work. On the other, it concerns the duties placed on an employer to ensure that they adhere to robust working practices, for the health and safety of all employees as well as any members of the public who might be affected by their actions. Finding this middle ground perspective in VR is important, because it would be unreasonable to expect an employer to contravene health and safety regulations, in order to comply with disability discrimination law, or vice versa.

Many occupational therapists may currently be unfamiliar with health and safety legislation, since it is seldom a core element of existing undergraduate programmes (Ross, 2006). However, you will see from the brief discussions above that there is an increasingly visible role for knowledgeable occupational therapists to assist employers to meet their obligations in this area.

OTHER ORGANISATIONS IN WORK, HEALTH AND DISABILITY

There are a significant number of other organisations which play a direct, or an indirect, role in aspects of workplace health and safety, or in disability and work matters, and it may be helpful for the occupational therapist who wants to gain an understanding of the wider picture, to familiarise themselves with just a few of them.

The Commission for Equality and Human Rights

This Commission is still in the planning stages, and is expected to be created in the autumn of 2007. It will include the Disability Rights Commission, which we read about earlier, as well as two other existing equality commissions.

The Office for Disability Issues

This new office was brought into being in 2005 and its purpose is to co-ordinate disability policy across government departments and drive forward the recommendations which were outlined in *Improving the Life Chances for Disabled People* (Department of Work and Pensions, *et al.*, 2005). For further information about their current priorities visit: http://www.officefordisability.gov.uk/ (accessed 11/05/07).

The Industrial Injuries Advisory Council

The Industrial Injury Disability Benefit Scheme is a state benefit which provides weekly compensation for people injured at work in industrial accidents and with certain prescribed diseases. Matters concerning the administration of the benefit scheme are dealt with by the Industrial Injuries Advisory Council (IIAC). It is a statutory body which was established in 1948. The IIAC's role is to provide independent advice to the Secretary of State for the Department for Work and Pensions, as well as to advise on the prescription of diseases. It monitors and reviews new scientific evidence about certain diseases which may have an occupational link, and then decides whether the list of prescribed diseases, for which benefit may be paid, should be expanded or amended. For interested readers, the full list of diseases covered by the Industrial Injury Disability Benefit may be found at: http://www.iiac.org.uk/prescribed_diseases/index.asp (accessed 28/04/07).

Advisory, Conciliation and Arbitration Service

The Advisory, Conciliation and Arbitration Service (ACAS) is a publicly funded organisation that was founded in 1975. ACAS provides independent, voluntary and confidential services to organisations which are intended to improve working life through creating better employment relations. They provide a range of training and work with employers and employees to resolve problems, such as disputes and disagreements at work. They will assist in the management of conflict, directed towards reaching an acceptable solution without involving, for example, an employment tribunal. They have produced recent guidance on age discrimination in the workplace (Advisory, Conciliation and Arbitration Service, 2006), and tackle discrimination and promoting equality (Advisory, Conciliation and Arbitration Service, 2005), which is concerned with any form of discrimination, including sex, race, disability, sexual orientation and religion. Further information about ACAS can be found at: http://www.acas.co.uk (accessed 19/07/07).

Trades Union Congress

The Trades Union Congress campaigns for a fair deal at work, as well as for social justice in the UK and abroad. It has 66 affiliated unions and represents about seven million working people. It advises people about their rights at work as well as being a major contributor to the national policy debate on the need for better access to occupational health services and the protection of workers' health and safety while at work. More information can be found at: http://www.tuc.org.uk (accessed 05/05/07).

Professional Organisations in Occupational Safety and Health

Professional Organisations in Occupational Safety and Health (POOSH) is an organisation which exists to promote the continuous improvement of the practice of occupational safety and health. It focuses in particular on education, communication and the encouragement of co-operation between all persons and agencies involved in the provision of a healthy and safe working environment. For the occupational therapist, the website www.poosh.org is a good resource for finding out about different professional groups and bodies within occupational health and safety in the UK. Organisations currently represented on POOSH include:

- Association of Occupational Health Nurse Practitioners (UK)
- British Occupational Hygiene Society
- Chartered Institute of Environmental Health
- Ergonomics Society
- Faculty of Occupational Medicine
- International Institute of Risk and Safety Management
- Institute of Risk Management
- Institution of Occupational Safety and Health
- Royal Environmental Health Institute of Scotland
- Royal Society for the Promotion of Health
- Royal Society of Chemistry
- Safety and Reliability Society
- Society of Occupational Health Nursing
- Society of Occupational Medicine.

10 Future Directions

This final chapter highlights current key issues which are of particular relevance to occupational therapists in vocational rehabilitation (VR), and also looks to the future. We will briefly consider the significant implications of impending policy changes, particularly with regard to benefits claimants with a disability. We will conclude by examining some of the challenges which may face occupational therapists in VR in the years ahead – paying particular attention to education, training and accreditation – and identify important areas which are in need of further research.

PLANNED WELFARE REFORMS

Earlier in the book we learned about how political and economic agendas have played a pivotal role in matters to do with work and disability. The current Government continues to drive forward welfare reform centred on this theme. The political spotlight remains firmly fixed on participation in employment as an integral part of an ongoing programme of welfare reforms. To this end, the Green Paper: *A New Deal for Welfare: Empowering people to work* (Department for Work and Pensions, 2006a), proposes a radical overhaul of the benefits system for new claimants. It builds on the changes introduced through the Pathways to Work programme, which, you may remember, includes Condition Management Programmes.

From 2008, incapacity benefit and income support for people with health conditions, will be replaced by a new employment and support allowance (ESA). This will be paid, in addition to the basic jobseeker's allowance, only to those people who agree to participate in work-related activity. These activities may include work-focused interviews with the personal advisor at the Jobcentre Plus, and participation in agreed programmes and activities which are work-related, or directed towards work return. Suitable activities may include attending a condition management programme or doing voluntary work.

A minority of people who are considered too unwell to work will receive additional benefits, over and above the ESA, which are not conditional on work participation. Expert practitioners suggest that the Welfare Reform Bill (Department for Work and Pensions, 2006a) will help create incentives for patients to return to work, increase the conditionality to benefit entitlement, stimulate VR through demanding that recipients show work-related activity, and offer programmes designed to help them manage their condition (Thurgood and Frank, 2007).

Attaching a financial inducement to promote return to work will, of course, have both advantages and disadvantages. On the positive side, it will remove some of the disincentives in the current system and prevent people becoming locked in a benefits trap. It also means that a far more pro-active approach will be pursued in supporting people back to work. These are both positive steps and disabled workers themselves have indicated that, despite existing strategies and support, they need access to more structured, formalised and appropriate support (Roulstone *et al.*, 2003). On the negative side, however, these planned reforms have significant resource implications if they are to be delivered effectively. The funding of these resources is yet to be clarified, although much of the provision will be out-sourced to the private and voluntary sector. In some parts of the country the infrastructure is not yet in place to deliver the agenda, therefore existing services may struggle to meet these targets. Additionally, details about the practical implementation of the reforms are currently limited.

The Disability Rights Commission (DRC) has raised concerns about this matter, and they are well placed to do so, since one of the Commission's top ten priorities is to close the employment gap between disabled and non-disabled people, including a successful outcome from welfare reform. In this regard, during its consultations, the DRC raises a number of vital questions about the implementation of the planned reforms (Disability Rights Commission, 2006), which include:

- With regard to eligibility, what is the best concept to underpin the ESA which avoids the rigidity of 'incapacity for all work'?
- In connection with assessment, what needs to be done to reform the personal capability assessment (the medical assessment which currently determines if someone is, or is not, capable of work) and other assessments, so that they are fit for purpose and consistent with the new concept?
- Concerning the conditionality element of the reforms, what is the appropriate level of responsibility that can reasonably be expected of ESA recipients, and should this vary by type of recipient, or activity?
- Regarding activities while on benefit, how can ESA rules ensure that people do not risk losing benefit when trying out work-related activities, volunteering or public appointments, while avoiding people being trapped in those activities without progressing to their full potential?
- In relation to the benefit structure, what is the best balance between means-tested and contributory elements for both the 'employment' and the 'support' group?
- How can existing recipients of disability benefits be enabled to take the risk of trying out work and related activities while ensuring that entitlement remains correct?
- Finally, what are the disability implications of longer-term reform?

The DRC followed up these questions with a number of possible alternatives and strategies in response to the Green Paper and also to the Welfare Reform Bill, and the interested reader can find out more at: http://www.drc.org.uk/disabilitydebate/priorities/documents/IB_Discussion_paper_March_2006.pdf (accessed 24/10/06).

The conditional element of programme participation that will be attached to benefit payments has particular relevance to occupational therapists. There are different viewpoints amongst members of the profession as to whether this will support or hinder the occupational therapist's role. You too will, no doubt, have your own views on the subject. Removing the voluntary aspect of participation does have the potential to undermine the success of existing successful programmes, because it means that the individual's personal control and choice are diminished. As a result, the person may feel compelled to attend therapeutic interventions, such as Condition Management Programmes, rather than being there through personal choice. This compulsion may counterbalance the therapeutic benefits which a number of occupational therapists currently attribute to the voluntary nature of participation within existing programmes.

The final point raised by the DRC concerns longer-term implications. It is important to reflect on the fact that these reforms are being delivered at a time when the economy is strong. History demonstrates that VR schemes have been swiftly dropped from the agenda during times of recession. On this note, it is interesting to see that in their latest departmental report, setting out a three-year target, the Department for Work and Pensions plans to 'increase the employment rate of disabled people, **taking account of the economic cycle**, and significantly reduce the difference between their employment rate and the overall rate, **taking account of the economic cycle**' (our emphasis) (Department for Work and Pensions, 2006b, p.70). What might the implications be, one wonders, for people with health conditions or disabilities who are expected to engage in work activity in a less than favourable economy?

Change is, of course, also taking place elsewhere in the domain of VR, beyond the welfare system. Employers (Tehrani, 2004), insurers (Association of British Insurers, 2005) and personal injury lawyers (Association of Personal Injury Lawyers, 2004) are increasingly looking to healthcare and rehabilitation to meet their particular objectives. Therefore the demand is rising for services and for practitioners with the necessary expertise. Encouragingly, this trend looks set to continue within these sectors. However, this increasing demand throws up issues about the knowledge and skills which are being sought by these respective parties, since a lack of suitably skilled and trained professionals is currently identified as a major barrier, preventing potential growth and service expansion within the field. A report for the Association of British Insurers, which examined the availability of rehabilitation resources in the UK, identified that occupational therapists with experience in VR were a key gap in rehabilitation resources (Wright et al., 2005). This concern brings us, in an opportune way, to examining salient issues with regard to the education and training of occupational therapists in VR.

EDUCATION AND ACCREDITATION

In the earlier days of the re-awakened political interest in VR, a British Society of Rehabilitation Medicine (BSRM) working party report recommended the need for further development of training programmes for health professionals in this field. They remarked that 'As work awareness is required in all NHS professions it needs to be part of the undergraduate training of all NHS staff. Those who need a greater input are undergraduate doctors, occupational therapists and physiotherapists' (British Society of Rehabilitation Medicine, 2000, p.63). Alongside the BSRM report, the College of Occupational Therapists undertook its own review of work rehabilitation and occupational therapy (OT). It concluded that 'while assessment of occupational performance is one of the core components of pre-registration occupational therapy courses, the demand for specific skills in work rehabilitation demands that this knowledge be extended,' and recommended that, 'work rehabilitation should ... be a stronger feature of pre-registration programmes' (Mountain *et al.*, 2001, p.54). More recently, a report by the Association of British Insurers called on the Government to 'establish a transparent accreditation system for rehabilitation qualifications and provide enough financial support to increase the number of rehabilitation specialists' (Association of British Insurers, 2005, p.10), although the Government has already acknowledged that some form of accreditation system is needed (Department for Work and Pensions, 2004).

Despite these clearly stated recommendation from key parties, progress towards addressing these proposals has been woefully slow. As a recent publication by the College of Occupational Therapists Specialist Section – WORK identifies, the lack of experience of many established clinicians and academics means that education and training in VR, at both undergraduate and postgraduate level, remains patchy, and, in the absence of an agreed pre- and post-registration core curriculum, the content of courses which are currently available shows considerable variation (Barnes and Holmes, 2007). The College of Occupational Therapists has consistently maintained the stance that occupational therapists have the skills to deliver VR, and yet potential employers have, anecdotally, on some occasions suggested otherwise.

This viewpoint is reinforced by findings from a recent study which examined the planned undergraduate OT curricula for 16 OT courses across England, Wales, Scotland and Northern Ireland. The intended aim of the research was to examine how work and VR were represented within the curriculum. A content analysis of each course document looked at the intended learning outcomes, module descriptions, reading lists, reference and bibliography lists, and any assignment details. Despite the obvious limitations raised by research of this kind, it is notable that just one out of the 16 course documents analysed made reference to VR and work rehabilitation, both within a mental health context. Terms such as occupational health, disability management, insurance sector and worker did not appear in any of the course documents. Few references were made to approaches and interventions associated with rehabilitation for work. Just one final year optional module included undertaking a worksite analysis (Ross, 2006). These findings suggest the need for further 'movement toward more occupation-based intervention [which] would be aided by greater inclusion of work and productivity issues in occupational therapy curricula' (Lysaght and Wright, 2005, p.216).

Occupational therapy education is not alone in these omissions. A study undertaken by academics in occupational medicine showed evidence that the number of hours spent teaching occupational medicine to undergraduate doctors had dropped from the levels reported in 1989. Of those courses that did offer some training in the subject, none included workplace visits (Wynn *et al.*, 2003). As has been stressed throughout this book, gaining an understanding of the workplace is a core element of any successful rehabilitation for work programme.

These concerns regarding education provision are shared by the Vocational Rehabilitation Association (VRA). The VRA is a small charitable organisation whose mission is to help members working in the field of disability and employment develop their professional practice and maintain their awareness of disability issues in this field. The VRA has highlighted the need for the accreditation of education and training in VR in the UK to ensure that standards are met and in order to produce competent practitioners who are fit for practice. They highlight a concern regarding the numbers of practitioners in the field with no professional qualifications whatsoever. Importantly, they emphasise the need for education to extend beyond purely theoretical knowledge, to support the transfer of this knowledge into the workplace, and to provide the means to measure the effectiveness of the intervention which is delivered (Vocational Rehabilitation Association, 2006). Further information about the VRA and membership can be accessed at: http://www.vocationalrehabilitationassociation.org.uk (accessed 09/11/06).

There are a number of complex reasons for these difficulties, not least the rapid rate of change in this sector, which has outpaced education. Consequently, there is now a need for much creative thinking to develop innovative learning opportunities for therapists in this field, particularly at an undergraduate level. Encouragingly, a recent survey of OT final year students at two UK universities found that over 60 per cent of respondents expressed an interest in pursuing a career in VR (College of Occupational Therapists, 2006). This is a positive shift and demonstrates that the work agenda is now filtering through to undergraduate students.

However, since much of VR is taking place outside of traditional service structures, there are presently insufficient opportunities for students to gain practical skills and experience in VR during their training. We are not alone in facing these difficulties. Even in those countries where the infrastructure is already well-established, sufficient placements are not always available (James and Prigg, 2004). Additionally, the focus of OT undergraduate education has been criticised for being directed more towards hospital-based practice, than towards meeting the needs of those wanting to work in occupational (work) rehabilitation (Thorpe, 2006). Furthermore, it has been suggested that the knowledge and skills learned in the undergraduate curriculum may not be sufficient for later needs when qualified (Strong *et al.*, 2003; Ahrens and Mulholland, 2000).

It is not unduly surprising that occupational therapists, or any other professional group, have been unable to hit the ground running. The complexity of the arena, as indicated in this book, can be considerable. Occupational therapists in the UK are fortunate to have a wealth of knowledge which they may draw upon from other countries where occupational therapists are already well-established in this field. The drawback of this is, however, that within the UK, much of the emerging sector remains heavily reliant on the skills and expertise of overseas therapists to deliver VR services. This workforce is often transient in nature, and therefore, perhaps too little investment is currently being made in creating a solid infrastructure for the future. In a number of regions, local initiatives, reflecting the breadth and uniqueness of VR activities in the UK, are sorely needed for the sustainable expansion and growth of this sector in the longer term.

CHALLENGES FOR OCCUPATIONAL THERAPISTS

To begin this section on a positive note, there is a wealth of exciting prospects within the current market for occupational therapists with the right skill set and expertise. To temper this enthusiasm however, ten years into the revival of VR we do not really seem to have made significant in-roads into capitalising on these opportunities. The OT literature recently challenged us to ask ourselves whether we may be complicit in the process of marginalising people with disabilities into special occupations and employment relations. We were also confronted about whether we were overly influenced by a traditional, Protestant work ethic and by political drives to reduce unemployment figures (Stewart, 2004). Running through these sentiments it seems there is a collective sense of frustration that may, perhaps, be shared by others as they read this book. Many occupational therapists will already know that they have a valuable contribution which they could, potentially, make within VR, but they are not sure where, or how, to set about doing it.

Perhaps, however, it may be timely to recognise and acknowledge that 'it takes more than a knowledge of occupational performance to convince policy makers of the value of occupational therapy in vocational rehabilitation. If knowledge is wisdom, then perhaps occupational therapists, with their collective wisdom and knowledge of occupational performance, require a major paradigm shift that integrates occupational performance and theories of career decision-making and career development' (McDonald, 1997, p.267). In addition, there is also a need for us to be able to demonstrate the ways in which we are effectively able to help others deliver their agenda – whether this be employers who want to reduce their rate of sickness absence, or Jobcentre Plus staff needing to meet their work entry targets. This is how demand for OT services will be sustained.

Some may, perhaps, feel that they lack the confidence or essential skills in VR (Shaw et al., 2006), others may have been powerless to persuade managers that this should form part of their current role. A reality which has become increasingly apparent in recent years is the fact that occupational therapists are not well-deployed for them to be able to effectively deliver rehabilitation for work interventions (Alsop, 2004; Joss, 2002). There are over 15,000 occupational therapists in the UK, however the vast majority of this number works in the NHS where they focus predominantly on discharge from hospital. It has been recognised that current practice has a very limited focus on rehabilitation of any form and even less on the vocational needs of clients. This is in spite of the fact that estimates suggest nearly a third of OT cases in the NHS involve individuals of working age (Wright et al., 2005), and yet more occupational therapists will be working with young disabled people who will soon be moving towards work.

This concern about the numbers of occupational therapists in VR is highlighted by the fact that, in 2002, there were thought to be just 400 occupational therapists undertaking VR as a primary part of their role in the UK (Wright *et al.*, 2005), although undoubtedly this number will have expanded significantly in the intervening years. This small number of rehabilitation practitioners must be seen within the context of the present situation, where over 2.5 million people are on incapacity benefits, of whom just under a third, roughly 800,000 people, are predicted to need specialist disability support to be able to work (British Society of Rehabilitation Medicine, 2003). Many more will, of course, be absent or struggling to stay in work because of a health condition or a disability. Despite calls to challenge existing organisational arrangements and to establish unified schemes that 'bridge the divide between health and occupation' (Alsop, 2004, p.525), at the moment regulation most certainly has the edge over legislation. Consequently, it seems that, in the foreseeable future at least, a major shake-up is unlikely.

In education we need to shift away from an over-reliance on sociological perspectives of work (Ross, 2006) and begin to consider how we may be able to expand our understanding of human occupation to provide us with an occupation-focused perspective of work. A number of OT courses will already be drawing in, and make use of, the expertise of practitioners, perhaps working as case managers or condition management practitioners, for example. Providing this theoretical knowledge is an important step forwards, but cannot replace the confidence and skill which are gained through experientially taking part in a worksite visit, for example. In a number of services, particularly within mental health, occupational therapists are acting as work champions, providing a focal point for others within the wider team. This may also be a useful model for education providers, who may want to ensure that work and VR become firmly embedded across both the length and breadth of their curriculum.

Returning to the literature, we can see that, in recent years, some demonstrable successes have been achieved, in spite of existing barriers. Throughout this book we have learned about examples of innovative practice. Others which we may find in the literature include: an out-patient OT service which is successfully supporting people to return to work or education, using early intervention and speedy placement into a familiar role when possible (Main and Haig, 2006), as well as an OT audit which highlighted how a successful return to work can be achieved when a co-ordinated multi-agency team is involved (Brewin and Hazell, 2004). Forging new partnerships with other agencies such as education, training, volunteering and employment is a highly effective way to move forwards (Devlin *et al.*, 2006). In this regard, an entrepreneurial approach towards service development is required.

Earlier, we discussed how calls have been made for education and training in VR to be accredited. It is to be anticipated that, in the future, practitioners themselves will be expected to obtain some form of accreditation too. This will ensure that therapists have the necessary skills and competencies to practice VR effectively and safely. In a number of other countries this is already mandatory. While there is currently no requirement for occupational health physicians or nurses to obtain a postgraduate qualification in this field, their respective professional bodies strongly recommend that this should be undertaken. What is our profession's stance on this matter to be? This question certainly needs to be a priority for debate and, hopefully, some consensus.

RESEARCH

There are a number of exciting avenues for researchers to follow in the field of VR. The Research and Development Strategic Vision and Action Plan (College of Occupational therapists, 2003) of The College of Occupational Therapists Specialist Section – WORK identified the following priority research areas:

- an exploration of the organisational policies which impact on occupational therapists and their remit to work across the total spectrum of self-care, productivity and leisure
- health and economic effectiveness of OT interventions
- standardised assessments and outcome measures
- glossary of terms by an international literature review
- relevant models of practice for VR
- perceptions of role and expectations of occupational therapists in this area of practice
- barriers and stigma which may impact on people with disabilities getting into work.

Reflecting the fact that this a key area of interest to occupational therapists across specialisms, several other specialist sections have also emphasised the importance of research in VR. While almost all of the areas identified above are concerned with gaining a better understanding of professional practice, other highly relevant areas include:

- Transitions – for example, how might we participate in planning for the future occupations and careers of young people with chronic illness, over and above focusing on the here and now of school (Shaw *et al.*, 2006)? In what ways may older people be actively supported to maintain a valued work role, if this is what they aspire to do?
- Timings – when is the right time for a therapist to begin VR? Despite a recognition of the fact that outcomes are greatly enhanced with early intervention, many existing services which address work support needs are reactive and therefore seem to be delivered too late. While on this point, how do we help the person recovering from a life-changing illness, perhaps requiring lengthy medical rehabilitation or convalescence, to successfully retain a worker identity?
- Effective targeting – how might we best identify who might benefit from return to work facilitation? Clearly, it is wasteful of an expensive resource to think that every person who is absent from work will need a therapist to facilitate their return. In the majority of cases this will be handled by an experienced employer. But there will be instances where additional support to re-enter work will be needed, to prevent unnecessary long-term absence or job loss. On this note, not all individuals will need the same level of support to return either. Are we able to identify those situations

where a simple or a more complex intervention is likely to be required? There are some suggestions that men achieve better outcomes from rehabilitation for work than women (Ahlgren and Hammarstrom, 2000). Are we confident that our services are designed to meet the needs of all who might benefit from them?

- Work and well-being at work – how can we further our understanding of the re-lationship between the occupation of work, health, and well-being? How might we measure the potential contribution of the workplace itself to work, health and well-being?

These, and many other questions, have raised themselves as worthy of research in the future. However, it is worth noting that finding the answers may not always be that straightforward. The researcher may have particular difficulty navigating his or her way around the electronic databases seeking out evidence on this subject, since search terms such as occupational health, are not particularly easy to locate. Furthermore, much of the literature on work is more likely to be found within sociological databases rather than health ones.

Conclusion

We have reached the end of our shared journey. It is now time to reflect on some of the things we have learned about vocational rehabilitation over the course of this book. Then, having done so, we need to step out into a world of work which is, perhaps, now a little more familiar, and take those ideas forward and integrate them into our work to benefit our clients.

References

Abberley, P. (2002) 'Work, disability, disabled people and European social theory', in Barnes, C., Oliver, M. and Barton, L. (editors) *Disability studies today*, Cambridge: Polity Press, Chapter 7.

Action for M.E. (2006) *M.E.: A guide* (information sheet), Bristol: Action for M.E. Available at: http://www.afme.org.uk/res/img/resources.M.E.%20A%20Guide.pdf (accessed 31/07/07).

Adam, S., Emmerson, C., Frayne, C. *et al.* (2006) *Early quantitative evidence on the impact of the Pathways to Work pilots* (research report no. 354), London: Department for Work and Pensions.

Advisory, Conciliation and Arbitration Services (2005) *Tacking discrimination and promoting equality*, London: ACAS. Available at: http://www.acas.org.uk/media/pdf/j/2/B16_1.pdf (accessed 28/04/07).

Advisory, Conciliation and Arbitration Services (2006) *Age and the workplace. A guide for employers*, London: ACAS. Available at: http://www.acas.org.uk/media/pdf/r/j/Age_and_the_Workplace.pdf (accessed 28/04/07).

Ahlgren, C. and Hammarstrom, A. (2000) Back to work? Gendered experiences of rehabilitation, *Scandinavian Journal of Public Health*, 28 (2), pp.88–94.

Ahrens, A. and Mulholland, K. (2000) Vocational rehabilitation and the evolution of disability management: an organizational case study, *Journal of Vocational Rehabilitation*, 15 (1), pp.39–46.

Aja, D. (1996) Finding a niche in job site analysis, *OT Practice*, July, pp.36–41.

Akabas, S.H., Gates, L.B., and Galvin, D.E. (1992) *Disability management: A complete system to reduce costs, increase productivity, meets employer needs and ensures legal compliance*, New York: AMACOM Books.

Alcohol Concern (2006) Impact of alcohol problems in the workplace, *Acquire*, February. Available at: www.alcoholconcern.org.uk (accessed 03/04/07).

Allaire, S.H., Li, W. and LaValley, M.P. (2003) Reduction of job loss in persons with rheumatic diseases receiving vocational rehabilitation: A randomized controlled trial, *Arthritis & Rheumatism*, 48 (11), pp.3212–3218.

Allen, R. (2005) 'Challenges of case management', in Whiteford, G. and Wright-St Clair, V., *Occupation & practice in context*, Sydney: Elsevier Churchill Livingstone, Chapter 9.

Allen, S. (1997) 'What is work for? The right to work and the right to be idle', in Brown, R.K. (editor) *The changing shape of work*, Hampshire: MacMillan Press Limited, Chapter 3.

Allen, V.R. (1986) Health promotion in the office, *The American Journal of Occupational Therapy*, 40, pp.764–770.

Alsop, A. (2004) Work matters (editorial), *British Journal of Occupational Therapy*, 67 (12), p.525.

Angers, M. (1995) Work and meaning conferring context of the clubhouse. Presented at the 8th International Seminar on the Clubhouse Model, Salt Lake City. Available at: http://www.iccd.org/iccd_library/8th/10angers.htm (accessed 06/04/07).

Anthony, W. (1994) Characteristics of people with psychiatric disabilities that are predictive of entry into the rehabilitation process and successful employment, *Psychosocial Rehabilitation Journal*, (17), pp.3–14.

Arksey, H., Thornton, P. and Williams, J. (2002) *Mapping employment-focused services for disabled people*, report no. 93, London: Department for Work and Pensions.

Armstrong, M. and Baron, A. (1995) *The job evaluation handbook*, London: Chartered Institute of Personnel and Development.

Arnetz, B., Sjögren, B., Rydéhn, B. *et al.* (2003) Early workplace intervention for employees with musculoskeletal-related absenteeism: A prospective controlled intervention study, *Journal of Occupational and Environmental Medicine*, 45 (5), pp.499–506.

Arthritis Care (2006) *Understanding arthritis*, London: Arthritis Care. Available at: http://www.arthritiscare.org.uk/AboutArthritis (accessed 10/04/07).

Arthritis Research Council (2002) *Arthritis: The big picture*, London: ARC. Available at: http://www.arc.org.uk/arthinfo/bigpic.asp#1 (accessed 10/04/07).

Association of British Insurers (2005) *Care and compensation*, London: ABI. Available at: http://www.abi.org.uk/BookShop/ResearchReports/careandcompensation.pdf (accessed 20/10/06).

Association of Personal Injury Lawyers (2004) *Best practice guide on rehabilitation*, Nottingham: APIL. Available at: www.apil.com (accessed 25/01/07).

Auerbach, E.S. (2001) The individual placement and support model versus the menu approach to supported employment: Where does occupational therapy fit in? *Occupational Therapy in Mental Health*, 17 (2), pp.1–19.

Australian Institute of Occupational Hygienists Incorproated (2005) *Occupational hygiene*, Melbourne: AIOH. Available at: http://www.aioh.org.au/about_occupHygiene.asp (accessed 02/05/07).

Backman, C.L., Kennedy, S.M., Chalmers, A. *et al.* (2004) Participation in paid and unpaid work by adults with rheumatoid arthritis, *Journal of Rheumatology*, 41 (1), pp.47–56.

Baker, N.A. (1999) 'Anthropometry', in Jacobs, K. (editor) *Ergonomics for therapists*, Boston: Butterworth-Heinemann, Chapter 3.

Baker, N.A., Jacobs, K., Tickle-Degnen, L. (2003) A methodology for developing evidence about meaning in occupation: Exploring the meaning of working, *OTJR: Occupation, Participation and Health*, 23 (2), pp.57–66.

Banks, M.H. (1995) Psychological effects of prolonged unemployment: Relevance to models of work re-entry following injury, *Journal of Occupational Rehabilitation*, 5 (1), pp.37–53.

Barnes, C. (1990) *"Cabbage syndrome": The social construction of dependence*, London: Falmer Press, Taylor & Francis Group.

Barnes, C. and Mercer, G. (2005) Disability, work and welfare: Challenging the social exclusion of disabled people, *Work, Employment and Society*, 19 (3), pp.527–545.

Barnes, M.P. (1999) Rehabilitation after traumatic brain injury, *British Medical Bulletin*, 55 (4), pp.927–943.

Barnes, T. and Holmes, J. (2007) *Occupational therapy in vocational rehabilitation: A brief guide to current practice in the UK*, London: The Executive Committee of the College of Occupational Therapists Specialist Section: WORK.

Barrett, L., Beer, D., Kielhofner, G. (1999) The importance of volitional narrative in treatment: An ethnographic case study in a work program, *Work*, 12 (1), pp.79–82.

Barris, R., Kielhofner, G. and Watts, J.H. (1988) *Occupational therapy in psychosocial practice*, New Jersey: Slack Incorporated.

Bassett, J. and Lloyd, C. (2000) Employment and young people with a mental illness: A review, *British Journal of Therapy and Rehabilitation*, 7 (11) pp.480–485.

Bassett, J., Lloyd, C., Bassett, H. (2001) Work issues for young people with psychosis: Barriers to employment, *British Journal of Occupational Therapy*, 64 (2) pp.66–72.

Beaumont, D.G. (2003) The interaction between general practitioners and occupational health professionals in relation to rehabilitation for work: A delphi study, *Occupational Medicine*, 53 (4) pp.249–253.

Becker, D.R. and Drake, R.E. (1993) *A working life: The individual placement and support (IPS) program*, Concord: New Hampshire-Dartmouth Psychiatric Research Center, cited in Bond, G.R. (1998) Principles of the individual placement and support model: Empirical support, *Psychiatric Rehabilitation Journal*, 22, pp.11–23.

Berg, M. (1987) 'Women's work, mechanisation and the early phases of industrialisation in England', in Joyce, P. (editor) *The historical meanings of work*, Cambridge: Cambridge University Press, Chapter 3.

Berg Rice, V.J. (1999) 'Ergonomics and therapy: An introduction', in Jacobs, K. *Ergonomics for therapists* (second edition) Boston: Butterworth Heinemann, Chapter 1.

Berridge, J., Cooper, C.L., Highley-Marchington, C. (1997) *Employee assistance programmes and workplace counselling*, Chichester: John Wiley & Sons Ltd.

Berthoud, R. (2006) *The employment rates of disabled people*, research report 298, London: Department for Work and Pensions.

Bertram, M. and Linnett, P. (1995) Empowerment through employment? An innovative work scheme for people with mental health problems, *British Journal of Occupational Therapy*, 58 (1), pp.7–8.

Bevan, S. and Hayday, S. (1998) *Attendance management: A review of good practice*, report 353, Brighton: Institute for Employment Studies Research.

Bevan, S. and Hayday, S. (2001) *Costing sickness absence in the UK*, report 382, Brighton: Institute for Employment Studies.

Beveridge, W.H. (1960) *Full employment in a free society* (second edition), London: George, Allen & Unwin.

Beyer, S., Grove, B., Schneider, J. *et al.* (2004) *Working lives: The role of day centres in supporting people with learning disabilities into employment*, research report no. 203, London: Department for Work and Pensions.

Birkholtz, M., Aylwin, L. and Harman, R.M. (2004) Activity pacing in chronic pain management: One aim, but whicj method? Part two: National Activity Pacing Survey, *British Journal of Occupational Therapy*, 67 (11), pp.481–487.

Black, M.M. (1976) The occupational career, *The American Journal of Occupational Therapy*, 30, pp.225–228.

Black, W. and Living, R. (2004) Volunteerism as an occupation and its relationship to health and well being, *British Journal of Occupational Therapy*, 67 (12), pp.526–532.

Blackhurst, C. (2005) Helping Remploy to march forward, *Evening Standard*, Wednesday, 2 March, pp.36–37.

Blackmore, P. (1999) A categorisation of approaches to occupational analysis, *Journal of Vocational Education and Training*, 51 (1), pp.61–78.

Bloom Hoover, J. (1996) Diversional occupational therapy in World War 1: A need for purpose in occupations, *American Journal of Occupational Therapy*, 50 (10), pp.881–885.

Bolchover, D. (2005) *The living dead*, Chichester: Capstone Publishing Limited.

Bond, G.R. (1998) Principles of the individual placement and support model: Empirical support, *Psychiatric Rehabilitation Journal*, 22, pp.11–23.

Bracegirdle, H. (1991) Two hundred years of therapeutic occupations for women hospital patients, *British Journal of Occupational Therapy*, 54 (6), pp.231–232.

Braveman, B., Robson, M., Velozo, C. *et al.* (2005) The worker role interview. Version 10.0. Chicago: MOHO Clearinghouse. Available at: http://www.moho.uic.edu/ (accessed 12/03/07).

Brewin, J. and Hazell, A. (2004) How successful are we at getting our clients back to work? The results of an audit, *British Journal of Occupational Therapy*, 67 (4), pp.148–158.

Bricher, G. (2000) Disabled people, health professionals and the social model of disability: Can there be a research relationship?, *Disability & Society*, 15 (5), pp.781–793.

Brief, A.P., Konovsky, M.A., Goodwin, R. *et al.* (1995) Inferring the meaning of work from the effects of unemployment, *Journal of Applied Social Psychology*, 25 (8), p.693.

Brisenden, S. (1986) Independent living and the medical model of disability, *Disability, Handicap and Society*, 1 (2), pp.173–178.

British Heart Foundation (2005) *Returning to work with a heart condition*, heart information series no. 21, London: BHF. Available at: www.bhf.org.uk (accessed 28/03/07).

British Heart Foundation (2007) Types of heart conditions. Available at: http://www.bhf.org.uk/living_with_heart_conditions/understanding_your_condition/types_of_heart_conditions.aspx (accessed 25/07/07).

British Occupational Health Research Foundation (2005) *Workplace interventions for people with common mental health problems: Evidence review and recommendations*, London: BORHF. Available at: http://www.bohrf.org.uk/downloads/cmh_rev.pdf (accessed 14/10/06).

British Occupational Hygiene Society (2007) *What is occupational hygiene?*, Derby: BOHS. Available at: http://www.bohs.org/standardTemplate.aspx/Home/AboutUs (accessed 02/05/07).

British Society of Rehabilitation Medicine (2000) *Vocational rehabilitation: The way forward*, London. BSRM.

British Society of Rehabilitation Medicine (2003) *Vocational rehabilitation: the way forward* (second edition). London: BSRM. Executive summary available at: http://www.bsrm.co.uk/Publications/Summary-Voc-Rehab.pdf (accessed 04/01/06).

British Society of Rehabilitation Medicine, Jobcentre Plus and Royal College of Physicians (2004) *Inter-agency guidelines for vocational assessment and rehabilitation after aquired brain injury*, London: Royal College of Physicians.

Brown, A., Kitchell, M., O'Neill, T. *et al.* (2001) Identifying meaning and perceived level of satisfaction within the context of work, *Work*, 16, pp.219–226.

Brown, R.K. (editor) (1997) 'Introduction: Work and employment in the 1990s', in *The Changing Shape of Work*, Hampshire: MacMillan Press Limited, Chapter 1.

Brown, P., Wright-St Clair, V. and Law, M. (2005) 'Economy as context: Evaluating occupation focused services', in Whiteford, G. and Wright-St Clair, V. (editors) *Occupation & Practice in Context*, Sydney: Elsevier Churchill Livingstone, Chapter 17.

Bumphrey, E.E. (1987) Occupational Therapy for People with Physical Dysfunction, *British Journal of Occupational Therapy*, 50 (10), pp.332–334.

Burchardt, T. (2000) *Enduring economic exclusion: Disabled people, income and work*, York: Joseph Rowntree Foundation. Available at: www.jrf.org.uk/knowledge/findings/socialpolicy/060.pdf (accessed 21/07/07).

Burchardt, T. (2005) *The education and employment of disabled young people: Frustrated ambition*, Bristol: Policy Press in association with the Joseph Rowntree Foundation.

Burton, L.F., Chavez, J.A. and Kobaska, C.J. (1987) Employability skills: A survey of employer's opinions, *Journal of Rehabilitation*, Jul/Aug/Sept, pp.71–74

Calman, K., Downie, R.S., Fyfe, C.E. *et al.* (1990) *Health promotion models and values*, Oxford: Oxford University Press.

Campaniello, J. (1988) When professional nurses return to school: A study of role conflict and well-being in multiple role women, *Journal of Professional Nursing*, 4 (2), pp.136–140.

Canadian Association of Occupational Therapists (2002) *Enabling occupation: An occupational therapy perspective*, Ottawa: CAOT.

Canadian Association of Occupational Therapists (2001) *Health promotion and disease prevention: A foundation for the Canadian health system*, Ottowa: CAOT. Available at: www.caot.ca (accessed 08/07/06).

Canadian Association of Occupational Therapists (2003) *Position statement: Everyday occupations and health*, Ottawa: CAOT. Available at: www.caot.ca (accessed 02/02/05).

Capo, L.C. (2001) Autism, employment and the role of occupational therapy, *Work*, 16 (3), pp.201–207.

Carman, S. (1999) *Work rehabilitation: A comparison of the services provided by three organisations*, unpublished Masters thesis, Sheffield Hallam University.

Case Management Society UK (2005) *CMSUK standards of practice*, Sutton: Case Management Society UK. Available at: www.cmsuk.org (accessed 21/03/07).

Cassileith, B.R. (1984) Hospice and the biopsychosocial model of healthcare: Will hospice be the mechanism for change in the American healthcare system?, *Journal of Hospice and Palliative Medicine*, 1, pp.18–20.

Castillo, J.J. (1997) Looking for the meaning of work, *Work and Occupation*, 24 (4), pp.413–425.

Chambers, R., Moore, S., Parker, G. *et al.* (2001) *Occupational health matters in general practice*, Oxon: Radcliffe Medical Press Ltd.

Chapman, C., Chantler, C., Harrison, J. and Saltrese, A. (2006) Best practice guidelines for case managers, Sutton: Case Management Society UK. Available at: http://www.cmsuk.org/documents/tmp70.pdf (accessed 22/07/07).

Chapparo, C.J. and Hooper, E. (2002) When is it work? Perceptions of six year old children, *Work*, 19 (3), pp.291–302.

Chappell, I., Higham, J. *et al.* (2003) An occupational therapy work skills assessment for individuals with head injury, *Canadian Journal of Occupational Therapy*, 70 (3) pp.163–169.

Charity Commission (2005) Charity working at the heart of society: the way forward 2005–2008, Liverpool: Charity Commission. Available at: http://www.charity-commission.gov.uk/Library/tcc/pdfs/StratReview05colour.pdf (accessed 22/07/07).

Chartered Institute of Personnel and Development (2006a) *Absence management*, survey report, London: CIPD. Available at: http://www.cipd/co.uk/surveys (accessed 14/11/06).

Chartered Institute of Personnel and Development (2006b) *Absence management factsheet*, London: CIPD. Available at: http://www.cipd.co.uk/ subjects/hrpract/absence/absncman.htm (accessed 15/11/06).

Chartered Institute of Personnel and Development (2006c) *Occupational health and organisational effectivness factsheet*, London: CIPD. Available at: http://www.cipd.co.uk/ subjects/health/occpnhlth/occhealth.htm?IsSrchRes=1 (accessed 15/11/06).

Chartered Institute of Personnel and Development (2007) *Job evaluation factsheet*, London: CIPD. Available at: http://www.cipd.co.uk/subjects/pay/general/jobeval.htm? IsSrchRes=1 (accessed 10/3/07).

Chartered Society of Physiotherapy (2005) *Fit to work*, London: The Chartered Society of Physiotherapy. Available at: http://www.csp.org.uk/uploads/documents/csp_leaflet_ fit2work1.htm (accessed 03/04/07).

ChildRIGHT (1998) *Facts revealed about child employment in Britain*, CR no. 145, London: Children's Legal Centre. Available at: http://www.childrenslegalcentre.com/ Homepage.asp?NodeID=89614 (accessed 12/01/07).

Christiansen, C. (1999) Defining lives: Occupation as identity: An essay on competence, coherence, and the creation of meaning, *American Journal of Occupational Therapy*, 53, pp.547–558.

Christiansen, C.H. and Townsend, E.A. (2004) *Introduction to occupation: The art and science of living*, New Jersey: Pearson Education Inc.

Christie, I. and Mensah-Coker, G. (1999) *An inclusive future?*, London: Demos.

Cockburn, L., Kirsh, B., Krupa, T. *et al.* (2004) Mental health and mental illness in the workplace: Occupational therapy solutions for complex problems, *Occupational Therapy Now*, 6 (5), pp.7–14.

College of Occupational Therapists (2003) *Research and development strategic vision and action plan for occupational therapy in work practice and productivity*, London: COT.

College of Occupational Therapists (2006) Vocational rehabilitation high on the agenda, *OT News*, May, London: COT, p.14.

Combs, I.A. and Omvig, C.P. (1986) Accommodation of Disabled People into Employment: Perceptions of Employers, *Journal of Rehabilitation*, April/May/June, pp.42–45.

Confederation of British Industry (2001) *Absence and labour turnover survey*, London: CBI.

Constantine, S. (1980) *Unemployment in Britain between the wars*, London: Longman Group Ltd.

Convery, P. (1997) 'Unemployment', in Walker, A. and Walker, C. (editors) *Britain divided: The growth of social exclusion in the 1980s and 1990s*, London: CPAG Ltd, Chapter 12.

Corcoran, M.A. (2004) Editorial: Work, occupation and occupational therapy, *The American Journal of Occupational Therapy*, 58 (4) pp.367–368.

Core, S. and Wilmer, S. (2003) Returning to work after a stroke: An important but neglected area, *British Journal of Occupational Therapy*, 66 (5), pp.186–192.

College of Occupational Therapists (2003) *Occupational therapy clinical guidelines for rheumatology*, London: COT.

Commonwealth Rehabilitation Service Australia (2004) *Journey to recovery: Mental health toolkit*, Canberra: Commonwealth of Australia.

Craddock, J. (1996) Responses of the occupational therapy profession to the perspective of the disability movement, Part 1, *British Journal of Occupational Therapy*, 59 (1), pp.17–22.

Creek, J. (2003) *Occupational therapy defined as a complex intervention*, London: College of Occupational Therapists.

Creighton, C. (1992) The origin and evolution of activity analysis, *American Journal of Occupational Therapy*, 46 (1), pp.45–48.

Cromwell, F.S. (editor) (1985) Work-related programs in occupational therapy, *Occupational Therapy in Health Care*, 2 (4) pp.9–25.

Crowther, R., Marshall, M., Bond, G. and Huxley, P. (2001) *Vocational rehabilitation for people with severe mental illness*, Cochrane Database of Systematic Reviews, issue 2, The Cochrane Collaboration.

Cullum, F.W.H. (1997) Managing health and safety: A role for occupational therapists, *British Journal of Occupational Therapy*, 60 (6), pp.259–262.

Curtis, J. (2003) Employment and disability in the United Kingdom: An outline of recent legislative and policy changes, *Work*, 20 (1), pp.45–51.

Dale, L., Barkley, A., Bayless, S. *et al.* (2003) Experience of cumulative trauma disorders on life roles of worker and family member: A case study of a married couple, *Work*, 20 (3), pp.245–255.

Danson, M. (2005) Old industrial regions and employability, *Urban Studies*, 42 (2), pp.285–300.

Davis, M. and Rinaldi, M. (2004) Using an evidence-based approach to enable people with mental health problems to gain and retain employment, education and voluntary work, *British Journal of Occupational Therapy*, 67 (7), pp.319–322.

Dean, D.H., Dolan, R.C., Schmidt, R.M. *et al.* (1999) Evaluating the vocational rehabilitation program using longitudinal data. Evidence for a quasiexperimental research design, *Evaluation Review*, 23 (2), pp.162–189.

Deem, R. (1988) *Work, unemployment and leisure*, London: Routledge.

Department for Work and Pensions (2001) *Neighbourhood renewal: Increasing employment amongst deprived areas and groups: Implementation strategy*, Annex D: Strategy for increasing employment rates for disabled people, London: DWP. Available at: http://www.dwp.gov.uk/publications/dwp/2001/nsnr/annex_d.htm (accessed 23/12/02).

Department for Work and Pensions (2002) *Pathways to work: Helping people into employment*, Norwich: The Stationery Office.

Department for Work and Pensions (2004) *Building capacity for work: A UK framework for vocational rehabilitation*, Norwich: HMSO.

Department for Work and Pensions (2006a) *A new deal for welfare: Empowering people to work*, Norwich: HMSO.

Department for Work and Pensions (2006b) *Departmental report 2006*, London: DWP. Available at: http://www.dwp.gov.uk/publications/dwp/2006/dr06/ (accessed 10/05/07).

Department for Work and Pensions, Department of Health, Department for Education and Skills, Office of the Deputy Prime Minister (2005) *Improving the life chances of disabled people*, London: HMSO.

Department for Work and Pensions, Department of Health, Health and Safety Executive (2005) *Health, work and well-being – caring for our future*, London: HMSO.

Department of Employment (1992) *Manual handling operations regulations (amended 1992)* (statutory instrument 1992, no.2793), London: HMSO. Available at: http://www.opsi.gov.uk/SI/si1992/Uksi_19922793_en_1.htm (accessed 24/03/07).

Department of Health (1992) *The health of the nation*, London: The Stationery Office.

Department of Health (1996) *Health survey for England 1994*, London: The Stationery Office.

Department of Health (1999a) *National service frameworks in mental health*, London: HMSO.

Department of Health (1999b) *The prevalence of back pain in Great Britain in 1998*, London: Department of Health Statistics Division.

Department of Health (2000a) *The national service framework for coronary heart disease*, London: DoH.

Department of Health (2000b) *Access to the medical records of some 100,000 miners and ex-miners seeking compensation for chronic obstructive pulmonary disease*, London: HMSO.

Department of Health (2001) *Valuing people: A new strategy for learning disability for the 21st century*, London: TSO.

Department of Health (2004) *Choosing health: Making healthy choices easier*, London: HMSO. Available at: www.dh.gov.uk (accessed 26/09/07).

Department of Health (2005a) *The national service framework for long term conditions*, London: HMSO.

Department of Health (2005b) *Independence well-being and choice: Our vision for the future of social care for adults in England*, London: DH.

Department of Health (2006a) *Caring for people with long term conditions: an education framework for community matrons and case managers*, document no. 6353, Nottingham: DH.

Department of Health (2006b) *Our health, our care, our say: A new direction for community services*, London: DH.

Department of Health (2007) *Coronary heart disease*, London: DH. Available at: http://www.dh.gov.uk/en/Policyandguidance/Healthandsocialcaretopics/Coronaryheartdisease/index.htm (accessed 23/07/07).

Department of Social Security (1998) *New ambitions for our country: A new contract for welfare*, Cmd 3805, London: The Stationery Office.

Department of Trade and Industry (2006) *Annual Small Business Survey 2005*, London: DTI. Available at: www.sbs.gov.uk (accessed 24/02/07).

Devlin, C., Burnside, L. and Akroyd, L. (2006) Mental health vocational rehabilitation: An overview of occupational therapy service provision in Northern Ireland, *British Journal of Occupational Therapy*, 69 (7), pp.334–339.

Dewson, S. (2005) *Evaluation of the Working Neighbourhoods pilot: Year one*, Research Report 297, Norwich: Department for Work and Pensions/HMSO.

Diasio, K. (1971) The modern era –1960 to 1970, *The American Journal of Occupational Therapy*, XXV (5), pp.237–242.

Di Bona, L. (2000) What are the benefits of leisure? An exploration using the leisure satisfaction scale, *British Journal of Occupational Therapy*, 63, pp.50–58.

DiMasso, J., Avi-Itzak, T. and Obler, D.R. (2001) The clubhouse model: An outcome study on attendance, work attainment and status, and hospital recidivism, *Work*, 17, pp.23–30.

Disability Rights Commission (2004) *Code of practice: Employment and occupation*, Norwich: The Stationery Office. Available at: http://www.drc.org.uk/library/publications/employment/code_of_practice_-_employment.aspx (accessed 28/04/07).

Disability Rights Commission (2006a) *Your rights at work: A guide for people with a learning disability and their supporters*, london: DRC. Available at: http://www.drc-gb.org/library/publications/employment/your_rights_at_work_-_a_guide.aspx (accessed 20/04/07).

Disability Rights Commission (2006b) *Definition of disability*, London: DRC. Available at: http://www.drc.org.uk/your_rights/are_you_being_discriminated_ag/definition_of_disability.aspx (accessed 05/05/07).

Douthwaite, J. (1994) Unemployment: A challenge to occupational therapy, *British Journal of Occupational Therapy*, 57 (11), pp.432–436.

Doyle, C.E. (2003) *Work and organizational psychology: An introduction with attitude*, Hove: Psychology Press.

Drake, R.F. (1999) *Understanding disability policies*, Hampshire: Macmillan Press Ltd.

Driver and Vehicle Licensing Agency (2007) *At a glance guide to the current medical standards of fitness to drive*, Swansea: Driver and Vehicle Licensing Agency. Available at: www.dvla.gov.uk (accessed 21/04/07).

DrugScope (2005) *Drug information*, London: DrugScope. Available at: www.drugscope.org.uk (accessed 03/04/07).

Ekberg, K. (1995) Workplace changes in successful rehabilitation, *Journal of Occupational Rehabilitation*, 5 (4), pp.253–269.

Ekdawi, M.Y. and Conning, A.M. (1994) *Psychiatric rehabilitation: A practical guide*, New York: Chapman & Hall.

Ekelman, B.A., Bazyk, S.S. and Bello-Haas, V.D. (2003) An occupational perspective of the well-being of Maya women in southern Belize, *OTJR: Occupation, Participation and Health*, 23 (4), pp.130–142.

Eldar, R. and Jelic, M. (2003) The association of rehabilitation and war, *Disability Rehabilitation*, 25 (18) pp.1019–1023.

Emerson, E., Malam, S., Davies, I. *et al.* (2005) *Adults with learning difficulties in England 2003/04*, London: NHS Health and Social Care Information Centre and National Statistics.

Engel, G.L. (1980) The clinical application of the biopsychosocial model, *American Journal of Psychiatry*, 37, pp.535–544.

Evans, J. and Repper, J. (2000) Employment, social inclusion and mental health, *Journal of Psychiatric & Mental Health Nursing*, 7 (1), pp.15–24.

Fabian, E.S., Waterworth, A. and Ripke, B. (1993) Reasonable accommodation for workers with severe mental illness: Type, frequency and associated outcomes, *Psychosocial Rehabilitation Journal*, 17, pp.163–172.

Faculty of Occupational Medicine (2006) Guidance on alcohol and drug misuse in the workplace, London: Faculty of Occupational Medicine.

Faculty of Public Health and Faculty of Occupational Medicine (2006) *Creating a healthy workplace. A guide for occupational safety and health professionals and employers.* Available at: www.fph.org.uk and www.facoccmed.ac.uk (accessed 10/02/07).

Faragher, E.B., Cass, M. and Cooper, C.L. (2005) The relationship between job satisfaction and health: A meta-analysis, *Occupational and Environmental Medicine*, 62 (2), pp.105–112.

Farnworth, L. (1995) An exploration of skill as an issue in unemployment and employment, *Journal of Occupational Science* (Australia), 2 (1), pp.22–28.

Farrell, C., Nice, K., Lewis, J. *et al.* (2006) *Experience of the Job Retention and Rehabilitation pilot* (research report no.339), Leeds: Department for Work and Pensions.

Fisher, G.S. (1999) Administration and application of the Worker Role Interview: Looking beyond functional capacity, *Work*, 12 (1), pp.13–24.

Floyd, M. (editor) (1996) *Vocational rehabilitation and Europe*, London: Jessica Kingsley.

Floyd, M. and Landymore, D. (2000) 'Vocational Rehabilitation Services', in *Fitness for work. The medical aspects* (third edition), Cox, R.A.F., Edwards, F.C. and Palmer, K. (editors) Oxford: Oxford University Press, Chapter 4.

Floyd, M., Pilling, D., Garner, K. *et al.* (2004) Vocational rehabilitation: What works and in what circumstances, *International Journal of Rehabilitation Research*, 27 (2) pp.99–103.

Foot, M. and Hook, C. (2005) *Introducing human resource management* (fourth edition), Harlow: Pearson Education Limited.

Frank, A.O. and Thurgood, J. (2006) Vocational rehabilitation in the UK: Opportunities for health-care professionals, *International Journal of Therapy and Rehabilitation*, 13 (3), pp.126–134.

Friedland, J. (1998) Occupational therapy and rehabilitation: An awkward alliance, *The American Journal of Occupational Therapy*, 52 (5), pp.373–380.

Furnham, A. (2005) *The psychology of behaviour at work*, New York: Routledge Press Inc.

Ganora, A. and Wright, G. (1987) Occupational rehabilitation: costs and benefits, *Journal of Occupational Health & Safety – Australia and New Zealand*, 3 (4), pp.331–337.

Garner, R. (1995) Pre-vocational training within a secure environment: A programme designed to enable the forensic patient to prepare for mainstream opportunities, *The British Journal of Occupational Therapy*, 58 (1), pp.2–6.

Garvey, J. (1995) 'Delivering training and education in occupational health for nurses', in Pantry, S. (editor) *Occupational Health*, London: Chapman & Hall, Chapter 11.

Gennard, J. and Judge, G. (1999) *Employee relations* (second edition), London: Chartered Institute of Personnel and Development.

Gibson, L. and Strong, J. (2003) A conceptual framework of functional capacity evaluation for occupational therapy in work rehabilitation, *Australian Occupational Therapy Journal*, 50, pp.64–71.

Glyptis, S. (1989) *Leisure and unemployment*, Milton Keynes: Open University Press.

Gould, A., De Souza, S. and Rebeiro-Gruhl, K. (2005) And then I lost that life: A shared narrative of four young men with schizophrenia, *British Journal of Occupational Therapy*, 68 (10), pp.467–473.

Gray, R. (1987) 'Languages of factory reform in Britain 1830–1860', in Joyce, P. (editor) *The historical meanings of work*, Cambridge: Cambridge University Press, Chapter 6.

Green, F. (2005) *Understanding trends in job satisfaction*, Swindon: Economic and Social Research Council. Available at: www.esrcsocietytoday.ac.uk/ESRCInfoCentre/research/WorkOrganisation/ (accessed 15/05/06).

Greenwood, R. and Johnson, V.A. (1987) Employer perspectives on workers with disabilities, *Journal of Rehabilitation,* 53, pp.37–45.

Gutman, S.A. (1995) Influence of the U.S. military and occupational therapy reconstruction aides in World War I on the development of occupational therapy, *The American Journal of Occupational Therapy*, 49 (3), pp.256–262.

Hackman, J.R. and Oldham, G.R. (1980) *Work redesign*, Reading: Addison-Wesley.

Hammel, J. (1999) The life rope: A transactional approach to exploring worker and life role development, *Work*, 12 (1), pp.47–60.

Hanson, C.S. and Walker, K.F. (1992) The history of work in physical dysfunction, *The American Journal of Occupational Therapy*, 46 (1), pp.56–62.

Harder, H.G. and Scott, L.R. (2005) *Comprehensive disability management*, Edinburgh: Elsevier Churchill Livingstone.

Hardy, A. (2001) *Health and medicine in Britain since 1860*, New York: Palgrave.

Harkness, S. (2005) *Employment, work patterns and unpaid work: An analysis of the trends since the 1970s*, research report, Swindon: Economic and Social Research Council. Available at: www.regard.ac.uk (accessed 15/09/06).

Harvey-Krefting, L. (1985) The concept of work in occupational therapy: A historical review, *The American Journal of Occupational Therapy*, 39 (5), pp.301–307.

Hatch, M.J. and Cunliffe, A.L. (2006) *Organization theory* (second edition), Oxford: Oxford University Press.

Hayday, S., Risk, J., Patterson, M. *et al.* (2004) *Current thinking on attendance management: A short guide for HR professionals*, research paper 4378RF, London: National Audit Office. Available at: www.employment-studies.co.uk/summary/summary.php?id=nao1204 (accessed 06/06/05).

Health and Safety Commission (2000) *Revitalising health and safety strategy*, London: HSC. Available at: www.hse.gov.uk (accessed 12/11/06).

Health and Safety Commission (2005) *Workplace strategy – moving to delivery*, London: HSC. Available at: http://www.hse.gov.uk/aboutus/plans/hscplans/janekennedy.pdf (accessed 13/11/06).

Health and Safety Commission (2006a) *Health and safety statistics 2005/2006*, London: HSC. Available at: http://www.hse.gov.uk/statistics/ (accessed 19/02/07).

Health and Safety Commission (2006b) *Statistics of fatal injuries 2005/2006*, London: HSE. Available at: http://www.hse.gov.uk/statistics/overall/fatl0506.pdf (accessed 01/11/06).

Health and Safety Commission (2006c) *The strategy in action: Report to ministers on the second year of the HSC Strategy*, London: HSC. Available at: http://www.hse.gov.uk/aboutus/hsc/strategyyear2.pdf (accessed 13/11/06).

Health and Safety Executive (2000) *Securing health together*, Norwich: HSE Books.

Health and Safety Executive (2002a) *The health and safety system in Great Britain*, Norwich: HSE Books.

Health and Safety Executive (2002b) *Upper limb disorders in the workplace* (second edition), Norwich: HSE Books.

Health and Safety Executive (2003a) *Heath and safety regulation*. A short guide, Suffolk: HSE. Available at: http://www.hse.gov.uk/pubns/hsc13.pdf (accessed 28/04/07).

Health and Safety Executive (2003b) *Aching arms (or RSI) in small businesses*, Suffolk: HSE Books. Available at: http://www.hse.gov.uk/pubns/indg171.pdf (accessed 29/09/07).

Health and Safety Executive (2004a) *Are you making the best use of lifting and handling aids?*, Suffolk: Health and Safety Executive. Available at: www.hse.gov.uk/pubns/indg398.pdf (accessed 29/09/07).

Health and Safety Executive (2004b) *Drug misuse at work: A guide for employers*, Suffolk: HSE Books. Available at: www.hse.gov.uk/pubns/indg91.pdf (accessed 05/04/07).

Health and Safety Executive (2004c) Managing sickness absence and return to work in small business, Suffolk: HSE Books. Available at: www.hse.gov.uk/pubns/indg399.pdf (accessed 21/07/07).

Health and Safety Executive (2005a) *Hand-arm vibration. Advice for employees*, Norwich: HMSO. Available at: www.hse.gov.uk/pubns/indg296.pdf (accessed 12/02/07).

Health and Safety Executive (2005b) *Tackling Stress: The management standards approach*. Available at: http://www.hse.gov.uk/pubns/indg406.pdf (accessed 24/07/07).

Health and Safety Executive (2006a) *Getting to grips with manual handling*. A short guide, Suffolk: Health and Safety Executive. Available at: http://www.hse.gov.uk/pubns/indg143.pdf (accessed 28/04/07).

Health and Safety Executive (2006b) *Workplace health, safety and welfare*. A short guide for managers, Suffolk: Health and Safety Executive. Available at: http://www.hse.gov.uk/pubns/indg244.pdf (accessed 28/04/07).

Health and Safety Executive (2006c) *Don't mix it – A guide for employers on alcohol at work*, Suffolk: HSE Books. Available at: www.hse.gov.uk/pubns/indg240.pdf (accessed 05/04/07).

Health and Safety Executive (2007a) *Self-reported work-related illness and workplace injuries in 2005–2006: Results from the Labour Force Survey*, Caerphilly: HSE Books. Available at: http://www.hse.gov.uk/statistics/lfs/lfs0506.pdf (accessed 24/07/07).

Health and Safety Executive (2007b) *What can lead to back pain in the workplace?*, Suffolk: HSE. Available at: http://www.hse.gov.uk/msd/backpain/wkp.htm (accessed 19/07/07).

Health and Safety Executive (2007c) *About COPD. Why is HSE interested in COPD?* Suffolk: HSE. Available at: http://www.hse.gov.uk/copd/aboutus.htm (accessed 30/07/07).

Heard, C. (1977) Occupational role acquisition: A perspective on the chronically disabled, *American Journal of Occupational Therapy*, 31, pp.243–247.

Henry, A.D. and Lucca, A.M. (2002) Contextual factors and participation in employment for people with serious mental illness, *Occupation, Participation and Health: The Occupational Therapy Journal of Research*, 22, supplement, pp.835–845.

Hermennau, D.C. (1999) 'Seating', in Jacobs, K. (editor) *Ergonomics for therapists*, Boston: Butterworth-Heinemann, Chapter 10.

Hignett, S. (2000) Occupational therapy and ergonomics: Two professions exploring their identities, *British Journal of Occupational Therapy*, 63 (3), pp.137–139.

Hill, M.A. (1967) The development of industrial therapy in Britain, *American Journal of Occupational Therapy*, XXI (3), pp.160–165.

Hocking, C. (2001) Implementing occupation-based assessment, *Australian Journal of Occupational Therapy*, 55 (4), pp.463–469.

Hodson, C. (2001) *Psychology and work*, Hove: Routledge.

Hoffman, M.A. (2000) Suicide and hastened death: A biopsychosocial perspective, *The Counselling Psychologist*, 28, pp.561–572.

Holmes, D. (1985) The role of the occupational therapist – work evaluator, *The American Journal of Occupational Therapy*, 39 (5), pp.308–313.

Honey, A. (2004) Benefits and drawbacks of employment: Perspectives of people with mental illness, *Qualitative Health Research*, 14 (3), pp.381–395.

Horton-Salway, M. (2002) Bio-psycho-social reasoning in GPs' case narratives: The discursive construction of ME patient's identities, *Health* (London), 6, pp.401–421.

Howard, G. (2000) 'Legal aspects of fitness for work', in Cox, R.A.F., Edwards, F.C. and Palmer, K. (editors) *Fitness for work: The medical aspects* (third edition), Oxford: Oxford University Press, Chapter 2.

Howard, G.S. and Cox, R.A.F. (2000) 'The Disability Discrimination Act 1995', in Cox, R.A.F., Edwards, F.C. and Palmer, K. (editors) *Fitness for work: The medical aspects* (third edition), Oxford: Oxford University Press, Chapter 3.

Hutchinson, D. (1982) *Work preparation for the handicapped*, London: Croom Helm.

Huyse, F.J., Lyons, J.S., Stiefel, F. *et al.* (2001) Operationalizing the biopsychosoical model: The INTERMED, *Psychosomatics*, Jan/Feb, 42 (1), pp.5–13.

Hyde, M. (1996) 50 years of failure: Employment services for disabled people in the UK, *Work, Employment & Society*, 10 (4), pp.683–700.

Inman, J., McGurk, E. and Chadw, J. (2007) Is vocational rehabilitation a transition to recovery?, *British Journal of Occupational Therapy*, 70 (2), pp.60–66.

Innes, E. (1995) Workplace-based occupational rehabilitation in New South Wales, Australia, *Work*, 5, pp.147–152.

Innes, E. and Straker, L. (2002) Workplace assessments and functional capacity evaluations: Current practices of therapists in Australia, *Work*, 18 (1), pp.61–66.

Innes, E. and Straker, L. (2003) Attributes of excellence in work-related assessments, *Work*, 20 (1), pp.3–76.

International Labour Organisation (1983) *International labour standards on vocational rehabilitation* (recommendation 168), Geneva: ILO.

International Labour Organisation (2001) *Code of practice on managing disability in the workplace*, Geneva: ILO.

International Labour Organisation (2005) *Introductory report: Decent work, safe work*, Geneva: ILO. Available at: www.ilo.org/public/english/download/glance.pdf (accessed 24/06/06).

International Labour Organisation (2006) *The ILO at a glance*, Geneva: ILO. Available at: http://www.ilo.org/public/english/download/glance.pdf (accessed 13/11/06).

International Labour Organisation (2007) *Equality at work: Tackling the challenge*, Geneva: ILO. Available at: www.ilo.org (accessed 13/05/07).

International Stress Management Association (2004) Working together to reduce stress at work: A guide for employees, London: Stress Management Association. Available at: http://www.hse.gov.uk/pubns/misc686.pdf (accessed 10/04/07).

Isernhagen, D.D. (2000) A model system: Integrated work injury prevention and disability management, *Work*, 15 (2), pp.87–94.

Jackson, M. (1993) From work to therapy: The changing politics of occupation in the twentieth century, *British Journal of Occupational Therapy*, 56 (10), pp.360–364.

Jackson, M., Harkess, J. and Ellis, J. (2004) Reporting patients' work abilities: How the use of standardized work assessments improved clinical practice in Fife, *British Journal of Occupational Therapy*, 67 (3), pp.129–132.

Jacobs, K. (1999) *Ergonomics for therapists* (second edition), Boston: Butterworth Heinemann.

Jahoda, M. (1982) *Employment and unemployment: A social-psychological analysis*, Cambridge: Cambridge University Press.

Jakobsen, K. (2004) If work doesn't work: How to enable occupational justice, *Journal of Occupational Science*, 11 (3), pp.125–134.

James, C. and Prigg, A. (2004) A self-directed fieldwork program to provide alternative occupational health placements for undergraduate occupational therapy students, *Australian Occupational Therapy Journal*, 51, pp.60–68.

James, P., Cunningham, I. and Dibben, P. (2003) *Job retention and vocational rehabilitation: The development and evaluation of a conceptual framework* (research report 106), Norwich: HSE Books.

Japp, J. (2005) *Brain injury and returning to employment*, London: Jessica Kingsley Publishers.

Johansson, U. and Tham, K. (2006) The meaning of work after acquired brain injury, *American Journal of Occupational Therapy*, 60 (1), pp.60–69.

Jolliffe, J.A., Rees, K., Taylor, R.S. *et al.* (2007) Exercise-based rehabilitation for coronary heart disease (issue 1), *The Cochrane Database of Systematic Reviews*, The Cochrane Collaboration, John Wiley and Sons Ltd.

Joss, M. (2002) Occupational therapy and rehabilitation for work, *British Journal of Occupational Therapy*, 65 (3), pp.141–148.

Joss, M. and Pratt, J. (2006) Occupational therapy in occupational health: Factors influencing referral, *British Journal of Occupational Therapy*, 69 (4), pp.177–181.

Julliard, K., Klimenko, E. and Jacob, M.S. (2006) Definitions of health among healthcare providers, *Nursing Science Quarterly*, 19, pp.265–271.

Kalina, C.M. (1999) Strategies in disability management: Corporate disability management programs implemented at the work site, *Annals of the New York Academy of Sciences*, 888, pp.343–355.

Kellard, K., Adelman, L., Cebulla, A. and Heaver, C. (2002) *From job seekers to job keepers: Job retention, advancement and the role of in-work support programmes* (research report no. 170), Leeds: Department for Work and Pensions. Available at: http://www.dwp.gov.uk/asd/asd5/rrep170.asp (accessed 22/07/07).

Kelly, G. (2004) Paediatric occupational therapy in the 21st century: A survey of UK practice, *National Association of Paediatric Occupational Therapy Journal*, Summer, pp.5–8.

Kemp, B. and Kleinplatz, F. (1985) Vocational rehabilitation of the older worker, *The American Journal of Occupational Therapy*, 39 (5), pp.322–326.

Kendall, E. (2003) Predicting vocational adjustment following traumatic brain injury: A test of a psychosocial theory, *Journal of Vocational Rehabilitation*, 19 (1), pp.31–45.

Kennedy, M.S. (1986) Able to work?, *British Journal of Occupational Therapy*, 49 (11), pp.354–356.

Kielhofner, G. (2002). Model of human occupation 3rd edition: theory and application, Philadelphia: Lippincott, Williams & Wilkins.

Keilhofner, G., Braveman, B., Baron, K. *et al.* (1999) The model of human occupation: Understanding the worker who is injured or disabled, *Work*, 12, pp.3–11.

King, P. (1993) Outcome analysis of work-hardening programs, *The American Journal of Occupational Therapy*, 47 (7), pp.595–603.

Kivimakaki, M., Leino-Arjas, P., Luukkonen, R. *et al.* (2002) Work stress and the risk of cardiovascular mortality: prospective cohort study of industrial employees, *British Medical Journal*, 325, p.857.

Koch, L.C. and Rumrill, P.D. (Jr) (2003) New directions in vocational rehabilitation: Challenges and opportunities for researchers, practitioners, and consumers, *Work*, 21 (1), pp.1–3.

Kreutzer, J.S., Marwitz, J.H., Walker, W. *et al.* (2003) Moderating factors in return to work and job stability after traumatic brain injury, *Journal of Head Trauma Rehabilitation*, 18 (2), pp.128–138.

Kumar, S. (2000) *Multidisciplinary approach to rehabilitation*, Boston: Butterworth-Heinemann.

Larson, E.A. (2004) Children's work: The less-considered childhood occupation, *The American Journal of Occupational Therapy*, 58 (4), pp.369–379.

Larsson, A. and Gard, G. (2003) How can the rehabilitation planning process at the workplace be improved? A qualitative study from employers' perspective, *Journal of Occupational Rehabilitation*, 13 (3), pp.169–181.

Law, M. and Baum, C. (2001) 'Measurement in occupational therapy', in Law, M., Baum, C. and Dunn, W. (editors) *Measuring occupational performance: Supporting best practice in occupational therapy*, Thorofare: Slack Inc., Chapter 1.

Lechner, D., Roth, D. and Straaton, K. (1991) Functional capacity evaluation in work disability, *Work*, 1 (3), pp.37–47.

Leontaridi, R. and Bell, D. (2006) *Informal care of the elderly in Scotland and the UK, health and community care research findings no. 8*, Edinburgh: Scottish Executive Central Research Unit. Available at: http://www.scotland.gov.uk/cru/resfinds/hcc8-00.asp (accessed 18/01/07).

Levitas, R. (1998) *The inclusive society*, Basingstoke: MacMillan.

Lloyd, C. and Waghorn, G. (2007) The importance of vocation in recovery for young people with psychiatric disabilities, *British Journal of Occupational Therapy*, 70 (2), pp.50–59.

Lobo, J.A.F. (1999) The leisure and work occupations of young people: A review, *Journal of Occupational Science*, 6, pp.27–33.

Locke, E. (1976) 'The nature and causes of job satisfaction', in Dunnette, M. (editor) *Handbook of industrial and organizational psychology*, Chicago: Rand-McNally, pp.1297–1349.

Loumidis, J., Stafford, B., Youngs, R. *et al.* (2001) *Evaluation of the New Deal for Disabled People Personal Adviser Service pilot* (research report no.144), Norwish: Department for Work and Pensions.

Low, J.F. (1992) The reconstruction aides, *American Journal of Occupational Therapy*, 46 (1), pp.38–43.

Lysaght, R. and Wright, J. (2005) Professional strategies in work-related practice: An exploration of occupational and physical therapy roles and approaches, *American Journal of Occupational Therapy*, 59 (2), pp.209–216.

MacDonald, E.M. (1970) *Occupational therapy in rehabilitation* (third edition), London: Balliere, Tindall & Cassell.

MacDonald-Wilson, K. (1995) Personal experiences: Negotiating reasonable accommodations, *The Journal of the California Alliance for the Mentally Ill*, 6 (4), pp.35–37.

MacDonald-Wilson, K.L., Rogers, E.S. *et al.* (2002) An investigation of reasonable workplace accommodations for people with psychiatric disabilities: Quantitative findings from a multi-site study, *Community Mental Health Journal*, 38 (1), pp.35–50.

Main, L. and Haig, J. (2006) Occupational therapy and vocational rehabilitation: An audit of an out-patient occupational therapy service, *British Journal of Occupational Therapy*, 69 (6), pp.288–292.

Marshall, E.M. (1985) Looking back, *American Journal of Occupational Therapy*, 39 (5), pp.297–300.

Marshall, A.N. (1995) A hope not yet fulfilled: People with psychiatric disabilities and the ADA, *Journal of the California Alliance for the Mentally Ill*, 6 (4), pp.41–43.

Mårtensson, L. (2001) Rehabilitation of patients with chronic pain in primary health care, *Scandinavian Journal of Occupational Therapy*, 8 (2), p.108.

Matheson, L.N., Ogden, L.D., Violette, K. *et al.* (1985) Work hardening: Occupational therapy in industrial rehabilitation, *American Journal of Occupational Therapy*, 39 (5), pp.314–321.

McClelland, K. (1987) 'Time to work, time to live: Some aspects of work and the reformation of class in Britain 1850–1880', in Joyce, P. (editor) *The historical meanings of work*, Cambridge: Cambridge University Press, Chapter 7.

McCluskey, A., Lovarini, M., Bennett, S. *et al.* (2005) What evidence exists for work-related injury prevention and management? Analysis of an occupational therapy evidence database (OTSeeker), *British Journal of Occupational Therapy*, 68 (10), pp.447–456.

McColl, M.A., Law, M.C. and Stewart, D. (1993) *Theoretical basis of occupational therapy: An annotated bibliography of applied theory in the professional literature*, New Jersey: Slack Inc.

McDermott, C., Richards, S.C.M., Ankers, S. *et al.* (2004) An evaluation of a chronic fatigue lifestyle management programme focusing on the outcomes of return to work or training, *British Journal of Occupational Therapy*, 67 (6), pp.269–273.

McDonald, R. (1997) Expanding the role of occupational therapy in vocational rehabilitation (letter to the editor), *British Journal of Occupational Therapy*, 60 (6), p.267.

McFadyen, A.K. and Pratt, J. (1997) Understanding the statistical concepts of measures of work performance, *British Journal of Occupational Therapy*, 60 (6), pp.279–284.

McKay, C.E., Johnsen, M., Banks, S., and Stein, R. (2006) Employment transitions for clubhouse members, *Work*, 26 (1), pp.67–74.

McNaughton, A. (1997) Occupational overuse syndrome/repetitive strain injury: The occupational therapist's role, *British Journal of Occupational Therapy*, 60 (2), pp.69–72.

Meager, N., Bates, P., Dench, S. *et al.* (1998) Employment of disabled people: Assessing the extent of participation (research report no. RR69), London: DfES Publications.

Mental Health Foundation (1999) *Mental health in the workplace: Tackling the effects of stress*, London: MHF. Available at: www.mentalhealth.org.uk (accessed 04/04/07).

Mentrup, C., Niehaus, A. and Kielhofner, G. (1999) Applying the model of human occupation in work-focused rehabilitation: A case illustration, *Work*, 12, pp.61–70.

Meredith, H.T.D. (1935) (editor) *The modern home doctor*, London: Daily Express Publications.

Mettävainio, B.I. and Ahlgren, C. (2004) Facilitating factors for work return in unemployed with disabilities: A qualitative study, *Scandinavian Journal of Occupational Therapy*, 11 (1), pp.17–25.

Meyer, A. (1922) The philosophy of occupational therapy, *Archives of Occupational Therapy*, 1, pp.1–10, reprinted in *American Journal of Occupational Therapy* (1997) 31 (10), pp.632–642.

Midford, R., Welander, F. and Allsop, S. (2005) 'Preventing alcohol and other drug problems in the workplace', in Stockwell, T., Gruenewald, J.W., Toumbourou, J. *et al.* (editors) *Preventing harmful substance use: The evidence based for policy and practice*, Sydney: John Wiley & Sons, Chapter 4.5.

Miller, W.R. and Rollnick, S. (1991) *Motivational interviewing – preparing people to change addictive behaviour*, Guilford: New York.

Modernisation Agency and Skills for Health (2005) *Long term conditions case management framework*. Available at: http://www.skillsforhealth.org.uk/view_framework.php?id=91 (accessed 05/03/07).

Molineux, M. (2004) (editor) *Occupation for occupational therapists*, Oxford: Blackwell Publishing Ltd.

Moll, S., Huff, J. and Detwiler, L. (2003) Supported employment: Evidence for a best practice model in psychosocial rehabilitation, *Canadian Journal of Occupational Therapy*, 70 (5), pp.298–310.

Monteath, H.G. (1983) Work assessment in the current economic climate, *British Journal of Occupational Therapy*, 46 (8), pp.223–224.

Montgomery, A.J., Panagopoulou, E.P., Peeters, M. *et al.* (2005) The meaning of work and home, *Community Work and Family*, 8 (2) pp.141–162.

Moore-Corner, R.A., Kielhofner, G. and Olson, L. (1998) *The work environment impact scale Version 2.0*, Illinois: MOHO Clearing House. Available at: http://www.moho.uic.edu/assess/weis.html (accessed 29/09/07).

Morgan, D. and Yongbloed, L. (1990) factors influencing leisure activities following a stroke: an exploratory study, *Canadian Journal of Occupational Therapy*, 57 (4), pp.223–229.

Morgan, K.O. (2000) *Twentieth century Britain. A very short introduction*, Oxford: Oxford University Press.

Morrison, E. (1990) 'A history of the profession', in Creek, J. (editor) *Occupational therapy and mental health: Principles, skills and practice*, London: Churchill Livingstone, Chapter 1.

Mosey, A.C. (1971) Involvement in the rehabilitation movement – 1942–1960, *The American Journal of Occupational Therapy*, XXV (5), pp.234–236.

Mosey, A.C. (1974) An alternative: The biopsychosocial model, *The American Journal of Occupational Therapy*, 38 (3), pp.137–140.

Mosey, A.C. (1986) *Psychosocial components of occupational therapy*, New York: Raven Press.

Mountain, G., Carman, S. and Ilott, I. (2001) *Work rehabilitation and occupational therapy. A review of the literature*. London: College of Occupational Therapists.

Nagle, S., Cook, J.V. and Polatajko, H.M. (2002) I'm doing as much as I can: Occupational choices of persons with a severe and persistent mental illness, *Journal of Occupational Science*, 9 (2), pp.72–81.

National Institute for Clinical Excellence (2002) *Core interventions in the treatment and management of schizophrenia in primary and secondary care*, London: NICE.

National Institute for Clinical Excellence (2004) *Chronic Obstructive Pulmonary Disease*, London: NICE.

National Institute of Disability Management and Research (2000) *Code of practice for disability management: Describing effective benchmarks for the creation of workplace-based disability management programs*, Ottowa: NIDMAR.

Neumayer, B. and Wilding, C. (2005) 'Leisure as commodity', in Whiteford, G. and Wright-St Clair, V. (2005) *Occupation and practice in context*, Sydney: Elsevier Livingstone Churchill, Chapter 19.

Newman, S., Steed, L. and Mulligan, K. (2004) Self-management interventions for chronic illness,*Lancet*, 364, pp.1523–1537.

NHS Centre for Reviews and Dissemination (2000) Acute and chronic low back pain, *Effective Health Care*, 6 (5), pp.1–8.

Nichols, P.J.R. (editor) (1980) *Rehabilitation medicine: The management of physical disabilities* (second edition), London: Butterworth.

Nice, K. and Thornton, P. (2004) *Job retention and rehabilitation pilot: Employers' management of long-term sickness absence* (research report no.227), Leeds: Department for Work and Pensions.

Neilson, W.R. and Weir, R.R.N. (2001) Biopsychosocial approaches to the treatment of chronic pain, *Clinical Journal of Pain*, 17 (4), supplement, pp.S114–S127.

Nippert-Eng, C.E. (1996) *Home and work: Negotiating boundaries through everyday life*, Chicago: University of Chicago Press.

Niven, K. (2004) *The potential for certification of incapacity for work by non-medical healthcare professionals* (Department for Work and Pensions research report no. 225), Norwich: HMSO.

Nolan, P., Orford, J., White, A. *et al.* (2003) Professional views on managing common mental health problems in primary care, *Primary Care Mental Health*, 1 (1), pp.27–36.

Noon, M. and Blyton, P. (1997) *The realities of work*, Basingstoke: McMillan Press

Oakley, F., Kielhofner, G., Barris, R. *et al.* (1986) The role checklist: Development and empirical assessment of reliability, *The Occupational Therapy Journal of Research*, 6, pp.157–169.

Occupational Health Working Group of the Faculty of Public Health and Faculty of Occupational Medicine (2006) *Creating a healthy workplace: A guide for occupational safety for health professionals and employers*, London: Faculty of Public Health and Faculty of Occupational Medicine.

Office for National Statistics (2003) *Better or worse: A longitudinal study of the mental health of adults living in private households in Great Britain*, London: The Stationery Office.

Office for National Statistics (2005) 'The labour market', in UK 2005: The official yearbook of the United Kingdom of Great Britain and Northern Ireland, Norwich: HMSO, Chapter 11. Available at: www.statistics.gov.uk/yearbook (accessed 07/06/05).

Office of the Deputy Prime Minister (2004) *Action on mental health: A guide to promoting social inclusion*, West Yorkshire: ODPM Publications.

Office of the Third Sector (2006) *Social enterprise action plan:scaling new heights*, London: HM Government. Available at: www.cabinetoffice.gov.uk/thirdsector (accessed 24/02/07).

O'Halloran, D. (2002) An historical overview of Australia's largest and oldest provider of vocational rehabiliatation – CRS Australia, *Work*, 19 (3), pp.211–218.

O'Halloran, D. and Innes, E. (2005) 'Understanding work in society', in Whiteford, G. and Wright-St Clair, V. (editors) *Occupation and practice in context*, Sydney: Elsevier Churchill Livingstone, Chapter 18.

Oliver, M. and Barnes, C. (1998) *Disabled people and social policy: From exclusion to inclusion*, Harlow: Addison Wesley Longman.

Olsheski, J.A., Rosenthal, D.A. and Hamilton, M. (2002) Disability management and psychosocial rehabilitation: Considerations for integration, *Work*, 19, pp.63–70.

O'Neill, P. (2006) Going strong, *Hazards*, 96, October/December. Available at: www.hazards.org/olderworkers (accessed 20/01/07).

Organisation for Economic Co-operation and Development (2003) *Transforming disability into ability. Policies to promote work and income security for disabled people*, Paris: OECD.

Oxley, C. (1995) Work and work programmes for clients with mental health problems, *British Journal of Occupational Therapy*, 58 (11), pp.465–466.

Park, A., Curtice, J., Thompson, K. *et al.* (editors) (2003) *British social attitudes: Continuity and change over two decades* (20th report), Thousand Oaks: Sage Publications.

Parlato, L., Lloyd, C. and Bassett, J. (1999) Young occupations unlimited: An early intervention programme for young people with psychosis, *British Journal of Occupational Therapy*, 62 (3), pp.113–116.

Parrish, J. (1991) Making reasonable accommodations under the A.D.A., *Focus Quarterly Newsletter of the National Mental Health Association*, spring.

Paterson, C.F. (1997a) 'A short history of occupational therapy in mental health', in Creek, J. (editor) *Occupational therapy and mental health*, New York: Churchill Livingstone, Chapter 1.

Paterson, C.F. (1997b) Rationales for the use of occupation in 19th century asylums, *British Journal of Occupational Therapy*, 60 (4), pp.179–183.

Paterson, C.F. (1998) Occupational therapy and the National Health Service 1948–1998, *British Journal of Occupational Therapy*, 61 (7), pp.311–315.

Paugam, S. and Duncan, G. (2004) The experience of unemployment: Elements for a European comparison, translated from L'experience du chomage: elements pour une comparaison europeenne (abstract in English), *Schweizerische Zeitschrift fur Soziologie*, 30 (2), pp.441–460.

Penrose Brown, J. and Blandford, S. (2002) An examination of the range of children's experience of work, *Support for Learning*, 17 (4), pp.193–200.

People Management (2004) UK is close to the top of EU long-term sick list, *People Management*, 10, 8 January, p.1.

Perkins, J., Simnett, I. and Wright, L. (editors) (1999) *Evidence-based health promotion*, Chichester: Wiley & Sons.

Perron, J. and McKay, M. (1997) 'Current models and trends in work practice service delivery', in Pratt, J. and Jacobs, K. (editors) (1997) *Work practice: International perspectives*, Oxford: Butterworth Heinemann, Chapter 39.

Pheasant, S. (1996) *Bodyspace: Anthropometry, ergonomics and the design of work* (second edition), London: Taylor & Francis Ltd.

Picone, P. (1999) 'Environmental design', in Jacobs, K. (editor) *Ergonomics for therapists* (second edition), Boston: Butterworth Heinemann, Chapter 7.

Pollet, S.L. (1995) Mental illness in the workplace: The tension between productivity and reasonable accommodation, *Journal of Psychiatry and Law*, 32 (1), pp.155–184.

Powell, A. (2002) *Taking responsibility. Good practice guidelines for services – adults with Asperger Syndrome*, London: The National Autistic Society.

Pratt, J. (1997) 'Work assessments', in Pratt, J. and Jacobs, K. (editors) *Work practice: International perspectives*, Oxford: Butterworth-Heinemann, Chapter 6.

Pratt, J. and Jacobs, K. (editors) (1997) *Work practice: International perspectives*, Oxford: Butterworth Heinemann.

Pratt, J., McFayden, A., Hall, G. *et al.* (1997) A review of the initial outcomes of a return-to-work programme for police officers following injury or illness, *British Journal of Occupational Therapy*, 60, pp.253–258.

Primeau, L.A. (1996) Work and leisure: Transcending the dichotomy, *The American Journal of Occupational Therapy*, 50 (7), pp.569–577.

Prospects (2007) *Occupational health nurse: Job description and activities*. Available at: www.prospects.ac.uk/cms/ShowPage/Home_page?Explore_ypes_of_jobs/Types_of_Job/p! eipaL?state=showocc&idno=719&pageno=1 (accessed 04/05/07).

Purdon, S., Stratford, N., Taylor, R. *et al.* (2006) *Impacts of the Job Retention and Rehabilitation pilot* (research report no.342), Leeds: Department for Work and Pensions.

Quiroga, V.A.M. (1995) Occupational therapy: The first 30 years 1900 to 1930, *The American Occupational Therapy Association*, Bethesda: AOTA.

Raper, J. (1995) 'Rehabilitation for work', in Pantry, S. (editor) *Occupational Health*, London: Chapman & Hall, Chapter 4.

Rebeiro, K. and Allen, J. (1998) Voluntarism as occupation, *Canadian Journal of Occupational Therapy*, 65, pp.279–285.

Reed, G. and Johnson, V.A. (1987) Employer perspectives on workers with disabilities, *Journal of Rehabilitation*, July/Aug/Sept, pp.37–45.

Rehab UK (2007) *About brain injury*, London: Rehab UK. Available at: http://www .rehabuk.org.uk (accessed 15/09/08).

Reker, T., Hornung, W.P., Schonauer, K. *et al.* (2000) Long-term psychiatric patients in vocational rehabilitation programmes: A naturalistic follow-up study over 3 years, *Acta Psychiatrica Scandinavica*, 101 (6), pp.457–462.

Rerek, M.D. (1971) The depression years – 1929 to 1941, *American Journal of Occupational Therapy*, XXV (4), pp.231–233.

Rethink (2005) *Recovery learning: A report on the work of the recovery learning sites and other recovery-orientated activities and its incorporation into the Rethink plan 2004–08*. Available at: http://www.rethink.org/living_with_mental_illness/recovery_ and_self_management/recovery/index.html (accessed 04/04/07).

Rick, J., Hillage, J., Honey, S. *et al.* (1997) *Stress: Big issue, but what are the problems?* (report 331), Institute for Employment Studies. Available at: http://www.employment-studies. co.uk/summary/summary.php?id=331 (accessed 20/09/02).

Robdale, N. (2004) Vocational rehabilitation: The enable employment retention scheme, a new approach, *British Journal of Occupational Therapy*, 67 (10), pp.457–460.

Roberts, S., Heaver, C., Hill, K. *et al.* (2004) *Disability in the workplace: Employers' and service providers' responses to the Disability Discrimination Act in 2003 and preparation for the 2004 changes* (research report 202), London: Department for Work and Pensions. Available at: www.dwp.gov.uk/asd/ (accessed 29/09/07).

Ross, J. (1998) The relationship between occupational roles and life satisfaction in young adults with serious mental disorders. Conference proceedings. Paper presented at the National Occupational Therapy Conference, Belfast. Abstract published in the *British Journal of Occupational Therapy* (2000) 63 (4).

Ross, J. (2006) *Meeting the challenge by mapping the curriculum: What do we learn about rehabilitation for work?* Conference proceedings. Paper presented at the 14th Congress of the World Federation of Occupational Therapists, Sydney, Australia, 23–28 July 2006.

Roulstone, A., Gradwell, L., Price, J. *et al.* (2003) *Thriving and surviving at work: Disabled people's employment strategies*, Bristol: The Policy Press in association with the Joseph Rowntree Foundation.

Royal College of Psychiatrists (2003) *Drugs and alcohol – whose problem is it anyway? Who cares?* Available at: http://www.rcpsych.ac.uk/pdf/whocares.pdf (accessed 05/04/07).

Royal Society for the Prevention of Accidents (1998–2007) Occupational safety: Facts and figures, Birmingham: RoSPA. Available at: http://www.rospa.com/occupationalsafety/facts.htm (accessed 02/10/07).

Royeen, C.B. (2002) Occupation reconsidered, *Occupational Therapy International*, 9 (2), pp.111–120.

Sandqvist, J.L. and Henriksson, C.M. (2004) Work functioning: A conceptual framework, *Work*, 23 (2), pp.147–157.

Saunders, R. and Piela, C. (1998) *Functional capacity evaluation: The Saunders Method*, Minnesota: The Saunders Group.

Sawny, P. and Challoner, J. (2003) Poor communication between health professionals is a barrier to rehabilitation (comment), *Occupational Medicine*, 53 (4), pp.246–248.

Schonebaum, A.D., Boyd, J.K., and Dudek, K.J. (2006) A comparison of competitive employment outcomes for the Clubhouse and PACT Models, *Psychiatric Services*, 57 (10), pp.1416–1420.

Schulman, B.M. (1994) Worklessness and disability: Expansion of the biopsychosocial perspective, *Journal of Occupational Rehabilitation*, 4 (2), pp.113–122.

Scott, A. (2006) *Vocational rehabilitation: The welfare reform context.* Presented on 14th June at City University, London.

Scriven, A. (editor) (2005) *Health promoting practice: The contribution of nurses and allied health professionals*, Hampshire: Palgrave Macmillan.

Secker, J. and Membrey, H. (2003) Promoting mental health through employment and developing healthy workplaces: The potential of natural supports at work, *Health Education Research: Theory and Practice*, 18 (2), pp.207–215.

Secker, J., Membrey, H., Grove, B. *et al.* (2002) Recovering from illness or recovering your life? Implications of clinical vs social models of recovery from mental health problems for employment support services, *Disability & Society*, 17 (4), pp.403–418.

Seebohm, P. and Secker, J. (2003) Increasing the vocational focus of the community mental health team, *Journal of Interprofessional Care*, 17 (3), pp.282–291.

Shamir, B. (1996) 'Meaning, self and motivation in organizations', in Steers, R., Porter, L.W. and Bigley, G.A. (editors) *Motivation and leadership at work* (sixth edition), New York: McGraw Hill International, Chapter 2.

Shaw, K.L., Hackett, J.L. and Southwood, T.R. (2006) The prevocational and early employment needs of adolescents with juvenile idiopathic arthritis: The occupational therapy perspective, *British Journal of Occupational Therapy*, 69 (11), pp.497–504.

Shaw, W.S., Robertson, M.M., Pransky, G. *et al.* (2003) Employee perspectives on the role of supervisors to prevent workplace disabilities after injuries, *Journal of Occupational Rehabilitation*, 13, pp.129–142.

Shrey, D.E., Hursh, N.C. (1999) Workplace disability management: International trends and perspectives, *Journal of Occupational Rehabilitation*, 9 (1), pp.45–59.

Silcox, S. (2006) Enabling rehabilitation: Beyond the medical model, *Occupational Health Review*, Jan/Feb, 119, pp.21–24.

Smigel, E.O. (editor) (1963) *Work and leisure: A contemporary social problem*, New Haven: College & University Press.

Smith, A. and Twomey, B. (2002) Labour market experiences of people with disabilities, *Labour Market Trends*, London: Office of National Statistics. Available at: http://www.statistics.gov.uk/articles/labour_market_trends/People_with_disabilities_aug2002.pdf (accessed 06/03/06).

Smith, A., Wadsworth, E., Moss, S. *et al.* (2004) *The scale and impact of illegal drug use by workers* (research report 193), Norwich: HSE Books.

Smith, D.E. (2003) Making sense of what people do: A sociological perspective, *Journal of Occupational Science*, 10 (1), pp.52–60.

Snashall, D. (1997) *ABC of work related disorders*, London: BMJ Publishing Group.

Spackman, C.S. (1968) A history of the practice of occupational therapy for restoration of physical function 1917–1967, *The American Journal of Occupational Therapy*, XXII (2), pp.67–71.

Spencer, J., Daybell, P.J., Eschenfelder, V. *et al.* (1998) Contrasting perspectives on work: An exploratory qualitative study on the concept of adaptation, *The American Journal of Occupational Therapy*, 52 (6), pp.474–484.

Stein, F., Söderback, I. Cutler, S. *et al.* (2006) *Occupational therapy and ergonomics: Applying ergonomic principles to everyday occupation in the home and at work*, London: Whurr Publishers.

Stewart, B. (2004) Vocational rehabilitation: Seeing the light (editorial), *British Journal of Occupational Therapy*, 67 (3), p.103.

Stokes, F. (1997) Using the Delphi technique in planning a research project on the occupational therapist's role in enabling people to make vocational choices following illness or injury, *British Journal of Occupational Therapy*, 60 (6), pp.263–267.

Strada, M.J. and Donohue, B.C. (2004) 'Substance abuse', in Thomas, J.C. and Hersen, M. (editors) *Psychopathology in the Workplace*, New York: Brunner-Routledge, Chapter 6.

Stroke Association (1996) *Younger people have strokes too. A survey of the experiences of younger people affected by stroke*, London: Stroke Association.

Stroke Association (2007) *What is a stroke?* (public information leaflet), London: Stroke Association. Available at: http://www.stroke.org.uk/information/what_is_a_stroke/index.html (accessed 31/07/07).

Strong, S. (1998) Meaningful work in supportive environments: Experiences with the recovery process, *The American Journal of Occupational Therapy*, 52 (1), pp.31–38.

Strong, S., Baptiste, S., Cole, D. *et al.* (2004) Functional assessment of injured workers: A profile of assessor practices, *Canadian Journal of Occupational Therapy*, 71 (1), pp.13–23.

Strong, S., Baptiste, S. and Salvatori, P. (2003) Learning from today's clinicians in vocational practice to educate tomorrow's therapists, *Canadian Journal of Occupational Therapy*, 70 (1), pp.11–20.

Summers, E. and Holmes, A. (editors) (2004) *Collins dictionary and thesaurus*, Glasgow: Harper Collins.

Sumsion, T. (1999) *Client-centred practice in occupational therapy*, Edinburgh: Churchill Livingstone.

Suto, M. (1998) Leisure in occupational therapy, *Canadian Journal of Occupational Therapy*, 65, pp.271–278.

Swain, J., French, S. and Cameron, C. (2003) *Controversial issues in a disabling society*, Buckingham: Open University Press.

Taggart, H.M., Arslanian, C.L., Bae, S. *et al.* (2003) Effects of T'ai Chi exercise on fibromyalgia symptoms and health-related quality of life, *Orthopaedic Nursing*, 22 (5), pp.353–360.

Takala, J. (1995) 'Worldwide view of occupational health and safety', in Pantry, S. (editor), *Occupational health*, London: Chapman & Hall, Chapter 1.

Tausky, C. (1995) The meanings of work, *Research in Sociology of Work*, 5, p.15.

Taylor, A. (2003) Access to work blocked as disabled people remain unaware of the initiative, *Community Care*, 21–27 August, pp.16–17.

Taylor, R.R. and Kielhofner, G.W. (2005) Work-related impairment and employment-focused rehabilitation options for individuals with chronic fatigue syndrome: A review, *Journal of Mental Health*, 14 (3), pp.253–267.

Taylor, S. (1998) *Employee resourcing*, London: Institute of Personnel Development.

Tehrani, N. (2004) *Recovery, rehabilitation and retention: Maintaining a productive workforce*, London: Chartered Institute of Personnel and Development.

Thomson, L., Neathey, F. and Rick, J. (2003)*Best practice in rehabilitating employees following absence due to work-related stress* (research report 138), Norwich: HSE Books.

Thorpe, K. (2006) How to better prepare our graduates for working in occupational rehabilitation: Occupational therapists' perspectives (abstract), *Australian Occupational Therapy Journal*, 53, p.62.

Thurgood, J. (1997) The Wexham Park experience: The work rehabilitation programme in one occupational therapy department following injury or physical illness, *British Journal of Occupational Therapy*, 60, pp.245–247.

Thurgood, J. (1999) The employment implications of the Disability Discrimination Act 1995 and a suggested format for developing reasonable adjustments, *British Journal of Occupational Therapy*, 62 (7), pp.290–294.

Thurgood, J. and Frank, A.O. (2007) Work is beneficial for health and well-being: Can occupational therapists now return to their roots? (editorial),*British Journal of Occupational Therapy*, 70 (2), p.49.

Toulmin, S. (1995) Occupation, employment and human welfare, *Journal of Occupational Science*, 2 (2), pp.48–58.

Towner, N. (2005) Hidden penury? Child Poverty, *Unison U magazine*, 13 (2), pp.20–21.

Townsend, E. (editor) (2002) *Enabling occupation: An occupational therapy perspective*, Ottawa: Canadian Association of Occupational Therapists.

Townsend, E. and Wilcock, A.A. (2004) Occupational justice and client-centred practice: A dialogue in progress, *Canadian Journal of Occupational Therapy*, 71 (2), pp.75–87.

Trades Union Congress (2001) *Class Struggles*, London: TUC. Available at: www.tuc.org.uk (accessed 10/09/05).

Trades Union Congress (2002) *Rehabilitation and retention: What works is what matters*, London: TUC. Available at: www.tuc.org.uk (accessed 10/09/05).

Trades Union Congress (2005) Countering an urban legend: Sicknote Britain?, London: TUC. Available at: http://www.tuc.org.uk/welfare/tuc-9208-f0.cfm (accessed 10/03/05).

Trades Union Congress (2006) *The hidden one-in-five – winning a fair deal for Britain's vulnerable workers*, London: TUC. Available at: www.tuc.org.uk (accessed 10/01/07).

Trades Union Congress (2007) *Real, but oh so slow, progress on long hours* (press release, 21 February), London: Trades Union Congress. Available at: http://www.tuc.org.uk/work_life/tuc-12970-f0.cfm (accessed 24/02/07).

Tsang, H., Lam, P., Ng, B. *et al.* (2000) Predictors of employment outcome for people with psychiatric disabilities: A review of the literature since the Mid '80s, *The Journal of Rehabilitation*, 66 (2), pp.19–31.

Tse, S.S. and Walsh, A.E.S. (2001) How does work work for people with bipolar affective disorder?, *Occupational Therapy International*, 8 (3), pp.210–225.

University of North Carolina (2006) *TEACCH Autism program: Mobile crew model*, Carolina: UNC. Available at: http://teacch.com/SE_Mobile.html (accessed 30/07/07).

Unruh, A., Versnel, J. and Kerr, N. (2002) Spirituality unplugged: A review of commonalities and contentions, and a resolution, *Canadian Journal of Occupational Therapy*, February, 69 (1), pp.5–19.

Unsworth, C. (1999) Living with epilepsy: Safety during home, leisure and work activities, *Australian Occupational Therapy Journal*, 46 (3), pp.89–98.

U.S. Department of Labor, Employment and Training Administration (1991) *Dictionary of Occupational Titles* (fourth edition) Washington DC: Government Printing Office.

Vasile, R.G., Samson, J.A., Bemporad, J. *et al.* (1987) A biopsychosocial approach to treating patients with affective disorders, *The American Journal of Psychiatry*, 144, pp.341–344.

Velozo, C. (1993) Work evaluations: Critique of the state of the art of functional assessment of work, *The American Journal of Occupational Therapy*, 47 (3), pp.203–209.

Verbeek, J., Salmi, J., Pasternack, I. *et al.* (2005) A search strategy for occupational health intervention studies, *Occupational and Environmental Medicine*, 62, pp.682–687.

Vierling, L. (1999) Four components for an improved return to work program, *Case Manager*, 10 (4), pp.52–54.

Vincello, L.A. (1999) 'Basic biomechanics', in Jacobs, K. (editor) *Ergonomics for therapists*, (second edition), Boston: Butterworth Heinemann, Chapter 4.

Vocational Rehabilitation Association (2006) *Recognising and accrediting education and training provision for the vocational rehabilitation professional*, Glasgow: VRA.

Vostanis, P. (1990) The role of work in psychiatric rehabilitation: A review of the literature, *British Journal of Occupational Therapy*, 53 (1), pp.24–28.

Waddell, G. and Aylward, M. (2005) *The scientific and conceptual basis of incapacity benefits*, London: The Stationery Office.

Waddell, G. and Burton, A.K. (2004) *Concepts of rehabilitation for the management of common mental health problems*, London: TSO.

Waddell, G. and Burton, A.K. (2006) *Is work good for your health and well-being?*, London: TSO.

Walker, A. and Walker, C. (editors) (1997) *Britain divided: The growth of social exclusion in the 1980s and 1990s*, London: CPAG Ltd.

Warr, P. (1987) *Work, unemployment and mental health*, Oxford: Oxford University Press.

Watson, T.J. (2003) *Sociology, work and industry* (fourth edition), London: Routledge.

White, S. (2006) *Social enterprise pathfinders*. Letter published on 9 October at: http://www.dh.gov.uk/PublicationsAndStatistics/LettersAndCirculars/DearColleagueLetters/DearColleagueLettersArticle/fs/en?CONTENT_ID=4139501&chk=bgJ4Vl (accessed 24/02/07).

Whiteford, G. and Wright-St Clair, V. (2005) *Occupation and practice in context*, Sydney: Elsevier Livingstone Churchill.

Wilcock, A. (1998) *An occupational perspective of health*, Thorofare: Slack Inc.

Wilding, K., Clarke, J., Griffith, M. *et al.* (2006) *The UK voluntary sector almanac: The state of the sector*, London: National Council for Voluntary Organisations. Available at: http://www.ncvo-vol.org.uk/uploadedFiles/NCVO/Research/AlmanacSummary2006.pdf (accessed 10/01/07).

Williams, C. (2001) *Overcoming depression: A five areas approach*, London: Arnold.

Williams, C. (2003) *Overcoming anxiety: A five areas approach*, London: Arnold.

Williams, R.M. and Westmorland, M. (2002) Perspectives on workplace disability management: A review of the literature, *Work*, 19 (1), pp.87–93.

Woodside, H.H. (1971) The development of occupational therapy 1910–1929, *The American Journal of Occupational Therapy*, XXV (5), pp.226–230.

Workcover NSW (2000) *Workplace assessment. Application for approval to provide occupational rehabilitation services*, New South Wales: WorkCover.

WorkCover NSW (2001) *Risk management at work guide*, Gosford: WorkCover.

Workcover NSW (2003) *Guidelines for employers' return to work programs*, New South Wales: Workcover.

World Health Organization (1986) *The Ottawa charter for health promotion*, International Conference on Health Promotion: The move towards a new public health, conference proceedings, November 17–21, 1986 Ottawa, Ontario: Canadian Public Health Association, Health and Welfare Canada, and the World Health Organization. Available at: http://www.who.int/hpr/NPH/docs/ottawa_charter_hp.pdf (accessed 02/02/07).

World Health Organization (1994) *Declaration on occupational health for all*, Beijing: WHO. Available at: http://www.who.int/occupational_health/publications/declaration/en/index.html (accessed 19/12/06).

World Health Organization (2001) *ICF: International classification of functioning, disability and health*, Geneva: WHO.

World Health Organization (2006) *Declaration on workers' health*, Stresa: World Health Organization. Available at: http://www.who.int/occupational_health/Declarwh.pdf (accessed 20/12/06).

Wright, M., Beardwell, C. and Marsden, S. (2005) *Availability of rehabilitation services in the UK: A research study for the Association of British Insurers*, Reading: Greenstreet Berman Ltd. Available at: http://www.abi.org.uk/BookShop/ResearchReports/Availabilty%20of%20Rehab.pdf (accessed 13/02/07).

Wynn, P.A., Aw, T.C. and Williams, N.R. (2003) Teaching of occupational medicine to undergraduates in UK schools of medicine, *Occupational Medicine*, 53, pp.349–353.

Index